A GIFT OF TIME

A Gift of Time

Continuing Your Pregnancy When
Your Baby's Life Is Expected to Be Brief

AMY KUEBELBECK AND DEBORAH L. DAVIS, PH.D.

THE JOHNS HOPKINS UNIVERSITY PRESS
Baltimore

The Johns Hopkins University Press
2715 North Charles Street
Baltimore, Maryland 21218-4363
www.press.jhu.edu

Library of Congress Cataloging-in-Publication Data

Kuebelbeck, Amy, 1964–
A gift of time : continuing your pregnancy when your baby's life is expected to be brief /
Amy Kuebelbeck and Deborah L. Davis.
p. cm.
Includes index.
ISBN-13: 978-0-8018-9761-0 (hardcover : alk. paper)
ISBN-10: 0-8018-9761-0 (hardcover : alk. paper)
ISBN-13: 978-0-8018-9762-7 (pbk. : alk. paper)
ISBN-10: 0-8018-9762-9 (pbk. : alk. paper)
1. Prenatal diagnosis—Psychological aspects. 2. Newborn infants—Death—
Psychological aspects. I. Davis, Deborah L., 1955– II. Title.
RG628.K84 2010
618.3'2—dc22——2010013273

A catalog record for this book is available from the British Library.

Special discounts are available for bulk purchases of this book. For more information, please contact Special Sales at 410-516-6936 or specialsales@press.jhu.edu.

The Johns Hopkins University Press uses environmentally friendly book materials, including recycled text paper that is composed of at least 30 percent post-consumer waste, whenever possible. All of our book papers are acid-free, and our jackets and covers are printed on paper with recycled content.

*To the many parents who shared their experiences for this book,
you have our deepest gratitude. Your generosity truly honors
your babies' lives. Every one of your stories is a love story.
You will be a beacon of hope to many.*

To all babies whose lives are brief—yet still a gift.

CONTENTS

Contents

INTRODUCTION

If you are reading this book because a prenatal diagnosis indicates that your baby likely will die before or after birth, or if you are reading this because your baby has already died, we are so sorry. Our hearts go out to you and your family.

If you are still pregnant: As you face this devastating news, you might be considering continuing your pregnancy and embracing whatever remaining time you have with your baby, even if that time is only before birth. You might be certain of choosing this option or you might be leaning toward terminating your pregnancy. You might wonder which is the kinder and more bearable course.

If your baby has already been born and died: You are mourning the death of your baby as well as the loss of the future you dreamed you would have together. You might be struggling to make sense of your experiences and emotions, and you might be searching for reassurance that you are not alone.

Whatever your baby's diagnosis or your personal circumstances, this book describes and affirms the wide range of experiences and emotions that can follow a life-limiting prenatal diagnosis. It offers encouragement and practical ideas for moving forward, including guidance for decision-making, strategies for coping with the remainder of your pregnancy, and ideas for nurturing and being with your baby, before and after birth and death.

This book also describes the concept of perinatal hospice and palliative care, which is a new way of supporting parents whose babies are expected to die before or shortly after birth. While this book is addressed to parents, it offers insight for caregivers as well.

Parents who have continued their pregnancies are quoted throughout this book, sharing their experiences, feelings, and insights. More than 120 mothers and fathers shared their stories with us through written questionnaires, in-person interviews, websites, journal entries, and e-mail correspondence. These parents are from across the United States, as well as from Canada, Europe, and Australia. Some of these parents received outstanding support from their caregivers, extended family, and friends. Others felt abandoned or even faced hostility. But all of them received a devastating prenatal diagnosis—a diagnosis of something expected to be fatal—and all of them chose to continue their pregnancies and embrace their time together with their babies.

We have generally chosen not to include the details of diagnoses, treatments, or circumstances, purposefully placing the focus on the emotional common ground you share with parents who have traveled this road before you. Their words can help affirm that you are not alone in your devastation and bewilderment. You are not the only one to feel terrified of continuing the pregnancy, to wish for a miracle, to be relieved that your baby will not have to live long with a debilitating condition, or to wonder what witnessing death will be like. Their words can help you establish realistic expectations for yourself and reclaim hope.

This book does not tell you how to feel, what to decide, or how to go about continuing your pregnancy. Rather, it supports your ability to make your own heartfelt decisions for your baby and see them through. Although these decisions may feel (or have felt) like an overwhelming burden and responsibility, they demonstrate your love for your baby and your concern for your child's best interests.

HOW TO USE THIS BOOK

It is not necessary to read this book through from beginning to end. You can skip around to the parts that speak to you and pace yourself. Take in whatever seems helpful and pass by whatever isn't. Return to the passages you find particularly comforting and try reading other parts later. Even if you do read it cover to cover and then put it away, we encourage you to revisit this book from time to time. What you need may stand out each time, and what you need each time might be different. This book is meant to be your companion.

You may even find it reassuring to start by first turning to the chapters about birth planning, spending time with your baby after birth, or reflecting in hindsight. That way, you can see that this is not a journey just of grief but also one that is full of treasures. Some of the voices of anguish that you will meet in the early chapters will reappear as voices of joy and overwhelming love in describing the birth of their baby, and they appear again near the end of the book, reflecting on their journeys with voices of gratitude and peace.

You also may find comfort in other parents' experiences of personal growth and previously unrecognized strengths. You can be reassured knowing that others have survived this journey, discovered its meaning, and eventually acquired a sense of peace. You too can survive—and emerge transformed. This transformation is part of your baby's legacy.

If reading this book moves you to cry, try to accept this reaction. These are healing tears of grief, joy, and strength that mix with those of other parents. You are not alone.

> Time is
> Too slow for those who wait
> Too swift for those who fear
> Too long for those who grieve
> Too short for those who rejoice
> But for those who love
> Time is eternity.
> — *Henry Van Dyke*
> (1852–1933)

A GIFT OF TIME

one

The News

Receiving Your Baby's Diagnosis

At first, I thought the reason the technician was having problems getting measurements was because our little guy was so active. That illusion was soon to be shattered, and my life became divided into "before" and "after." This was truly a defining moment for me. Perhaps it was *the* defining moment of my life. *—Annette G.*

When you discover that you are pregnant, you expect a certain kind of journey. You wonder if your child is a boy or a girl and begin searching for the perfect name. You may imagine fitting into maternity clothes, preparing a nursery, and enjoying a baby shower. You may picture what your baby's birth will be like. You may look farther into the future and think about how your baby will fit into your family, perhaps envisioning holidays and the simple pleasures of daily life together.

But now prenatal testing has revealed serious problems, problems so serious that your baby is not expected to survive.

This is not the journey you planned. It isn't even on the map. Babies aren't supposed to die, especially in this era of prenatal care, vaccines, antibiotics, and newborn intensive care. How do parents cope with such stunning news? How do parents figure out the best way to proceed? How is it possible that your only options are terminating the pregnancy or continuing the pregnancy—*and that your baby likely will die, no matter what you do?*

When prenatal test results indicate that your baby has catastrophic problems, your dreams and expectations are shattered. Your devastation is as real as your baby. Your pregnancy, and perhaps your life, has been sheared into "before" and "after."

BEFORE THE DIAGNOSIS

We were thrilled. We were ecstatic. We told everyone right away. We were, like, four minutes pregnant or something, and we told the whole world. *—Jessica*

I was nauseated, bloated, and most of all deliriously happy.
—Jamie

Perhaps your pregnancy was planned and you conceived easily. Maybe you endured grueling treatments for infertility and rejoiced that a baby finally was on the way. This may be your first baby, or you may already have a busy house full of children. Perhaps you needed to adjust to an unexpected pregnancy or to news that you were expecting more than one baby, and you may have thought that you had already faced the biggest challenge that this pregnancy would present. Whatever the circumstances, your hopes for your baby have already begun taking shape.

Before the diagnosis, my pregnancy was wonderful. I was so ready to have a baby. I had been preparing for this time in my life since I was a little girl. *—Chelsea*

I'd so wanted this little one. I had maternity leave all arranged, the room started. *—Tracy*

I was looking forward to all the fun things you can do with your kids. I wanted an excuse to go to the zoo. I wanted to take him to the fair and have him ride the Ferris wheel with Mommy and Daddy. I wanted him to play in the backyard that is always empty. I wanted to buy all the toys that would have scattered the yard. *—Rachel*

The idea that I could possibly be pregnant seemed impossible. I was dragging my feet at this renewed prospect: to start it all over, diapers, baby bottles, sleepless nights. But it also meant reliving first smiles, first words, and first steps and savoring the complete abandonment newborns have in the arms of their parents. Little by little, the perspective that was drawn on the horizon began to take form in my head; my heart was already endeared by this little one who had forced through our door. —*Isabelle*[1]

Family and friends may have been looking forward to this baby too. If you have older children, you may have already shared with them the exciting news that they were going to have a baby brother or sister.

I could hardly wait any longer to tell our daughter. I said to her that Daddy and I have a surprise for her. She said, "Am I going to be a big sister?" My husband and I laughed and I said, "Yes, Mommy is having a baby." Her little face lit up as she gave me a big hug and said, "Thank you!" with a squeal. As if we had just given her the world. It made us so happy to be able to tell her that a baby was on the way. —*Greta*

Along with high hopes and happy anticipation, you may have held the common assumption that if you take prenatal vitamins, don't drink alcohol, eat your broccoli, obtain obstetric care, and generally take care of yourself, the result after nine months will be a healthy baby. Most of the time, that is what happens. So it's only natural if you never imagined anything could go wrong with your pregnancy. Still, some parents worry or even have an intuition that something is not right. You may have felt a sense of foreboding or in hindsight be able to see that there were ominous signs.

Looking back, I should have known there was something wrong. If I knew my dates beyond a shadow of a doubt, why wasn't my baby's growth on schedule? But I was naïve, believing that every pregnancy ends in a healthy baby. And I guess, in my defense, it was my first pregnancy—what did I know? —*Alaina*

The News

⌐ I felt like something wasn't right. I was extremely afraid and paranoid that I was going to have a miscarriage or something. I wanted to be excited, but there was always that nagging feeling that something wasn't right. —*Deanna*

⌐ Somehow I feel I knew at a soul level that my baby was sick.
—*Elle*

⌐ The week before we got the news, my wife and I went on vacation in the mountains of Georgia. One night, a big storm blew through. Tornadoes, hail, the works. It woke my wife out of her sleep. She said she sat up in bed and heard the strangest sound. She said that in the middle of the thunder, in the middle of the lightning, in the middle of all the banging trees against the roof, she heard the sweetest sound of some baby birds singing as loud as they could. She said at the same moment God spoke to her heart and said, "I will have you doing this same singing in the storm." She woke me up the next morning and told me this story. I had no idea what would be so terrible. I prayed for God to spare us from the storm, but I received no answer. —*Scott*

If you or family members have a history of medical problems or if you have endured the death of another baby previously, your awareness of possible problems may have already been heightened.

Whether you were blissfully optimistic or had nagging feelings of unease, your outlook did not cause your baby's problems. Some parents are grateful for having been able to enjoy the pre-diagnosis time without worries, while others who felt apprehensive believe that their anxiety or intuition in some way helped prepare them for what was to come.

UNDERSTANDING DIAGNOSTIC PRENATAL TESTING

Even though you've already been through a battery of tests, you still may have questions about the testing process. Like many parents, you simply may have been following your caregivers' lead for routine care. But now you may want more information about how the doctors came to their conclusions, especially if you or the people around you are doubting or questioning the results. It seems that everyone knows parents who had alarming test results but their baby was just fine. How do you know that isn't the case for your baby?

Diagnostic prenatal testing is a relatively recent development in obstetric care. Before the 1980s, when fetal exam by ultrasound and amniocentesis became a routine part of prenatal care, babies were complete surprises at birth. Folk tales and superstitions were offered as questionable indicators of gender, and if a mother's belly was especially big, the doctor or midwife would feel for multiple babies. But if a baby had anatomical or chromosomal differences, this was revealed only after birth.

Testing offers an increasingly clear window into the womb, enabling parents and their health care practitioners to learn much about a baby before birth. Some parents are simply curious, eager to know more about their little one, and ultrasound offers a noninvasive way to "see" the baby. Others seek testing because they want reassurance that all is well, so in addition to ultrasound they may opt for invasive but definitive tests such as amniocentesis or chorionic villus sampling, which look at the baby's chromosomes. Of course, even though normal test results are no guarantee, parents anticipate gaining some peace of mind for the rest of the pregnancy. Most parents do get welcome reassurance that their baby is healthy and developing normally.

Some parents decline diagnostic prenatal tests because they are committed to bearing the baby they've conceived and dealing with whatever comes. Other parents, even if they would not end a pregnancy based on test results, accept testing because it can offer critical information for making decisions on behalf of their baby.

When prenatal testing is chosen, the process starts with noninvasive screening, such as a combination of maternal blood tests and ultrasound. Routine lab tests detect substances in the mother's blood that indicate the statistical possibility that the baby *might* have certain anatomical or chromosomal problems. Unfortunately, blood tests can yield "false positive" results, meaning that some mothers who receive a positive (abnormal) result are carrying a baby who is perfectly healthy. Abnormal results can be caused by factors including misjudging the date of conception, the mother's weight, and if there is more than one baby.

Routine ultrasounds can also show hints of certain chromosomal or anatomical problems, but they are not necessarily conclusive, especially if they are done by a practitioner who is not a specialist.

If any of these screening tests yield irregular results, more detailed diagnostic testing is offered so doctors can try to determine the baby's actual condition. For example, if a Level 1 screening ultrasound reveals "markers," or clues, that suggest possible chromosomal anomalies, a more-detailed Level 2 ultrasound exam might then be done. Some suspected anatomic problems also require a Level 2 ultrasound with a specialist, and in the case of heart defects, a fetal echocardiogram with a pediatric cardiologist. If abnormal results are confirmed, parents may then be offered an amniocentesis, in which a sample of amniotic fluid is removed from the mother's womb, using a long needle through the mother's abdomen under the guidance of ultrasound to avoid hurting the baby. The fluid contains fetal cells, which can be tested for genetic information. While waiting for the amnio test results, which can take ten days or more, a preliminary test is sometimes performed on a portion of the fluid sample. These results may come back in a few days but are not definitive.

Because of the wide net cast by screening tests, frightening initial results sometimes prove unfounded by further testing and the baby is indeed healthy. That's why your doctor or midwife may have initially told you not to worry when your results came back indicating a possible problem. Sadly, as further diagnostic testing and perhaps second opinions have confirmed, a false alarm does not appear to have been the case for your baby.

RECEIVING THE NEWS

⌐ I remember bombarding my husband with a thousand questions while driving the hour-long trip to the doctor's office. I said things like, "Oh, I just can't wait! I so want to know if we are having a boy or girl!" "Aren't you excited? How can you control your excitement?" I was so nervous, I couldn't eat that morning; I could barely sit still during the car ride. We had plans to go shopping for a baby crib, clothes, etc., that afternoon. I couldn't wait. Within minutes our world was turned upside down—our hopes and dreams crushed. —*Chelsea*

If your baby's problem happens to be identified with routine ultrasound, you're probably coming to this appointment expecting nothing more than a standard exam. You may even bring your baby's siblings or grandparents to share in the excitement of this first viewing. Instead, you receive terrible news in a darkened room, with grainy images of your baby on a computer screen. The quiet, protracted exam, the long wait for a doctor's appearance, and a storm of physical and emotional sensations make for an agonizing experience.

We watched his tiny black-and-white body move around on the screen. I was mesmerized by the miracle growing inside me. Then something just felt wrong. The sonographer just lingered a little too long on certain parts of his body. I asked her if something was wrong, and she said that she would be right back and left the room. I think that was the longest and most terrifying moment of my life. We did not know anything, and nobody was there to answer any questions. When she came back, we were moved to another room far removed from the rest to wait some more. About forty-five minutes later, the doctor came in and our world came crashing down. —*Brooke*

In the middle of our excitement, the sonographer interrupted us and said she was observing some very worrisome features on the baby. It was like our bubble of exuberance burst right then. My husband said he felt nauseated, and I started shaking uncontrollably on the bed for the rest of the ultrasound. —*Heidi*

I'm sure, in retrospect, that the ultrasound technician must have seen it outright, but she kept up the conversation until time came to take the measurements. Then she told us to stay in the room for a moment. I sat up and chatted to my husband about how well that had gone. And then the technician returned with another radiologist. I went totally cold. I asked if something was the matter.

He said no, just lie back and he'd retake the measurements. When he turned on the machine again, he went right for the head. When I couldn't take the tension any longer, I said to the radiologist, "What is it?" He said, "Anencephaly." I whispered, "No brain?" My husband gasped and turned around. I went utterly numb. I don't really remember what happened immediately after that, but I asked how sure he was. He said 100 percent sure. When was the last time a medical person said "100 percent" about anything? I knew something about anencephaly. I knew it was incurable. I knew there was no danger to me. I knew it meant our baby would die. —*Jane T.*

It didn't take long to figure out that something was definitely wrong with the baby. My 3-year-old daughter was whispering her innocent questions about the gel and the equipment in the room. I tried to keep her quiet as I stared at the words "abnormal" and "irregular" being typed onto the screen. The technician was very quiet, just doing her job. I remember so clearly a tightening in my throat, heaviness on my chest, and pressure in my head. This can't be happening to my baby. —*Greta*

The ultrasound tech began to move the wand around my belly. He asked me, "Are you hoping for a boy or a girl?" and I responded with (and I quote), "I don't mind if I have a boy or a girl, I just want to have a healthy baby." Just then, he stopped the wand on my belly for a second, looked at me, and then continued to focus the wand on one area. He did not say much anymore. He then informed me that he was finished but that he had to run a few things by the doctor on shift. I began to become uneasy, and my husband told me not to worry. When the doctor came in, I could not comprehend what he was telling us. I wanted to throw up, I cried very hard, and my heart was pounding out of my chest. I felt weak and faint, very faint. —*Jenny A.*

I knew by the look on the sonographer's face that something was wrong. She was so nervous when she walked out of the room that she forgot to tell me that we were done. She did not offer me a photo of my baby either. In fact, as she was running out the door, a picture fell to the floor; I picked it up and put it in my purse. —*Elizabeth B. P.*

A Gift of Time

If further tests are necessary or if you seek a second opinion, this can stretch the uncertainty over days and even weeks. As you wait, you may hold onto optimism, cling to denial, or be filled with anxiety.

⌐ When I went in for a routine ultrasound, everything seemed normal except my doctor told me that the baby might have a cleft lip. In my heart and soul my baby was fine; a cleft lip is no big deal. Anything worse cannot happen to *my* baby. I decided to go ahead with the high-resolution ultrasound but still thought nothing could be wrong with *my* baby. I met with a genetic counselor first who explained to me the multitude of reasons behind cleft lips; I listened and smiled and thought, *none of that applies to me.* —*Azima*

⌐ It was a very emotional time. We were told that the baby had a heart defect, but they weren't sure what it was. An appointment was scheduled two weeks after the ultrasound for an echocardiogram to determine the severity. Both of us were clueless. I remember searching on the Internet for congenital heart defects, and it scared me so I stopped. I wanted to stay positive and keep a positive energy. My husband wanted the facts first, before jumping to any conclusions. —*Christine*

⌐ The first test indicated we had a one in nineteen chance of delivering a baby with Trisomy 18. That phone call was really shocking. I remember thinking, "Well, since I have never even heard of Trisomy 18, there is no way I will have a baby with this condition." I stayed up very late that night finding out online what exactly Trisomy 18 was. My husband and I both cried ourselves to sleep that night. —*Jenny D.*

⌐ It seemed like we were being dropped from the top of the stairs by stages. First, at my Level 2 ultrasound, they found that Katherine had a diaphragmatic hernia. Then I had an amnio test, then that same day our doctor sent us to an infant cardiologist, who found Katherine's heart condition. Then three days later, we were hit with the Trisomy 13. —*Lizabeth*

⌐ It was this progression of going from "We're going to have this happy healthy baby" to "We're going to have this baby with mild disabilities and coordination problems" to "We're going to have a Down syndrome baby" to "We're going to have a baby that's not going to survive and we probably shouldn't have any more babies." It was like every turn was another left. —*Jill N.*

⌐ At first, the doctor thought that maybe I wasn't drinking enough water, and that was the reason for the low amniotic fluid. I drank so much in the following two weeks I felt like my brain was drowning. Then a nurse told me that too much water can be harmful too. Our third and final visit with the doctor confirmed that our baby either didn't have kidneys, or if she did they were too small to see and not going to work. —*Chelsea*

When amniocentesis is offered, some parents decline because it carries a small risk of causing miscarriage. But because there can be value in learning more information in order to make decisions on the baby's behalf, some decide that the benefits to their baby outweigh the possible risks.

⌐ We told the genetic counselor that we would not terminate our pregnancy no matter what the outcome of the amniocentesis was. She told us that there would be other decisions that could be made with the information that the amniocentesis provided, such as delivering in a hospital with a good neonatal intensive care unit, having our family members all around us for the birth, and being able to learn about all possible interventions that may be done for a critically ill infant and making those decisions before birth. With this information we changed our minds about the amniocentesis.

—*Jenny D.*

⌐ It was hard for me because they were jabbing a big needle into my wife's abdomen, and it was really painful for her. I watched it on the ultrasound screen, and that was hard for me to watch, to see her in pain, to see the needle go in the amniotic sac, to see the baby reacting. Later that day my wife was still leaking amniotic fluid from the amnio, and so we thought we screwed everything up by doing that test because we couldn't wait. But it stopped leaking. —*James*

You may be given the news with professionalism but also compassion. One mother recalled her doctor saying gently, "I feel like I'm a traffic cop who's coming to your door in the middle of the night to tell you that your child was just killed in a car accident."

⌐ The genetic counselor was very sweet to us on the phone, and I even heard her voice shake a time or two as if it was as hard for her to give this news as it was for us to receive it. —*Jenny D.*

⌐ The ultrasound technician was wonderful. She cried right along with us and gave us lots of extra pictures. —*Kathleen*

Unfortunately, too many parents are met with uncomfortable silence, a terse recommendation, or clinical insensitivity. This lack of empathy only amplifies your anguish.

⌐ The doctor informed us that he didn't see any kidneys, and he said, "This baby wouldn't be worth getting up for." I think everything went quiet at that point. My mind was racing: What does this mean, what do we do? I didn't respond to him. I was speechless. —*Deanna*

⌐ The tech got really quiet and turned the screen away. She asked another nurse to have a doctor come into the room. As soon as she said this my heart dropped, and I knew that something wasn't right. The doctor came in and within seconds they turned the light on and said that there was something wrong with the baby's head and we would have to terminate. —*Annette H.*

⌐ The doctor shook our hands and introduced himself. He sat down behind his desk, folded his hands, and told us that the ultrasound we had just finished had confirmed the results of the first ultrasound and that we needed to terminate our pregnancy immediately. My husband and I were shocked. Once I found my voice, I said, "But we thought our baby was just going to need surgery." The doctor looked at me like I was crazy, then picked up the reports in front of him and said, "This baby should never have made it through the first trimester—you should have miscarried this preg-

The News

nancy. I don't know why you didn't, but we'll go ahead and terminate it now." Both my husband and I silently started to cry—we had no idea that our baby had so many problems. —*Alaina*

⌐ The sonographer covered my stomach with the towel and left me lying there upset and wondering what it was. I don't know how long it took for the doctor to show up. It could have been five minutes or fifteen, but it felt like a lifetime. When the doctor came in, I will never forget what he did. I was lying there with my pants down, feeling about as vulnerable as I'd ever felt in my life, and the man walks in with a sympathetic smile on his face. What he did as the sonographer was taking her pictures is something I will never forget. His body language will haunt me forever. I could tell he was excited. When I say excited I mean the kind of excited that geologists get when they discover a fossil. The doctor was covering his fist over his mouth to hide the smile I know I saw. He pointed to the screen as it scanned over David's heart, and before he could help himself he said, "Oh, get that shot of the heart. That's a beauty." He realized instantly that he'd put his foot in his mouth. He looked at me and dug even deeper by saying to me, "I'm so sorry. I meant the picture, not your baby." So my baby isn't a beauty. Is that what you mean? My baby is freakishly deformed. Is that what you are proclaiming to me? I wanted to say this, but I was silent as I concentrated on the screen, trying to push back tears. —*Rachel*

For some parents awaiting conclusive results, the terrible news comes not during a doctor's visit but over the phone.

⌐ We saw that we had a message on our answering machine. It was our genetic counselor, and she left her home number and told us that we could call her any time before 9:30 p.m. My husband and I looked at each other with a knowing stare that seemed to freeze time. We were unable to move, to speak, or maybe even breathe for a full minute. We each grabbed an extension for the phone and settled into a bedroom with the door closed to call her back. Then came the news we knew must be coming. "Your amniocentesis results are in. Your son does have Trisomy 18." —*Jenny D.*

We were sent home to wait for amnio results, and I think we were mostly in shock. A familiar feeling, which I now know must have been grief, started creeping up on me. A week and a half later I called the genetics clinic out of desperation. I knew the results were most likely not back, but I had to check. When the genetics counselor told me the preliminary results, Trisomy 18, I began to cry. I was alone with my daughter and my tears scared her. I will never forget the look on her face as I stood in the kitchen and cried. —*Kristi R.*

I got a phone call from the genetic counselor. She said that 100 percent of the baby's cells have Trisomy 13. Initially I felt relieved to finally know exactly what was wrong with the baby. I called my husband and told him. And then I carried on with my mundane chores. The news slowly dawned on me. As I was washing our dishes, my tears started to roll down my cheeks. I started weeping from the bottom of my heart. —*Azima*

I was alone at home when the call came. As soon as I hung up the phone I collapsed onto the floor and just fell apart. I am still haunted by the sounds that came out of me. They didn't even sound human. —*Kathleen R.*

Whether you receive the news about your baby's diagnosis during an ultrasound, at a follow-up visit, or over the phone, you're being thrust onto an unknown path and swept away in an unintended direction.

THE IMMEDIATE EMOTIONAL STORM

Feelings of confusion and disbelief may be your first reaction. What is occurring around and inside of you may seem unreal.

I could barely comprehend what I was hearing. Everything seemed to move in slow motion. I had to tell myself to breathe. —*Annette G.*

～ We were in disbelief. I remember thinking the doctor had made a mistake. It seemed like I was sitting in on someone else's appointment. *—Delsa*

～ I remember my husband curled in a ball in the corner of the room sobbing. I continued to look back and forth between him and the doctor who seemed to be saying absolutely nothing in a Charlie Brown voice. She recommended that we go to a children's hospital to get further testing and apologized before she left the room. I do not know how long we sat there in silence with a mountain of used tissues surrounding us. Once we were able to leave, we went to my mother's house to pick up the boys. I asked her to sit down and proceeded to tell her what the doctor said. The rest of that day is a blur. *—Brooke*

～ The more the doctor talked, the harder it was to hold back the tears. It felt like the room was slowly spinning around me; time stood still for me as I tried to comprehend what he was trying to tell me. I tried not to get too upset; it would make it real. I wanted to give the doctor a chance to tell me not to worry, that he could be wrong. I remember turning my head and seeing my husband sitting in the chair wringing his hands with this solemn, scared look on his face and my mom sitting there as well, just as terrified. *—Chelsea*

～ I stopped listening to the doctor, despite all the questions I had to ask. We were discussing a hideous future, and it was that of our child. Like a game of billiards that has gotten out of hand, words banged into each other in my head to the point that nothing made any sense at all. *—Isabelle*

You may feel plunged into an unknown world. What happens next? If you received the news at a doctor's office, even getting out the door and going home feels surreal.

～ In the first minutes of getting the news that there was a serious problem, I didn't know what I was going to do. I just looked at the calendar on the doctor's desk and flipped the pages through four more months, not knowing what I would do. I was sobbing. We were given no hope, no resources. I didn't know how I was going to make it through the next five minutes, let alone the next four months. —*Chris*

⤳ We went out into the hall, and my husband collapsed to the floor in tears. We had to walk by a bunch of other pregnant women who were on their way to the doctor's office, who looked at us with such terror. —*Erin*

⤳ The only thing I could think to do was to call my mom while I was sobbing in the parking lot. No one was with me. Then I had to drive home alone, and for the life of me I don't know how I did that and not kill myself along the way. —*Rachel*

⤳ It was incredibly difficult—what was there to say to one another? Our baby was dying and there was nothing that my husband and I, two Ph.D. scientists, could do about it. We left the doctor's appointment in numb shock. I remember standing in the parking lot and just crying. —*Jane G.*

⤳ All that was left for us was to leave. We found ourselves alone on the sidewalk, like two shipwrecked victims on the shore, annihilated. I was sobbing in my husband's arms, stabbed in the heart by such an alarming first announcement. How could our little one, who had forced destiny to come and live with us, be wounded to this extent? —*Isabelle*

⤳ As we were waiting for the train, I was so tempted to jump onto the tracks and let it hit me. I could not handle the intensity of the pain that I was being forced to feel. If it was not for my children back at home, I can honestly say that I would not be writing this. —*Brooke*

A sense of confusion may hang on for days. It takes time for your mind to process such a seismic shift in reality. You know it's true, and yet, how could it be?

⤳ I just could not process what they had told us. How could this beautiful child of mine be fatally ill? Why is this happening to us? I just couldn't understand it. —*Jessie*

The News

⌐ All I wanted to do was crawl into bed and wake up again hoping this was all a bad nightmare. —*Amy*

⌐ I couldn't believe it—and yet I could. I don't know what I was feeling, if I even felt anything. I was scared and desperate and terrified—but not in denial. For some reason, I never doubted it was all happening. —*Jane T.*

Particularly if you are a religious person, this news can cause immediate spiritual anguish.

⌐ I started asking, "God, is this a test? Why are you testing me? Why do I need to be tested?" We felt so alone, and so completely terrified. —*Jennifer*

⌐ The day we found out about the complications of this pregnancy, it was an indescribable agony. The darkness that surrounded my heart was suffocating. Time stopped, and I felt forsaken. I count heavily on my faith to carry me through trials. That day, a mocking thought was repeated over and over in my mind: "Where is your God now?" —*Kelly G.*

⌐ It was complete and utter darkness, the darkest moment of my life, complete disbelief and anger. —*Jo*

⌐ After the crushing news, my wife and I were walking down what seemed like a five-mile-long hallway, and I turned to her and said, "We are going to hold hands, trust God, and sing in the storm." We had a promise from God that we could not afford to let go of.
—*Scott*

Your relationship with your partner may also be tested. How will you handle this as a couple? Will you be able to reach out to each other? At times, you may feel alone, even together.

⌐ As we ended the phone conversation with the genetic counselor, my husband and I looked into each other's eyes and both saw for the first time the deep pain of a parent whose child is fatally ill.

We were completely, utterly devastated. We went to our bedroom to sob. We held each other for hours and just cried. —*Jenny D.*

— We didn't sleep at all that night, just lay in silence. —*Erin*

During the first days and weeks after receiving your baby's diagnosis, you have much to learn about your baby and important decisions to make about your pregnancy. The next chapter explores the decision-making process, normalizes the wide variety of emotions, and suggests how to deal with the pressures. Then, if you decide to continue your pregnancy, the rest of this book provides you with a supportive context for braving the emotional journey of parenting your baby during pregnancy and beyond.

two

⌒

What Now?

Making Decisions about Continuing Your Pregnancy

⌒ We were in shock and at a loss for what the "right" thing to do was. Terminate the pregnancy? Carry to term and let him die then? Nothing seemed "right." It all seemed wrong. —*Susan E.*

Now that you know your baby's diagnosis, you have critical decisions to make. Some of them are literally about life and death. It's difficult enough to make a decision of this magnitude, and you are being asked to make it while your head is spinning and your heart is broken.

If you are still sorting through the diagnostic tests and reviewing your options, this chapter offers clear information and guidance on the decision-making process and affirms your ability to make an informed decision on behalf of your baby. You'll also find insights from other parents, some of whom were initially ambivalent about continuing, others who were sure from the beginning. If you've already made your decision to continue your pregnancy, this chapter can offer you validation.

FACING THE DECISION

After an unborn baby is found to have a life-limiting condition, parents often are expected to decide quickly whether to continue the pregnancy or end it. Continuing the pregnancy would raise many other questions to be decided later, but the question whether to terminate or continue is usually the first and most urgent choice parents are asked to make.

It's unfathomable that your baby will die, and yet you are being asked to accept this reality and choose between what seems to be "terrible" and "horrible." Your baby's existence may seem so broken and futile that you may want it to end sooner rather than later.

You might search and hope for a way out of this dilemma. You may get second opinions, hoping that the first evaluation was mistaken. You may wish for a miracle—or a miscarriage—to make the decision for you.

⌐ Making a decision was heart-wrenching. I had never been put in a position before to make a decision so significant. I did not want to have to make any of the decisions. At one point I felt like I wanted to just have a miscarriage, and then it would have been out of our hands. —*Christine*

Before you can wrap your mind around the choice between terminating or continuing the pregnancy, you must first confront the fact that modern medicine has no cure for your baby's condition. This represents yet another layer of violated expectations—that even though medical breakthroughs grab the headlines, there are many conditions for which medicine has no fix.

⌐ We were hoping for a miracle. Modern medicine could perform miracles, right? It had to for our baby—she couldn't die. —*Pam F.*

You may become primarily focused on uncovering any options for giving your baby life. You may spend hours on the Internet researching your baby's condition and sorting through medical studies, anecdotal reports of individual children, and sometimes-contradictory information. You may spend even more hours being evaluated by doctors, poring over whatever information they are able to offer and looking for any ray of hope that your baby can thwart death. Still reeling from your shattered dreams for a blissful pregnancy and a healthy baby, it can be simply too much to comprehend that your baby will die.

Gradually, as your shock wears off and your baby's prognosis sinks in, your perspective can shift. When you can accept that there is nothing you can do to change your baby's diagnosis, you can carefully

What Now?

consider how to proceed in the face of it. Instead of trying to fight your baby's impending death, you can put your energy toward embracing your baby's life. Instead of thinking about giving your baby a long life, you can start considering how to give your baby a *good* life. Instead of hoping that your baby can be cured, you can hope that your baby can experience a peaceful death. You can decline aggressive medical intervention and tests or treatments that might extend life without improving its quality. Thoughts of intensive care turn to palliative care. This shift in perspective is an integral part of making that first decision about whether to terminate or continue because it allows you to rethink your dreams for this child and focus on the hand that was dealt.

Even more significant, in this situation that feels so out of control, you can see that there is still a great deal you can control. You still have a profound opportunity to protect, welcome, and love your baby for as long as your baby is able to live.

OPTIONS PRESENTED

Options typically offered to parents are to end the pregnancy—by conventional abortion methods or by inducing labor prematurely— or to continue the pregnancy and "let nature take its course."

Some parents feel they were given their options compassionately and fully and that they weren't pressured in either direction.

⸺ The social worker really presented us with answers to all our questions (would the baby suffer if she was born alive, could her organs be donated, would she feel pain if we terminated, etc.) with enormous sensitivity. I really felt like she wanted us to have as much information as we could so that we would feel good about any choice we made. The respect she showed for us—and for our daughter—was both comforting and empowering. She was marvelous. —*Alessandra*

Some caregivers may not intend to express an opinion but may be unintentionally directive simply by their choice of words. Telling parents that their choices are to terminate the pregnancy or to "do nothing" and let the baby die after birth raises terrifying images in parents' minds about what it would be like to stand by helplessly and abandon their baby to death. As devastating as it would be to end the pregnancy, when it is presented as taking appropriate action and entails familiar concepts such as scheduling an appointment and going to a clinic, this option can seem much more imaginable.

Unfortunately, termination is sometimes the only option offered or recommended. Some practitioners mention the option of continuing the pregnancy but characterize it as a pointless and futile choice. While these practitioners may be giving what they believe to be their best recommendation, many parents resent the pressure and feel abandoned.

The only option that my doctor presented us with was termination. Even after we adamantly refused, he kept bringing it up. He just could not understand why we would want to continue the pregnancy. He saw no purpose in us continuing. —*Kathleen*

The doctor at the ultrasound didn't present any hospice options. He said that the best course of action was to "fix me up right away" so that I could "start over." He did mention that "some people" chose to deliver, but he made that sound like a ridiculous choice. —*Katharine*

My husband and I both sensed a strong push from the genetic center to terminate the pregnancy. They kept reiterating the "incompatible with life" aspect of his diagnosis. —*Heidi*

The doctors just told us to terminate. They didn't say anything else but terminate, even though we still didn't know what the baby's condition was or what was going on. Really, all we heard was TERMINATE. I hated that word. —*Annette H.*

Sometimes the vague language used to describe termination—and even the word itself—can mask that the procedures being recommended are actually types of abortion. This lack of clarity can lead parents to feel manipulated rather than informed.

What Now?

⌐ I felt numb from hearing the diagnosis, and my reaction was to do anything to get out of this pain. In my shock, I couldn't understand what they were talking about when they mentioned "termination." There is only so much the mind and the heart can take in an hour's time. Finally it hit me what they were trying to say: that "termination of the pregnancy" meant aborting my baby. —*Sue*

⌐ I don't want to say the perinatologists and gynecologists pushed, but they encouraged me to terminate my pregnancy. They never used the word "abortion" when they talked about that procedure. —*Missy*

⌐ When the doctor looked at my chart and realized what the diagnosis was, he said, "We need to talk." He immediately launched into discussing termination. We were adamant: No. At some point he came back with this other option that we could do, and he started describing it. With my nursing background, I quickly caught on to what he was talking about, and he was talking about a late-term abortion. The way he said it still makes me angry. At some point he had to leave the room, and my husband looked at me and said, "Well, that sounds pretty good." I looked at him and said, "Do you know what he's talking about? This is what he's talking about." My husband was appalled because the doctor was making it sound like it was nothing. He was so misrepresenting the truth. I was very grateful that I had some medical background to know what he was talking about, because I think we may have been talked into that option, and that wasn't at all what we wanted. —*Kathleen*

Some practitioners justify being vague because they want to protect parents from painful realities. But being vague about termination procedures also sidesteps the reality of what happens to your baby. Vagueness invites future agony if you later discover that what you consented to was not what you would have chosen if you had been fully informed. As painful as the details might be, when a compassionate practitioner can offer complete information and have these difficult conversations with you, this is far more helpful than shielding you or avoiding you. Then you can truly exercise informed consent.

A Gift of Time

Some parents are surprised that even as termination is being recommended, some abortion options aren't available at their own hospital or from their own physician. Availability can depend on hospital policies, physician willingness, and laws that vary from state to state.

Parents also may feel the added pressure of time constraints. Some hospitals and clinics perform terminations only up to 24 weeks of pregnancy, so parents who receive a diagnosis close to that limit may need to decide quickly or else travel to a physician who is willing to perform third-trimester abortions.[1]

When There Is Pressure to Terminate

The only option offered was termination. In spite of us insisting we wanted to continue this pregnancy, the medical personnel that handled us that day didn't offer us any other help. They kept emphasizing that "no one carries a baby with this condition" and how terrible it would be. They kept saying that Trisomy 18 is "incompatible with life." The pressure to terminate was tremendous. —*Chris*

If abortion is presented to you as the only option available or the only rational choice, your practitioner may base this recommendation on the belief that continuing a pregnancy and giving birth presents greater risk to the mother's physical and emotional health than termination. (This assumption is not supported by the evidence; see "Researching Possible Risks to the Mother" later in this chapter.) Parents can also perceive that their baby is being judged unworthy of nurturing, a life unworthy of life—a painful message to hear.

Our baby's life was under attack, and it was disguised as compassion. After watching our baby swim happily inside me, suck her thumb, and move her little feet, the doctor put her hand on my knee and said in a loving voice as I wept, "You know, you can terminate this pregnancy for good reason by inducing labor, and this is indeed a very good reason." I was sobbing. Our baby was going to die and she asked me if I wanted to end her life now! I felt as though no one in the medical profession valued our baby because of her genetic makeup, and I could do nothing but sit there and cry. I wanted to love and honor the life of our little girl, and I wanted everyone else to do so too. —*Courtney*

The doctor firmly believed terminating was best for us. We told him again we were not going to terminate—obviously this specialist didn't care at all about us, or what we were going through, or what would happen to us. How I hated that doctor for his treatment of us. —*Alaina*

The geneticist strongly seemed to recommend termination, either immediately at their hospital (I was already 23 weeks and they were willing to do it up until 24 weeks) or at a center willing to do later terminations. It wasn't really a value judgment; I just think he was totally unable to see this sick little baby as a person with a potential to experience and provide love. —*Alessandra*

Some advice to terminate is rooted in outdated thinking about miscarriage, stillbirth, and infant death. For decades, the subject was taboo. In a misguided attempt to protect parents from grief, doctors and nurses typically refused to allow parents to see a baby who was stillborn or dying, and parents were advised to forget about the baby and have another one. Perhaps caregivers meant well, but for many parents this approach caused long-lasting grief and emotional harm. Fortunately, most hospitals have now adopted more enlightened practices.[2] Caregivers offer parents the opportunity to see and hold their baby,[3] collect keepsakes such as handprints and footprints, and take photographs. The baby's body is treated with respect, and caregivers acknowledge the parents' emotional need to affirm this baby's existence. Those who automatically recommend termination may not understand that this is a real baby whose death is a real loss, and they are at risk of repeating the mistakes of the past.

Advice to terminate a pregnancy is also sometimes rooted in outdated practices regarding neonatal intensive care. From the 1960s through the 1990s, when neonatal intensive care technology was being developed and first implemented, nuanced medical decisions lagged behind. When parents wanted to continue a pregnancy after a fatal prenatal diagnosis, they were typically forced to hand over their newborn to the neonatal intensive care unit (NICU), where their baby would suffer through aggressive interventions before dying. Termination was seen by some as the lesser of two evils, a way to avoid futile, painful, and sometimes protracted medical intervention. This landscape has changed dramatically, with modern standards in neonatology including taking a more holistic view about the burdens and benefits of aggressive treatment and allowing comfort care instead when a baby's condition is life-limiting. Today, parents who receive their baby's terminal diagnosis during pregnancy have the humane option of planning a gentle birth and delivering their dying baby into palliative care instead of intensive care.

In addition, some practitioners recommend termination because they are unsure how to monitor a pregnancy expected to end in the baby's death. They went into obstetrics to work with the joyful beginning of life, not the end. There is a natural aversion to dealing with death and grief and often a lack of training. Aware that they cannot fix what is wrong, some practitioners perceive the death of a baby as a professional failure, their skills rendered useless by this situation. Doctors are accustomed to *doing* something, and waiting doesn't feel much like "doing." Finally, many practitioners are not yet aware that there are documented benefits, ways of supporting parents, or programs to which they can refer parents who wish to continue the pregnancy.

If you are feeling pressured to terminate, it is up to you to seek the additional information and support you need. You can start by talking with your caregivers, who may be open to helping you continue. If they remain resolutely closed to the idea, ask to be referred to someone else who will support you. You deserve to receive compassionate care that fits your needs.

When Support Is Lacking

I was shocked at how little information and little guidance we were given regarding the options we had and support for either choice. I asked if there were any support groups for people who continued their pregnancies. She said no. I asked what people did if they terminated their pregnancies. She said they had someone they would send me to who dealt with things like that, the sooner the better. —*Kristi R.*

What Now?

Regrettably, it is common for parents to feel cast adrift upon receiving their diagnosis. You may find that there is more emotional and practical support for terminating a pregnancy than there is for continuing. Caregivers may be troubled by this and wish they had more to offer to you.

⌐ We left that day devastated and alone. I asked if there was a support group for moms who continue a pregnancy like this. They said no, but there was support if I terminated. I asked to speak to any other mom who had a baby with a condition like this; they said there are none. I was sent away from the hospital with no support, resources, or hope. What a dark day that was. I had to find help on my own. —*Chris*

⌐ My genetic counselor apologized when Colm was diagnosed and said, "I am so sorry, I have nothing to give to you for support."
—*Pam M.*

PERINATAL HOSPICE AND PALLIATIVE CARE

Perinatal hospice, also sometimes called perinatal palliative care, is an innovative and compassionate model of support that can be offered to parents who find out during pregnancy that their baby has a life-limiting condition. "Perinatal" means around the time of birth; perinatal hospice incorporates the philosophy and expertise of hospice into the care of pregnancies and babies like yours. Perinatal hospice is not a place; it is a way of thinking about your pregnancy and your baby.[4] This practical and empathetic approach supports you through the rest of your pregnancy, through decision-making before and after birth, and through your grief. It is a continuum of supportive care that honors your baby as well as your role as parents.

Perinatal hospice support begins at the time of diagnosis, not just after the baby is born. It can be thought of as "hospice in the womb," including prenatal care and birth planning to fit your special situation, as well as preliminary decision-making about medical care for your baby after birth. If your baby lives longer than a few minutes or hours after birth, perinatal hospice also incorporates more conventional hospice care such as managing symptoms and easing any possible discomfort.

Palliative care is another term you might hear. This is a broader concept that aims to relieve suffering, address pain and other symptoms of a condition or disease, and care for the patient as well as the family. It affirms life and regards dying as a normal process, intending neither to hasten nor postpone death.[5] The goal is to enable the person who is terminally ill to have the best possible quality of life, by providing comfort and dignity to the patient and by offering support to the grieving family. Palliative care can be provided while also pursuing medical treatments that might benefit your baby. Palliative care is an umbrella that includes hospice, which focuses on end-of-life support. Ideally, perinatal hospice and palliative care involves a comprehensive team approach that includes obstetricians, maternal-fetal medicine specialists, midwives, labor and delivery nurses, neonatologists, NICU staff, chaplains and pastors, doulas, social workers, genetic counselors, pediatricians, therapists, childbirth educators, trained parent advocates, and traditional hospice professionals.

As knowledge spreads about perinatal hospice and palliative care, practitioners have begun offering this option, or parents find out about it on their own.

Our perinatologist arranged for perinatal hospice to contact us. This helped a lot, just knowing that there was support out there for us. —*Behka*

I called my sister, who is a NICU nurse in another state. She told us how we could work with Noah's diagnosis. She told me about hospice care and comfort measures as part of the birth plan.
—*Jenny A.*

We were told nothing by the perinatologists, but we learned about a local perinatal hospice from about five people within a forty-eight-hour period. We learned about this service soon after we sent a mass e-mail to friends, family, and acquaintances, requesting prayers and referrals to any resources for those coping with infant loss. My OB also had just learned about perinatal hospice and told us about it. —*Jennifer*

If you have not had experience yet with hospice, the idea may seem frightening and morbid. But hospice is not about dying. It's about living fully during the time remaining. As Dame Cicely Saunders, a British physician who is considered the founder of the modern hospice movement, famously said: "You matter because you are you, and you matter to the last moment of your life."[6]

Or you may fear that choosing hospice means giving up and losing hope. But hospice and palliative care are about providing a different kind of medical care, with different kinds of hope. When your baby is expected to die, your original wishes and dreams for your child's long life are dashed. But as you adjust to the reality of your baby's impending death, your hopes can change direction: for your baby to be born alive, for your baby to be held, for your baby's life to be filled with love. These are profound kinds of hope. Parents who have chosen perinatal hospice have said that this kind of care helped their hopes be fulfilled.

It is also natural to fear choosing hospice and palliative care if you are worried that the diagnosis might be wrong. You might worry that if your baby isn't as sick as doctors say, you should have chosen intensive care instead. It is true that prenatal diagnosis is not perfect. At birth, some babies' conditions are less—or more—severe than predicted. Sometimes the diagnosis was ambiguous all along. On very rare occasions a diagnosis was wrong or the baby's condition improves over the course of the pregnancy. Perinatal hospice and palliative care encompasses all these scenarios. A baby might be born stronger than expected and seeming to say that she's able to fight to stay awhile longer. In this case, upon further testing, doctors may be able to offer a better prognosis, and parents may decide that medical intervention is warranted. Another baby might be born weaker and sicker than expected, seeming to say more urgently that all he needs is comfort and love, and parents can change their plans accordingly. If a baby is born healthy, hospice will be joyfully excused. Even if your baby's prenatal diagnosis is uncertain, that's a reason to explore perinatal palliative care, not avoid it. It can help you make sense of what your baby's possible scenarios might be. Decisions and plans can always be adjusted as the baby's needs are made known. You—and your caregivers—can let your baby lead you.

For an up-to-date list of perinatal hospice and palliative care support programs, visit www.perinatalhospice.org. But you don't need an established program to get this kind of care. You simply need a caregiver who understands this approach and is willing to help coordinate this care for your baby and family.

GATHERING INFORMATION

As you work to decide whether to terminate or continue, your first task is to gather information. You might be receiving medical information from medical professionals such as a perinatologist or genetic counselor, and you might also be seeking or receiving information from family, friends, clergy, the Internet, and other sources. You may be learning more than you thought possible about medical conditions you didn't even know existed. You might be getting a crash course in physiology, neurology, pathology, genetics, obstetrics, medical ethics, and end-of-life care. You might feel overwhelmed by statistics, options, and possibilities.

It's like trying to drink out of a fire hose. You just can't take in all that information. —*Bianca*

In spite of the mountain of shocking detail before you, you may feel desperate for information. This doesn't make you morbid—this is your quest for mastery. By mastering what lies before you, you can feel more oriented, better able to ask the questions you couldn't articulate earlier, and more confident about the choices you make. Or perhaps you take a different approach and don't want a lot of details. Maybe all you need to know is that your baby will die, and you rely on your values or gut feelings to make your decision. However you go about gathering facts and weighing your options, you benefit from having access to as much information as you feel you need.

Absorbing shocking medical information takes time. If your doctor tells you your baby's diagnosis and then launches into an explanation of medical details and options, you'll likely not be able to take it all in. Your emotional shock can make it impossible for you to hear, much less remember, what you've been told.

⟶ On the day of the diagnosis we were told to take time to think about things, and that if we had any questions the staff were available. The problem was that I had no recollection of that, until I reread my journal. I was a walking zombie. We walked out of the hospital and we literally could have walked under a bus. I wouldn't have known any different. I didn't hear anything. I could barely see. —*Elle*

Because you're in shock, you may believe that you've received scant information, while your practitioner's perception is that you're now well-informed. This disconnect may be remedied by your caregiver first giving you a chance to process your emotions and disbelief. Whether it's ten minutes in the exam room or coming back for another appointment the next day, you may be able to calm down enough to take in the critical details. If you feel you weren't able to absorb the information the first time, it's entirely appropriate to request another appointment to discuss details again.

Researching Your Baby's Condition

⟶ I learned through hours of Internet research and discussions with my doctors and my genetic counselor that there was a possibility that our baby would live up to an hour after birth. I decided that even five minutes with my baby alive in my arms would be worth it.
—*Chelsea*

Learning more about your baby's condition and prognosis can help you decide whether to continue or terminate. Perhaps you have a specific diagnosis but aren't sure what it entails. To find out more, your prenatal caregivers can be good resources. However, given the rarity of some conditions, it's possible they have not had any firsthand or recent experience. You can ask for a consultation with a neonatologist, pediatrician, or other specialist regarding your child's condition. You also may find it helpful to contact another kind of true expert:

other parents whose infants shared your baby's condition. It can be reassuring to get a parent's perspective as well as details on what your baby's future might hold.

⁓ My doctor introduced us to another couple who had a little girl with the same condition two years earlier. We met with them, learned about their experience with their daughter, and decided to carry our son to term. We were especially impressed with the memories they had of her and getting to spend time with her after she was born. Our doctor had also shared that time with them, and he assured me that carrying Nathaniel and giving birth to him could be far more beautiful and healing than I could imagine or currently understand. —*Annette G.*

If you are pregnant with two or more babies, your decision is complicated further. You must consider the condition and best interests of all your babies. Fortunately, in most cases a healthy baby is unaffected by the presence of a sick baby, and you can carry both or all safely to term, even if one is not likely to survive much longer.

⁓ Our options were to attempt a selective reduction, with a 5 percent chance of miscarriage of the presumably healthy baby, or to carry both babies as close to term as possible, with the intrinsic risks of a twin pregnancy and increased risks due to the anencephaly. Our primary concern was for the best outcome for our presumably healthy child, and the 5 percent risk of miscarriage seemed way too high. —*Jane G.*

Concerns about Suffering

A major concern for most parents is whether their baby will suffer during the pregnancy or after birth.

⁓ We wanted to know if having Trisomy 18 would be painful and if terminating the pregnancy could prevent that pain. And the nurse said, no, there's no reason this baby will be uncomfortable. —*Jill K.*

What Now?

Even parents who happen to be physicians or other medical professionals may need to consult with people who have more expertise. Said one father, a physician himself:

⟜ I knew the geneticist well. One of my questions to him was, "Is there any suffering involved in our daughter's existence?" He said, "No, not really." That was a big point. It very quickly became obvious to me that having an extra chromosome is not a capital crime. —*David D.*

To find out more about whether your baby might suffer after birth because of his or her condition, you can consult a palliative care specialist or an anesthesiologist to ask whether a baby with this condition might need pain relief and, if so, how it could be provided. If pain is a possibility, it can be treated aggressively and effectively, and some pain can be avoided altogether by careful decisions about which medical interventions you want or don't want for your baby. A terminally ill baby does not need to be rushed to intensive care, surgery, or a ventilator. Instead, you can envelop your baby in comfort and love.

If you have not been assured of adequate pain control or comfort care for your baby after birth, you might be wondering if termination would be the kinder choice. Fortunately, great strides have been made in both palliative care and neonatal medical ethics. Now it is considered permissible, even commendable, to forgo medical intervention that is experimental or will only prolong dying and to provide active comfort measures instead. In addition, palliative care has become a medical specialty in its own right.[7] It includes pain control and attending to the patient's unique needs for comfort and nurturing. Perinatal hospice draws on both the movement to create humane conditions in the care of tiny newborns as well as the movement toward palliative care. (For more discussion of palliative care and medical decisions for the baby after birth, see Chapter 5.)

⟜ I did not even know if it were medically possible to continue my pregnancy. A dear friend, a professor of genetics whom we called in urgently, confirmed that it was possible to carry out the pregnancy with such a diagnosis and told us how to go about it. By "being there" for this baby, I could take him to the end of his little life, as it had been programmed, without putting my own life in jeopardy, without the risk of making him suffer (no relentless therapeutic measures at birth, rather palliative care as necessary). He would just live out his entire life, carried by our tenderness and softly fall asleep in the afterlife—in his own time. —*Isabelle*

An Overview of the Termination Option

As you research your options and evaluate what's best for your baby, especially if you are weighing whether termination would be more compassionate, you also may need more information about what would be involved in ending your pregnancy. There are two basic options: surgical abortion and premature induction of labor. (Drug-induced abortions, such as with RU-486, are not an option because prenatal tests cannot yet detect problems soon enough after conception for those drugs to work.)

Surgical Options

If you received your diagnosis very early, during the first trimester, the most common procedure would be a vacuum-aspiration surgical abortion.[8] Another first-trimester procedure is dilation and curettage (D&C),[9] which uses a curette to scrape the inside of the uterus, the same procedure that's used if tissue remains after a miscarriage. In the second trimester, through about 24 weeks of pregnancy, the most common method is an outpatient dilation and evacuation (D&E) abortion.[10] Because the baby is larger, the woman's cervix is dilated during appointments typically over more than one day, and during the final procedure surgical instruments are used to remove the baby in pieces, so parents are not allowed to see the remains afterward. Another procedure used late in the second trimester or in the third trimester is intact dilation and extraction (D&X), a controversial method commonly known as "partial-birth" abortion. As in a D&E, the process of dilating the cervix typically is done on an outpatient basis and can take several days. Then the baby is partially delivered breech, or feet first, and the head is collapsed with a scissors or forceps and the brain matter is removed before the head is delivered so the cervix doesn't need to be dilated fully.[11] The U.S. Supreme Court has upheld a ban on using this method on a live fetus, so clinics that still perform this procedure or similar late-term procedures often administer a lethal injection of potassium chloride or an intentional overdose of the heart medication digoxin into the baby's heart in the womb first.[12] The injection is performed like a reverse amniocentesis, under the guidance of ultrasound, except unlike an amniocentesis in which the needle is kept away from the baby, in this procedure the needle pierces the baby's chest and the injection causes the heart to arrest. More than one injection is sometimes needed.[13] Alternatively, some practitioners cut the umbilical cord in utero before beginning the extraction process.[14] For parents who are concerned about the baby's suffering, details about the injection and subsequent surgical procedures to remove the baby's body can be very disturbing but essential to their decision-making.

Premature Induction

Terminating a pregnancy soon after diagnosis by inducing premature labor in a hospital is much closer to a normal birth experience. The mother would be admitted and given drugs to start labor. This process can take more than a day because the mother's body is physiologically not ready to go into labor. Depending on the baby's condition and stage of development, he or she might not survive the birth process or might die soon after birth of complications of prematurity, particularly immature lungs and an inability to breathe, in addition to the fatal condition. Some centers also require a lethal injection into the baby before inducing labor, to avoid the legal obligations associated with a live birth. When hospital ethics guidelines prohibit termination by induction or other methods, some doctors circumvent this policy by administering the lethal injection at a clinic so the hospital will treat the situation as a natural fetal death.[15] Some hospitals treat induction terminations with the same sensitivity as a natural stillbirth or infant death, offering parents the opportunity to spend time with their baby, helping parents collect keepsakes, and treating the baby's body with respect.

Even when parents decide to continue their pregnancy, circumstances can change and labor may need to be induced prematurely. If you are unable to go full-term, you can still approach your pregnancy and your baby's birth, life, and death in the spirit of perinatal hospice, not abortion.

Researching Possible Risks to the Mother

As you make this profound decision, one important consideration is whether this pregnancy could cause harm to you—physically, emotionally, or perhaps affecting your future fertility.

Physical Health

If you are told that your pregnancy threatens your health, you can ask for clarification about whether you are actually facing a greater risk. Some physicians feel that even the normal risks of pregnancy become too great if the baby is expected not to live. But terminal conditions in the baby typically do not pose any greater physical risk to you than the normal risks of pregnancy. The risks involved in carrying a baby with anencephaly, for example, are still low.[16] And in small studies of mothers who continued their pregnancies with babies who had lethal conditions, there were no maternal physical complications.[17] It's important to note that abortion also carries physical risks, which increase as pregnancy progresses. The maternal mortality risks of abortion after 21 weeks are slightly greater than the normal risks of pregnancy and childbirth.[18]

If there are possible side effects related to the baby's condition, such as a larger-than-usual amount of amniotic fluid (polyhydramnios), some parents conclude that those are risks they are willing to take in order to protect and meet their baby. Physicians, especially maternal-fetal medicine specialists, are trained to watch for complications and to treat both the baby and the mother.

It is rare for a pregnancy to pose a direct threat to a woman's life. If a threat to the mother is so severe that the baby must be delivered too prematurely to survive, the mother can receive urgent medical care while the baby can still be provided with comfort and treated with respect.

You can ask for specifics about your own and your baby's particular risk factors for pregnancy, labor, and birth.

What Now?

We decided that if this baby and pregnancy weren't going to harm me or any future babies, we would carry to term. When they told us that everything would be fine with me, we knew that we had made the right decision. —*Annette H.*

Fertility

If your doctor says that continuing your pregnancy poses a risk to your fertility, you can ask for clarification about this too. While you may fear damage to your uterus or reproductive system, the reality may be much more benign. Some physicians reason that a pregnancy like this affects your fertility because you can't get pregnant with a healthy baby while you are "stuck on hold" with this one. You will be another six to twelve months older by the time you can try to conceive again. If you are a younger mother and have conceived easily, this may not be a major concern. But if you have struggled with fertility or if you are an older mother nearing the end of your childbearing years, this can be a terrible dilemma. Which baby do you focus on: the one you carry now or a future healthy child you *might* conceive? Ask for specifics about any possible impact on your fertility so you can weigh the costs and benefits for yourself.

Emotional Health

Especially if your pregnancy is expected to be otherwise normal, your emotional well-being may be the most pressing worry for you and for those who care about you. How could you possibly walk around for the rest of your pregnancy, watching your belly grow and feeling your baby move, all the while knowing your baby will die? How could a mother do that and survive emotionally? How could a father stand by helplessly and watch his baby die? What about the baby's siblings?

Many caregivers assume that terminating the pregnancy is easier on parents psychologically than carrying to term a baby who is not expected to live. They believe that continuing the pregnancy unnecessarily allows feelings of devotion to grow, so letting go becomes more difficult and grieving more profound. Some practitioners also believe that termination is a shortcut through pain and grief, allowing you to achieve "closure" and put this behind you sooner. Another line of reasoning is that you can alleviate your sorrow by having another baby who is healthy.

But these assumptions discount the bond that you already feel with your baby by the time the diagnosis is made. Terminating the pregnancy doesn't terminate the bond, and it does not alleviate your pain. There is no shortcut through grief. And having another baby—assuming parents are able to conceive again in the first place—is no magic cure either. Babies are not interchangeable; many parents continue to honor, remember, and grieve for their deceased baby long after they bear another. Termination also requires parents to take invasive action that violates the protective urges that accompany a wanted pregnancy.

A counselor advised me not to go through the pregnancy because I had a history of depression, and he was worried about my mental and emotional health. But what about my mental and emotional health if I went against everything I believed in and had to live my life with the knowledge that I consented to kill one of my children? —*Sue*

It's important to note that there is no research to support the presumption that aborting the pregnancy is easier on the parents psychologically. In fact, studies to date suggest the opposite: that women who terminate grieve as much or more than women experiencing a spontaneous death of a baby[19] and that aborting a baby with birth defects can be a "traumatic event . . . which entails the risk of severe and complicated grieving."[20] One long-term study found that "a substantial number . . . showed pathological scores for post-traumatic stress."[21] Another study found that fourteen months after termination for fetal anomaly, nearly 17 percent of women were diagnosed with a psychiatric disorder, such as posttraumatic stress, anxiety, or depression.[22] In contrast, parental responses to perinatal hospice are "overwhelmingly positive."[23] As the parents' stories in this book attest, continuing the pregnancy for as long as they can and embracing their baby's brief life can be a beautiful, profoundly meaningful, and healing journey.

A crisis such as this can test your values in ways you never would have imagined. It can crystallize—or force you to reexamine—your beliefs about life, death, and what is most important to you. You may be revisiting philosophical questions that now hold urgent meaning for you. You may be questioning your religious or spiritual beliefs.

A crisis such as this can also test your decision-making skills. If you normally make important decisions with your rational mind, you may be newly aware that your heart also wants to be consulted on this one.

— When I allowed myself to pay attention to what my body and heart really wanted, to listen to my gut, eventually I was able to let go of my need to know all of the facts. And now that I think about it, I see that this was the first step toward my decision to carry my baby to term rather than inducing labor: By letting go, I was able to accept. I started to love Frankie fully as he was, and I could be very present with him. —*Susan E.*

Meditation, prayer, journaling, or talking with your partner or trusted friends can help you tap into your intuition about what is best for you and your baby.

Spiritual, Religious, and Ethical Considerations

Prenatal tests and technology are modern developments, and the dilemma of whether to terminate or continue a pregnancy based on test results is a recent phenomenon. But the life-and-death issues being raised are quite old: Is it ever permissible to take a life? What are my obligations to a fellow human being? When does life begin? These are profound questions that in many forms have challenged philosophers and theologians for thousands of years. It's no wonder that this decision can feel overwhelming.

Because this decision can have spiritual, religious, and ethical implications, you may want to consult professional clergy. You might hear a perspective that helps you decide—and cope.

⟶ Our priest told us that this would only be six months of my life, in reality not very long. It seemed like an eternity to me, though. —*Annette H.*

⟶ Spiritual guidance was the *only* thing that kept my pregnancy going. Our priest said that this baby is meant to die from her condition, and anything else would be a different cause of death. I told him how I felt and that I was praying for God to take this baby to heaven now, but I also trusted my faith to guide me. We did what the priest told us to do. I think if he had said it was OK to let go early, we would have. I also didn't think that terminating the pregnancy would "make it all go away." I wanted my heartache to go away, not my baby. —*Jo*

Just like advice from people in other professions, religious advice might be contradictory or unhelpful. You may ultimately look for guidance and inspiration by examining your own beliefs or retreating into private prayer.

⟶ One religious leader told us that if our baby did survive, she would be a "living doll" and take over our lives. It still didn't feel right to me. Another religious leader told us the choice was up to us, but if we carried to term her life would be worth it—whether it lasted a second or a century. We both knew he was right and our decision was made from there on out. —*Erin*

⟶ Our faith played a huge part in our decision. We had prayed and prayed to become pregnant. How could we terminate this pregnancy and then pray to God to become pregnant again? With a perfect baby next time, please. It did not seem right. Even though I am making it sound like the decision and our trust in God was easy, it was anything but that. I could not sleep. I was beside myself. I was overwhelmed with grief. —*Kristi R.*

⟶ I prayed for an answer. I read my Bible night and day. One night, just before we had to make the decision, it became clear. I had to leave it up to God. It couldn't be on our hands. —*Kelly G.*

What Now?

⌒ I prayed that the pregnancy would come to an end very soon naturally. We have always professed that the dignity and worth of all human life, from conception to natural death, must be upheld. So even though we couldn't imagine how we would survive, we submitted to our belief that we needed to uphold the dignity of our baby's life to the fullest degree by carrying the pregnancy to term. This was a very difficult decision because emotionally we really wanted the pregnancy to end very quickly. —*Jennifer*

You may find it helpful to know that religious teachings can accommodate early induction in certain cases. For example, in the rare situation in which the baby must be delivered prematurely to save the mother's life, even religions with strong traditions of protecting the unborn consider this to be tragic but morally acceptable because the intent is not to directly cause the death of the baby.[24]

Early induction can be ethically or morally justified under other circumstances too. For example, if the mother's health is deteriorating, the baby's health can deteriorate too. Or sometimes the baby's condition leads to a higher risk of stillbirth, and inducing after viability but before the due date may offer a better chance that the baby will be born alive. Even if the baby might die sooner in terms of date, early delivery can give baby and parents a chance to meet before death. Again, the intent is not to cause the baby's death but to plan for a gentle birth and enhance the baby's quality of life.

You also may wonder about spiritual matters that are beyond the realm of medicine, questions such as whether your baby has a soul. It can be reassuring to consider that although your baby's physical body may not be suited for this life, the spiritual essence of your baby is perfect and eternal.

⌒ Our priest said that in God's eyes, this baby is nothing less than perfect. This baby is completely alive and with a soul but just imperfect from a medical science standpoint. —*Jo*

⌒ A shift in my own consciousness became more apparent as I dealt with people who reported that they were praying for Frankie. I remember that when others would tell me specifically that they were praying that God would heal Frankie by giving him kidneys, I would focus on their use of the word "heal." My heart would question: How can you heal something or someone that is already perfect? Frankie had become perfect and even complete to me. —*Susan E.*

Besides turning to religion and philosophy, you also could evaluate the ethics of your options by reading about medical ethics or consulting with a hospital ethics committee. You can draw on your beliefs about life and death and strive to determine the best interests of your child.

Whether your decision is based on religious belief, intellectual analysis, or your gut feeling, you can come to some of the same conclusions that philosophers, theologians, and ethicists have spent years honing.

Your Beliefs about Abortion

Being faced with the very real option of termination can challenge abstract opinions that you may have had about abortion. If you'd always thought you could easily decide "yes" or "no," you may be surprised if it's not a simple decision for you after all. In fact, many parents with strong convictions against abortion find themselves considering it.

I have always been pro-life under any circumstance and always said I'd never waver—but I never had to walk the walk I was walking. I am ashamed to say that I considered the termination of my baby, but it is true, I considered it. —*Jo*

Given that I am a pro-life Christian, one would expect this decision to be easy for me. But it wasn't. Worried that my choice could cause my baby to experience discomfort every day I carried him, I considered the options. Also weighing heavily on my mind was our first child, who was 4 at the time, and my husband. Could I make their grief easier if I just ended this quickly? —*Kelly G.*

If you are disturbed by your willingness to consider termination as an option, remember that the diagnosis itself forced you to think about issues you never imagined you'd face. To make the best decision, you needed to carefully weigh your options.

Others who support legalized abortion may surprise themselves by their firm rejection of terminating their pregnancy. But your convictions about social policy need not dictate what you would choose for yourself. Whatever your beliefs or background, your decision is about your baby, not about political opinions.

⌐ When the doctor said the word "terminate," I knew he was talking about a late-term abortion. I never thought I would have to make a decision like this. I always said that I was pro-choice. But I didn't give it more than a second's thought: I chose *life*. —*Rebecca J.*

⌐ I probably would consider myself pro-choice. So we were dealing with the dilemma of, first of all, are we going to have the baby or not? We decided to let Alaina decide. We wouldn't intervene. We thought, let's just let Alaina, and divine intervention if there is any in this case, determine this. She'll be with us as long as she wants to, and we'll support her and love her. —*James*

⌐ I'm very much a pro-choice person, but for me, the right choice was to complete the pregnancy. —*Missy*

MAKING DECISIONS WITH YOUR PARTNER

It may help to be aware of how you typically make decisions as a couple. Does one of you tend to make decisions instinctively, while the other one researches every last detail and then some? Do you comparison-shop until you can't compare any more and then experience buyer's remorse afterward anyway? Do you make firm decisions and never look back? Does one of you tend to defer to the other, or do you have a collaborative style?

Not surprisingly when more than one person is involved, not all couples initially agree about which path to take.

⟿ I just felt that this baby was still alive and it was not my decision to make, to end its life. My husband wanted to end the pregnancy at first just to be done with it and not have to go through all that lay ahead. This did cause some problems between us. After I explained to my husband that this would be the only time we would have with this child, he changed his mind, and we decided to make the most of the time we had. —*Sherry*

⟿ My husband considered terminating. I told him that I felt this baby move; I looked into the eyes and face at the sonogram—there was no way I would terminate. So that was the end of conversation over the weekend. I was very scared that we would not agree. At our next appointment with the doctor, my husband spoke up and said we would not terminate. In spite of the situation, I never felt so much peace as I did that afternoon. —*Angel*

It is normal for a father's primary concern to be for the mother's emotional and physical health, and he may question the mother's wish to continue out of concern for the burdens this places on her. The mother is the one who would have to carry the baby, but of course it's the father's child too. This can provoke a delicate dance of attempting to express an opinion while also trying to defer to the mother, who might not even know yet what she wants to do.

⟿ My husband said it was my decision as I was carrying this baby and he couldn't ask me to do anything I wasn't comfortable with. I told him that it wasn't fair that he was putting all this on me as our decision would be felt by both of us and our kids, and if I carried to term I would need him as never before. —*Sue*

⟿ My husband told me right away that he did not want to go out of state for a late-term abortion. However, he realized I had to make the decision. —*Tracy*

Some couples find themselves pretty much on the same wavelength. Whether friends, family, or practitioners affirm your decision or not, your partner can be your best ally and advocate. You may

What Now?

---

huddle up, relying on each other as sounding boards and coming to a decision together.

⌐ As I lay on the ultrasound table, I sobbed and sobbed and said to my husband that I couldn't go through with a termination. He confidently said, "You don't have to." He didn't want to terminate our baby's life either. *—Katharine*

⌐ My husband told me, "Chris, if we terminate this pregnancy, you won't sleep another night. We will have regrets. We will take this one day at a time, and in the end we will get over this." I knew that we were together on this, and that whatever was ahead we had each other. I didn't have the support of the medical people, but I had the support of my husband. *—Chris*

⌐ After a few weeks of late-night talks, we knew we were in for the long haul. Our child would not have very much time here on Earth and we were not going to rob him of the precious time he had left. *—Donna*

CONSULTING WITH PEOPLE YOU TRUST

⌐ I remember feelings of confusion and isolation that made it very difficult to see the situation clearly and to make decisions confidently. We leaned on our family and friends to help navigate this overwhelming information. *—Missy*

Although it's unlikely that you know anyone who has experienced what you're going through, with a decision of this magnitude it is natural to turn to others for support and guidance. Your shock and grief can make it difficult for you to think clearly, and you may have friends, family members, or others you trust who can provide insights.

⌐ I had some helpful advice from my mom: She said not to resist some of the plans that God has for you in your life. She just felt that we should not be tempted to go the way that some of our friends and doctors might suggest, that we should see it through and allow that experience in our lives. That was great advice. —*Missy*

For some parents, however, advice from friends and family can feel like pressure. If their recommendations don't feel right to you, their advice only makes you feel alone. Outnumbered, you may cave to their way of thinking. Or you may decide to trust your own instincts and forge ahead anyway. Especially if you're deciding to go against strong opinions, this may further isolate you.

⌐ I prayed and cried and agonized. I asked every person I could find what they would do. Most everyone told me that they would terminate. It felt wrong to me. I already loved her so much. —*Jamie*

⌐ We immediately decided against terminating, but after talking to our parents, religious leaders, and friends we decided to terminate. Our parents felt it was cruel to make me carry to term knowing I couldn't take her home. —*Erin*

⌐ At the beginning I actually sought out people who thought terminating would be best because I thought that would justify my feelings of wanting to be done with the pregnancy. After I decided to continue, I stopped sharing many things with the people I felt did not support our decision, just for fear of hearing "I told you so."

—*Jo*

What you may need more than anything else is someone who will listen and be a sounding board, without trying to fix or advise you. If you can find even one person, this support can be a lifeline. It can also help to remember that this is your life, your pregnancy, and your baby. It's also your decision.

⌐ Everyone had an opinion on what we should do about this. Some people informed me, "You need to just get it taken care of; there is no sense carrying on with a pregnancy like that." My OB never pushed me one way or another. I even asked him what other people do, and he said that I needed to do what was best for me not what other people would do. I felt at peace when we came to

What Now?

the point that we realized we needed to make this decision and just forget about what everyone else had to say. —*Deanna*

⟶ Regardless of our family members' and friends' beliefs, each person held back his or her opinion and allowed us the space to make our own decision. All of our loved ones were available to listen or help out however we needed. We were very blessed with this. —*Susan E.*

DECIDING TO CONTINUE

Some parents decide immediately to continue. Others take longer to reach a decision, watching the days after the diagnosis tick by, feeling the baby moving while being aware of a looming deadline for ending the pregnancy. The time comes to make a decision.

For many parents, making the decision to continue isn't easy or automatic. Your first impulse may be to end the pregnancy.

⟶ For a minute or two, sitting in the genetic counselor's office, I was crying a lot, and there was definitely a piece of me that thought, you know, maybe termination is the answer. Let's just end this nightmare right now. —*Jill N.*

⟶ At first I thought termination might be the best route. It could be done right away, and then it would be over with and then we could move on. However, I had already felt the baby move around, and I knew that it wouldn't be that easy. I felt that because we did have to make the decision on behalf of our baby, and if we did want the least pain and suffering for her, we would have to go full-term. The baby inside of me was not suffering. She was OK, and I had already grown attached to her. I couldn't bear the thought of having her removed from me. —*Christine*

This impulse to try to get out of the situation is a normal reaction to normal fears about dying and death. Before you learn about the positive aspects of continuing your pregnancy and parenting a dying baby, these scenarios can be terrifying to contemplate.

⟿ I harbored a real fear and sense that "I do not want to do this" when Lucy was first diagnosed. —*Jane G.*

⟿ My initial reaction was to recoil from the broken baby growing inside me. There was no doubt in my mind that abortion was still not a moral option. Yet I had to cling to my resolve so I would not be swept away by the sheer panic that gripped my heart. —*Kathy*

Some parents initially choose termination, even to the point of making an appointment. But then something happens that changes their minds. Sometimes circumstances fatefully intervene, and sometimes they simply have time to reconsider.

⟿ My initial reaction was to terminate. I thought the classic, *Let's just be done with it, we can move on and we can start over.* But I woke up the next morning feeling completely different. We'd already made an appointment with perinatal hospice for the next day. We were still trying to figure things out. When we walked out of that appointment, I remember we were both sitting in the lobby, and we both said, "Yeah, this is what we need to do." —*Bridget*

⟿ An abortion date was scheduled, but because of some twist of fate, all of the rooms were occupied on that day. My wife and I immediately changed our decision and went for broke: We were going to have our baby. —*David W.*

⟿ It seemed that since there was no hope for our baby, what was the point in prolonging the inevitable outcome, his death? Once we decided that we would induce, we had set our minds on it. It was such a difficult decision to make that we couldn't undo it. On the other hand, it never felt like we made the decision to induce; it was out of our hands from the get-go, and as we were in shock we couldn't decide any other way. It seemed that not just the doctors, but society, had decided for us. So when the doctors recommended that I postpone the induction for almost a month because of placenta previa, it seemed like a cruel joke. But it turned out to be a stroke of luck or good fate or Providence at work. During that next month while we waited for me to be induced, my husband and I each privately contemplated our baby's life and its meaning to himself, to us, and to the world. One day I said to my husband, "What if we carried this pregnancy through to its natural end? And let Frankie live out his life as it is?" My husband responded that he had been thinking the same thing. We each had pondered the same philosophical questions concerning Frankie's little life and inevitable death: All of us have an inevitable death in the offing. Frankie was no different from the rest of us. We began to see that we could not measure the value of our baby's life in terms of years or even months or days. We simply needed to be present with this baby while he was with us, to let him have his life as it was intended. —*Susan E.*

Some parents decide to continue not so much out of a desire to carry to term but because the alternative is something they cannot bring themselves to do.

Since everyone told us to terminate, that is all that we thought about at first. I thought about having to go into that office and know that I was killing my baby, and that thought just killed me. It made me feel worse and worse. My husband eventually told me that he couldn't live with himself if we terminated, and if this pregnancy wasn't going to harm me or keep me from having healthy babies we should carry to term. When he told me this, all the horrible weight on my shoulders just lifted. We knew that we would still have hard times, but we could live with this decision. —*Annette H.*

At one point, it seemed like termination was the best choice. We lived with that decision for about a week—not really doing anything about it, but that seemed like the logical choice with all the issues we were facing. After a bit, my husband and I talked to each other about it. We had each separately decided that we couldn't live with that decision. We felt bad enough that we were probably going to be facing the death of a child, but we didn't want to also live with the guilt of a termination on top of it. —*Janel*

My husband's family was really pushing me to get an abortion, but honestly, I just could not. My baby was alive! He was alive inside of me and moving! He was not an "it" or a "fetus." He was a real live human being. He was my son! —*Brooke*

As you weigh the option of continuing and assess all that it entails, you may begin to reconsider your initial rush toward death. You may realize that emotionally, termination could be just as difficult, for different reasons. Consenting to end your baby's life may bring added burdens of regret and guilt. Abortion does not shield you from enduring—and grieving for—your baby's death, and you may receive less support in your grief if those around you perceive your baby as merely a disposable and unseen accident of nature.

As you face your fears, you may be greeted with a sense of calm as you reconsider. Even though death is inevitable and soon, why bring it on sooner than necessary? Particularly if your baby won't suffer and there are no risks to the mother's health, why not hold on until you absolutely must let go? There is freedom in letting your baby's death be completely beyond your control. Your heart is going to break either way; why not embrace the opportunity to fill your heart first?

I felt deep within me that rushing these things would not have resolved anything. We also wanted to give ourselves the means to mark a pause in the vicious chain of events. Leave him his little life so that he could discover our love. Catch our breath from having to face this death to which we were irredeemably tied. Push back the final deadline, or rather let it arrive naturally. Give me the time to tame the unacceptable idea that I was going to lose my little one. Give us the time to get to know him and to build memories with him. —*Isabelle*

For some parents, the decision is so instinctive and immediate that it almost feels like no decision at all. They move forward, feeling purposeful and confident about continuing the pregnancy.

There was no decision to make. Amaya was our baby, and an ultrasound that showed her anomalies did not change that. —*Gina*

What Now?

The genetic counselor asked us if we wanted to terminate the pregnancy. My husband and I in unison said, "That is not an option for us." We had never had a conversation to reach that decision; we both felt it strongly and spoke it strongly at that moment. —*Jenny D.*

It did not take us long to make our decision. After hearing the final diagnosis and all of our options, we left the doctor's office walking hand in hand down this never-ending hallway to the elevators. While waiting for the elevator, my husband turned to me, and when our eyes met we both knew what we would do. We would be bringing our son home and hold him every minute that was granted to us. —*April*

My husband and I both knew right away we would continue. We didn't really feel like there was a decision to be made. Our son was our son from the moment he was conceived. The only discussion was regarding how much intervention we wanted for our son after he was born. —*Kathleen*

Some parents find confidence when they compare this decision to one they might make about another loved one diagnosed with a terminal illness.

At the time, my father was facing death with dignity with the help of a hospice program. It seemed that I could provide my own hospice of sorts for our baby. —*Missy*

To us, it seemed that inducing early would be a form of euthanizing our unborn baby, and we knew that if we were told that either of our sons wasn't expected to live beyond the next five months, we certainly wouldn't desire to end his life early. —*Jennifer*

My husband compared having a baby with a terminal illness to having cancer or running a race. Even though Rose wouldn't finish the race, we weren't about to trip her and make her stumble. Or if one of our parents had a diagnosis of cancer, we wouldn't just say, "Might as well kill her now; she's going to die anyway." —*Debbie*

Perhaps you make a formal declaration to your doctor, or perhaps you simply throw away the phone number for scheduling an abortion. Whether you are feeling confident or ambivalent, you are now embarking on a new journey with your little one.

Once you have decided to continue, you may have feelings of peace that validate and reinforce your choice.

When we decided to carry our baby until term, we both had such a strong peaceful feeling come over us. It was the first time throughout our tragic news that we felt good about something. —*Allison*

Immediately after we decided to continue the pregnancy, I felt some peace that we finally had a plan. Amid all the bad news and things that felt very out of our control, I felt a sense of relief that one important decision had been made and we could move forward reconciling ourselves to the outcome. —*Alessandra*

For us, in the end the decision to continue was the only one that made us feel OK. Anytime we even talked about the other option my heart would pound, and I would get very anxious and nervous. As soon as I said we were continuing I felt relief and comfort. —*Camille*

However, it is normal to also feel anxious about what is yet to come. Continuing your pregnancy may bring a sense of purpose and resolve, but it can still feel like a burden to be endured. You may feel that this is actually the more difficult path for you, even if you believe it is the right one for your baby.

Even though carrying the baby was the hardest choice, it was the choice that held blessing and peace at the end. We would not carry guilt with us the rest of our lives. But it was also the choice that allowed me to remain pregnant with a baby who would not live. It was the choice that allowed me to watch my belly swell with life that would end before it started. It was the choice that allowed me to wake up each morning knowing that I would never hold a crying baby in my arms, I would never kiss a soft head as he nursed, and he would never be a sibling to my older son. It was a hard, un-fair, and heartbreaking choice. —*Karla*

These mixed feelings are common and natural. It can help to re-mind yourself that fears and doubts don't mean you've made a bad decision; they simply mean you're in a painful and unfamiliar situa-tion. Keep in mind that as your pregnancy continues over time, you can adjust and settle into this path. The unknown becomes known, and you realize it isn't so scary after all.

Your decision to continue your pregnancy is a significant mile-stone in parenting your baby—not a milestone you had expected, back when you were dreaming of a healthy baby. But as every loving mother and father learns eventually, parenting sometimes means ad-justing to who your child is and responding to what this child needs. The best person in the world to provide that is you.

This knowledge of your baby's diagnosis is a gift that allows you to make the most of your pregnancy, which may be the only time you will have with this baby. With this knowledge, you can opt for another gift—the gift of time.

three

The Emotional Journey

Grieving and Adjusting to Your New Path

Time, indifferent to what was happening, continued at its usual rhythm. The days brought their batch of appointments and activities to do, all done with a sovereign and calm appearance, despite the fact that a volcano of suffering was erupting in my heart. Scolding, overwhelming, then suddenly appeased, quieted, it was there, waiting with me for what was to happen next. —*Isabelle*

As you turn toward the path of continuing your pregnancy, you may feel overwhelmed by emotions and the uncertainty of how this journey will unfold. On the outside, your condition may look unchanged, but your mission has been utterly transformed.

Tentatively moving forward, you may be surprised by the power of your emotions. You may be struck by the utter contrast of what you expected—joyful preparation for new life—and where you are now: grief-stricken and bracing for death.

But continuing your pregnancy is not only a journey of grief. It is also a journey of discovery and gratitude. In fact, it is important for you to experience both the sorrow and the joy. Your grief enables you to adjust to your baby's reality, and your joy guides you forward in positive ways that will nurture your baby, your family, and yourself. Though the roller coaster of conflicting emotions can be bewildering at times, there are no "wrong" feelings. You are entitled to experience your entire range of emotions without apology. Learning to cope with your many intense emotions is key to your adjustment.

While this may be the most heart-wrenching time you've ever experienced, you may also find that, as it unfolds, this experience can lead you through a metamorphosis. You are embarking on a profound journey that can lead you to richer ways of being and loving. You will tap into your strengths and perhaps discover some you didn't know you had. You'll grow confident that you can survive. And you will learn that what matters most is not what tragedy you face, but how you choose to respond.

This chapter offers you a supportive context for braving the complex emotional journey of parenting your baby during pregnancy, after birth, and into death. It focuses on anticipatory grief, which you'll experience before your baby dies, and offers a framework for understanding and managing the complicated mix of feelings that you may experience throughout your pregnancy and your baby's life. You'll acquire realistic expectations and strategies for coping. You'll also hear from other parents and find that your feelings are shared by many.

ANTICIPATORY GRIEF

Naturally, people grieve after a loved one dies. But even before death, when you know that death is probable or imminent, it is normal to start grieving. This is called anticipatory grief, and it will continue throughout your pregnancy and your baby's short life. (After your baby dies, your grief will change orientation; that part of your journey is covered in Chapter 9.)

Anticipatory grief can have psychologically positive aspects. For instance, knowing that your baby will die can enhance your appreciation of your baby and the time you have. Anticipatory grief can sharpen your focus and help order your priorities. It presses you to attune to your baby and be mindfully present during precious moments with your little one.

Another positive aspect of anticipatory grief is that you can experience a more gentle, gradual goodbye. Instead of having to meet death suddenly and let go of your baby now, you can begin to grieve while you still have the comfort of your baby's presence. As you adjust to the prospect of letting go, you still get to hold your baby close. When your letting go must begin in earnest after death, recalling these memories of holding your baby close can help you continue to adjust.

⟶ Many times I couldn't sleep and I'd just go sit and cry. During those moments she'd always kick me. It was always that reminder that she's still there, not to be so sad yet. —*Bridget*

AN OVERVIEW OF THE GRIEVING PROCESS

Anticipatory grief is an early and integral part of your grieving process, which will occupy a significant portion of your emotional energy for many months to come. Because grief is so agonizing, many people believe that grieving is something bad to be avoided or gotten over as quickly as possible. But grieving, whether before death or after, is a painful and necessary process that enables you to come to terms with loss and move forward in spite of it. Grieving is ultimately a constructive process whereby you gradually let go of what might have been and adjust to what is.

In general, the deeper the investment in what might have been, the deeper the grief. Even before your diagnosis, you already were invested in your baby. Bereaved parents commonly report that their baby's death is the most significant grief they've ever experienced.

Understanding the grieving process doesn't spare you from its ravages, but when your emotions make sense, it can be easier to cope. Instead of drowning in a seemingly endless sea of pain, you can remember that grieving is a natural and important process. Instead of thrashing aimlessly and exhaustingly, you can identify your emotions and move through them toward solid ground. You can also move toward safe harbor by expressing your grief through purposeful action that honors your baby's life.

Informed about grief, what you're grieving, and how you're grieving, you can respond constructively instead of destructively, with intelligence rather than desperation. More important during this pregnancy, understanding grief can motivate you to be present with your baby and gather the memories and keepsakes that will carry you toward healing beyond the end of your baby's life.

Your grief will have many layers, as you gradually realize every-thing you are losing. You're losing the chance to raise this child, and you may be grieving for the milestones you'll miss—the first tooth, the first step, the first day of school. You're losing what could have been experienced together, such as sharing your favorite stories, play-ing at the beach, or camping in the woods. These losses are real.

⌒ He or she will never be able to have the life that we all have been able to experience. All of the images that I had in my mind will never come true. We will never be able to give him or her a ride in the bike trailer like our older son has been planning. Our son will never be able to change the baby's diaper. We will never see our baby walk or talk. The list goes on and on. —*Katharine*

⌒ Realizing the broken dreams is one of the hardest things I've had to face. All the mental images of the ideal family of four on vacation or hiking in the mountains reverted back to just the three of us. —*Heidi*

⌒ I cried and cried and cried. I cried for the loss of life, the utter waste, the utter shame, and the complete and utter loss of poten-tial. I could have had a daughter. She could have been amazing. We would have given her an amazing life, loved her beyond love. She would have had a lovely life, with us. —*Elle*

There are also many related losses you may be acutely experiencing right now. For example, you may grieve for your dreams of a blissful pregnancy, a joyous birth, a healthy newborn, and an uncomplicated homecoming.

⌒ I was very angry at first that I had to know about my daughter's condition. I felt like I was cheated out of a happy pregnancy. I never wanted to know something like that. The knowledge was a heavy burden. —*Monika*

All these losses are mixed into your mourning, and it can help to identify them. When you know what you are grieving for, the depth of your feelings and reactions makes sense.

Moving through Grief

By moving through your grief, you free yourself to experience the joy of your baby's life. While this may sound contradictory, it rests on the fact that emotional repression is not selective: If you repress your painful emotions, you suppress your pleasurable emotions as well. So if you avoid grief, you end up avoiding joy as well. This is a high price to pay, particularly while your baby is alive.

When you're in the midst of grief, it's difficult to believe that the hard work of moving through this pain leads to joy or healing. Grief can be distressing—even frightening—in its power, but making sense of the turmoil can help you tolerate it. Here are a few facts about grief to light your way.

Grieving during your pregnancy is a normal and healthy process. Grief is an integral part of this journey. Whatever your situation, your grief will continue throughout your pregnancy and your baby's life, but your grief can coexist with your loving preparations for meeting and nurturing your baby after birth.

Grief encompasses many emotional and physical feelings. For instance, you may experience shock, disorientation, irritability, guilt, failure, sorrow, withdrawal, hopelessness, anxiety, and yearning. You may also experience an array of physical symptoms, including fatigue, tightness in the throat or chest, or changes in appetite or sleep. Your expression of grief is as unique as you are.

Any emotion in the dictionary would probably apply: anger, confusion, denial, fear, sadness . . . the list goes on and on. —*Shayla*

I experienced every emotion under the sun: love for my baby, tremendous fear of the unknown, deep sadness over the loss of the healthy baby I had dreamed of, and anger that the medical professionals provided me no support. —*Chris*

Grief can be chaotic, and there are no timetables or deadlines. It is never a neat set of stages, but a fluid mix of feelings. You will experience ups and downs, periods of despair and periods of respite. You may cycle through feelings many times over. Progress can even be one step forward and two steps back. Still, you are strengthening your adjustment and making an overall movement toward renewed purpose. Know that it's OK to feel caught up in a process that is beyond your control.

My circle of emotions went through sadness, shock, grief, acceptance, a desire to celebrate our baby's life and give him or her as much love as possible in what little time I had, and back to sadness that we wouldn't have our baby for very long. It is amazing how many tears a person can generate. Just when I thought that I had cried about as much as I could, more tears came. —*Katharine*

There is no single best way to grieve. You may experience a wide range of emotional and physical feelings or just a narrow range, with feelings of varying intensity. You may express your grief openly or only privately. While all grieving parents experience some similar emotions and behaviors, your path will be unique and likely very different from your partner's. (You will find more on this relationship later in this chapter.) Expect to find your own way and do what you need to do.

Sometimes I wondered if we were dealing with this OK. Many people would say, in giving me a compliment, that they could not believe how positive we were about this. Then, I would wonder, am I going *nuts*? —*Jennifer*

I was often moody, depressed, and distracted. It was a challenge to do the mundane tasks of the day. We ate out a lot during those months, partly because I never had the desire to cook and partly we needed to just escape reality for a few moments. —*Heidi*

I knew it was OK to cry in front of people, but I couldn't cry all day long, so I kept my tears inside and would let them all out while alone. —*Annette H.*

～ My shower became my safe place to cry. This happened some-times uncontrollably; I was alone with my thoughts, and I often succumbed to tears. —*Kristen*

～ My husband was withdrawn and quiet. My emotions were all over the place. —*Kelly G.*

Grief evolves over time. While grief is generally chaotic, you can also feel a sense of progress as your emotions evolve. You may feel your-self adjusting to your situation and thinking, "OK, now what?" And as you settle into this pregnancy, you may come to realize that you want to be able to see past your pain and also experience positive mo-ments with your baby.

EVOLVING EMOTIONS

As your emotions evolve throughout your pregnancy, there is a natu-ral progression from shock and disbelief toward facing reality, coping with it, adjusting to it, and moving forward with it. This progression isn't steady but rather an ebb and flow. This allows you to gradually face and cope with what you can handle without overwhelming you.

As you move your energy from fighting reality to accepting it, you can figure out ways to move forward in the face of it. You can embrace the rhythm of this special pregnancy and find yourself captivated by the wonder of this budding life. As your energy turns toward your baby, you may feel inspired to fill your baby's life with love, eager to welcome your baby into your arms, and determined to help your baby die a dignified natural death. You can make a concerted effort to reap as many positives as you can for as long as your baby is with you.

The following sections address some of the evolving emotions par-ents may face, including the following:

- Shock, numbness, and denial
- Conflicting thoughts and feelings
- Guilt, failure, and anger

Shock, Numbness, and Denial

Since learning your baby's condition, you may have moments where you're not feeling much of anything. You may find it hard to believe that you're even in this position and you may question whether the prognosis is as grim as the tests indicate. You find it difficult to absorb the shocking news and to come to grips with all that your baby's diagnosis—and this pregnancy—entails. You may feel like you spend periods of time in a daze.

I think I became numb for the rest of the pregnancy. I didn't know how to cope. I wanted so badly to enjoy my pregnancy and talk about the little experiences I had, but I felt like I wasn't supposed to talk about it. —*Chelsea*

Feeling numb is a reasonable reaction to an intensely painful reality. So is wishing away this bereavement. You may wish you'd never conceived this child, only to face this agonizing pregnancy. You may hope to miscarry or deliver prematurely, especially if your doctor is saying that your baby won't survive much longer anyway. For this entire experience to be over quickly may seem preferable to being stuck in the limbo of prolonged anticipation.

We were initially told our baby would die in utero within two weeks of the diagnosis. Incredibly, he lived for sixteen weeks. At the time—and to this day—this aspect of the experience is the most troubling: I knew my baby was going to die and so I wanted it to happen because every kick was a painful reminder that this life could not be. —*Missy*

I hoped that I would miscarry my baby soon. I struggled as I read accounts of women who talked about how they hoped and hoped that their babies would be born alive, and treasured each day of pregnancy as a day that they were able to be with their child. I did not want to terminate, but I did not feel this love. I wanted to grieve and move on, not to be faced with grief again. —*Jane G.*

You may begin this journey with a desperate intent to keep your distance from this baby, believing that it would make your baby's death less devastating. Some mothers resist wearing maternity clothes, normally a proud and visible marker of pregnancy. You may feel unworthy or want to remain invisible. But trying to keep your distance not only saps your energy, it can rob you of feeling the fullness of love.

⟶ I didn't really want to love Lily, not in a deep way, anyway. I was pretty sure I didn't want to feel the pain of losing Lily (this turned out to be unavoidable). So sometimes I sort of tried to forget that she was on the way. It was hard to think about it, and hard to tell people about it. I'm especially glad my wife did such a good job of communicating, because I'm sure my own efforts along these lines were not impressive. Sometimes I felt guilty about wanting to avoid things. —*Mark*

⟶ The pain was so great, the anger was great, and the disbelief was great. Getting out of bed was a struggle. It took me a long time to realize that I was actually carrying a baby who needed me. I didn't feel worthy of maternity clothing for about a month until my size gave me no choice. —*Jo*

⟶ As I slowly began to grow and "pop out," I became determined to not wear maternity clothes. I guess in the beginning I was just trying to be practical. If the doctors were right and I would soon lose her, then why bother. And as time went on I think I didn't want to draw any more attention to the fact that I was pregnant. It was supposed to be an exciting time. I didn't want to pretend that everything was OK, especially to strangers. —*Greta*

Conflicting Thoughts and Feelings

As your numbness and shock wear off, you'll begin to feel the force of your grief. But your grief won't be straightforward. Because you are facing this incomprehensible fusion of new life and impending death, you can expect to experience wild swings of joy and sorrow, celebration and dread.

⌒ Some days I was terrified to lose her; others I wanted her to stop moving so this would be over. I wanted her to live but was so terrified to raise a severely disabled child. Sometimes I prayed she would be stillborn, sometimes that she would take a breath and pass away in my arms. It was a roller coaster. —*Erin*

As you prepare to welcome, you also prepare to let go. Vacillation is the nature of anticipatory grief and a normal part of continuing this pregnancy. Most parents swing back and forth between conflicting emotions and thoughts.

⌒ Every emotion that there is would course through my body on a daily basis. Even good things like kicks would eventually lead to sadness. Would that be the last time I ever felt her move? —*Jamie*

⌒ I did have a few times that I thought things would be better if Noah would just come already! The daily anticipation was wearing. I wished that we could just start to move on, and yet I knew I wanted to cherish each day I had to feel him move, kick, punch, and just be. —*Kristin*

⌒ I had gotten over the initial shock, and I oscillated between acceptance and self-pity (with a lot of fear and anxiety mixed in).
—*Jane G.*

⌒ Some days I was overcome with a mother's love for him, protective and nurturing. Other days, I tried hard not to think about him, to not think of losing him. —*Karla*

It is also normal to resist appreciating and celebrating your baby. Why should you invest your heart only to have it broken?

⌒ I should treasure this life, treasure the bulge of my abdomen, knowing that life still existed inside of me. I should cherish every kick, knowing that this is the relationship that I would have with this little one. But how do you purposely fall in love knowing the pain increases when love is present? —*Karla*

⁓ I think my husband and I were both struggling to see the good that can come out of so short a life. —*Jane G.*

⁓ At first, we did not want any photos of our baby. We did not want to see our son if he was stillborn. At one point we decided to take the baby's presents out from under the Christmas tree, and my husband removed them. But through the night we sobbed together, and those early pronouncements melted away in our tears as we realized we would want to have as many photos as we could of our son, and we realized we would want to hold him and kiss him whether he was born alive or dead. We decided the presents belonged under the tree with the gifts for the rest of the family, and my husband put them back. We decided that we would cherish every moment we had with our baby now, while he was very much alive and kicking inside of me. —*Jennifer*

Conflicting feelings are in especially stark relief if you are expecting more than one baby and only one is sick.

⁓ I was really struggling with grief and having the risks of a twin pregnancy without any of the "cuteness" of actually getting to bring home twins. —*Samantha*

Everyone's mix of conflicting thoughts and emotions is different, and you'll likely experience different mixes from day to day or month to month. While this discord can be taxing, the moments of positive thinking and feeling give you respite from your grief. You may even make a concerted effort to focus on the positive and remind yourself that, for the present, your baby is alive and with you.

⁓ I didn't want to be sad all the time. I needed to laugh, I needed be able to just be "normal." —*Monika*

⁓ We didn't want to be the sad couple, we wanted to be normal. And deal with it when it comes. —*James*

⁓ It wasn't that we were showing strength; it was that we'll have plenty of time to cry. Now is not the time. —*Jill K.*

The Emotional Journey

⟶ I thought trying to grieve at that point would really get in the way. I was a happy dad, and she was a happy mom. —*Brad*

It can help to remind yourself that whatever your mix of feelings, that mix is what is right for you. It is part of your process of coming to terms with your pregnancy and your baby's condition. As long as you feel like you're in touch with your grief and moving through it, however slowly, you are continuing to adjust.

Guilt, Failure, and Anger

Feelings of guilt, failure, and anger arise from the belief that you have control over what happens to you. No one has complete control over their reproductive fortunes, but at first you'll protest this reality. Anger is a way to lash out at the unfairness of this twist of fate; guilt and failure stem from your feelings of responsibility.

Even if you recognize you don't have complete control, it is normal to feel responsible for your baby's condition or to worry that you may be seen that way. After all, you may reason, this child was conceived by you and carried by you. You or others may wonder if there are aspects of your genetic makeup, medical history, or lifestyle that contributed to your baby's condition. You may feel responsible for disappointing those close to you who were eagerly anticipating your baby's arrival. Even if you know your baby's condition was due to random chance, it is normal to feel some sense of responsibility and the attendant feelings of guilt and failure.

 ⟶ I was frightened that I had done something to make my baby sick, even though I knew I had done everything right. —*Chelsea*

 ⟶ I pulled out the little piece of paper that I had folded away in my pocket to show my husband all the things I'd written down that were wrong with David. And once I told him that they said David was going to die, he started bawling and turned his head from me. He asked me if it was his fault. I remember telling him that the doctors said this is nobody's fault. They told me that sometimes these things just happen. Even now I wonder if I can ever truly believe that, as I've had that very thought several times. I wonder if I could ever believe that it isn't in some way my fault. The last thing in the world that I would ever want is to hurt my little boy. —*Rachel*

⟶ My husband and I felt as if it was our fault that this happened, that we were being punished, because we had been very apprehensive about having this child to begin with. —*Shayla*

⟶ I felt guilt—I should be able to save her. I was letting everyone in my family down by not being able to protect her and bring her safely into this world. —*Alaina*

⟶ I was more worried about my parents. As a parent already, I could imagine what it would be like for my child to be going through this. I wanted to be strong for them and let them think I was OK. Who wants their parents to worry about them?
—*Kimberly Anne*

⟶ I worried about the pain and confusion our older son would experience, if he thought this was what pregnancy was like. I worried about the pain my husband experienced every day he looked at me. And I carried guilt because I couldn't give them a normal healthy pregnancy and a normal healthy baby. —*Kelly G.*

If you've struggled with infertility or if a previous child had the same or another life-limiting condition, you may rage at the unfairness. It is normal to feel especially despondent if you've been down this road before.

⟶ It's happening again. The pain is happening again. We are going to have another baby who will suffer and die. Why is this happening again? —*Pam F.*

⟶ After the ultrasound, it took us weeks before we were able to admit that it hurt, and we started grieving. The thought of losing another child was unbearable. —*Behka*

Anger is a natural reaction to feeling like your life is spinning out of control. You may feel angry at the situation, your body, fate, Mother Nature, or God. You may be irritable or feel angry at people for not

The Emotional Journey

knowing how to support you. You may feel incensed at parents who take their fertility for granted or who neglect their children.

    I struggled with the unfairness of this; I wanted this baby. All I wanted was one more child to love, to raise, to be a part of the family that I had always dreamed of having. One day at the swimming pool, I saw a young expectant mother smoking a cigarette in the parking lot. My rage at her and at the injustice of my situation almost undid me. —*Karla*

    Some days I was angry at everything. Anything my husband did was wrong, from dishes to dinner, to how he drives the car. I was short with my son and had no patience for his 2-year-old-ness.
                                          —*Janel*

You may even feel angry at your baby for putting you through this ordeal. This also can add to your guilt.

    I was angry and hurting. I struggled with my feelings toward my baby. I was angry at him for changing my body, angry at him for still being alive two weeks after our diagnosis. I wanted to be done. The guilt set in when I thought about his innocence and contemplated his life, the life that I was being blessed to share a part. —*Karla*

    These feelings are common and natural aspects of grief, part of the process of coming to terms with the injustice of your situation. The key is to not get stuck in destructive self-recrimination. It may help to remember the following:

- Sometimes bad things happen to good people.
- Your baby's condition is not a punishment that you deserve; it is a fluke of nature and a tragic, unexpected detour.
- You did not knowingly cause or choose this fate for your child.
- Feeling guilty is not the same as being guilty.
- Feeling a sense of failure is not the same as being a failure.

It can also help to remember that part of coming to terms with your baby's condition is to realize that you cannot control every aspect of your life. This realization can help you take charge of what you *can* control.

⌒ I did everything possible to be a good mom. I could only control so much. That was one of the hardest things for me, was losing control. —*Chelsea*

⌒ If I was in control, I'd have a healthy baby. But once we found out he wasn't going to live, we thought, we'll just make the most of what we *can* do. —*Greg*

CONFRONTING FEARS

⌒ We always feared the next step. When we first received the diagnosis, we were afraid of the coming eleven weeks. When we had a few more weeks to go, my husband worried about labor complications. I was afraid of giving birth, not because of the pain. I wanted to stay pregnant forever because Anya would be alive. —*Delsa*

Fear can arise from many sources. You may have many worries about how everything will unfold. You may worry about physical and emotional suffering for your baby, for yourself, or for your family members. You may fear the process of childbirth or be afraid of what your baby will look like. You may be afraid of your baby's death and at the same time afraid that your baby might live in spite of his or her condition. Your fears and worries may seem endless.

⌒ I was honestly worried that she wouldn't be as loved because she would be different. I was worried that she would die; I was worried that she would live and I would not be good enough or strong enough to deal with what came with that. —*Jamie*

⌒ I was afraid of the death experience, that he would resist that. As completely irrational as it sounds, I was also afraid that—because he had defied everything else—he would live and just be a very, very sick baby. There was a lot of fear I was coping with. —*Missy*

⌒ I was dreadfully afraid of postpartum depression. With my two boys, I had the typical "baby blues" from the hormonal changes, and I was really terrified that since I wouldn't physically have a little newborn to nurture, it would be harder to kick that sadness and it would turn into depression. —*Jennifer*

⌒ I was afraid of the grief, of never being able to move on. I was afraid for my mom; she took it all very hard. —*Erin*

Fears of the Unknown

Continuing your pregnancy naturally poses many unknowns that can cause anxiety. You likely don't know anyone who has done this before you, and you won't find the reassurances you need in the typical pregnancy guidebooks. This journey is largely uncharted. How long will your pregnancy last? What kind of labor and birth can you expect? Will your baby be born alive? What will happen after your baby's birth? Your caregivers may have little experience with babies like yours, and any predictions may be merely educated guesses.

⌒ The worst part was not knowing what would happen. I was preoccupied with trying to know what would happen to Rose; would she die at birth? Would she live a day, a month, a year? How would we cope with what would she might look like? —*Debbie*

⌒ Every day I would wonder if it was going to be the day. I had read that it is typical for babies with this condition to be born anywhere from 28 to 40 weeks. I was able to cope by enjoying the life I felt inside of me, but that didn't mean I wasn't full of anxiety every day. It was by far the most difficult thing I have ever done and probably will ever do. —*Deanna*

⌒ I did not know when the baby would come, although we'd been told that 33 weeks was average. I pretty much had to take it day by day. Sometimes hour by hour. —*Tracy*

As this mother discovered, one technique for dealing with fears of the unknown is to try to take one day, even one hour, at a time. For example, if you are anxious about not knowing when your baby will be born, ask yourself whether you are in labor right now. No? Then you can let go of that worry for now. You can also simply observe this worry as part of your process for preparing to meet your little one.

Fears that Your Baby Will Suffer

Another common source of anxiety for parents is the possibility that their baby might experience pain. Even though you likely considered your baby's potential for suffering when you made the decision to continue, those fears may still haunt you. After all, how can your baby have a life-limiting condition and not suffer? Don't fatal diseases and deformities hurt? Could labor or birth be traumatic? Is death painful? And what if your baby survives for a while—will his or her quality of life be so poor that your decision to continue inadvertently causes undue suffering?

I worried that my baby was in pain, due to the lack of amniotic fluid. I thought that I was squishing her if I coughed or sneezed. I worried that she would suffer during the birth. —*Chelsea*

I was afraid my baby would be born alive and then struggle for life in my arms. I was afraid that this baby who was so very, very sick would not find a peaceful death. —*Missy*

I was deeply worried about any deformities and disabilities he would have for the time he would live. I didn't want for him to suffer or be in any pain. —*Kimberly Anne*

I worried that he would be in pain, especially toward the end as his body "realized" that something wasn't right and would begin to shut down. My medical caretakers assured me that he wouldn't be in pain. My husband agreed with them and even compared Frankie's dying phase to his own deceased father's, which appeared pretty peaceful to us. But how can anyone know that for sure? So I remained concerned. —*Susan E.*

The overriding worry was whether or not, if she were born alive, she would have pain. The only reason I ever questioned carrying her to term was that I was petrified she would be in pain and I couldn't bear that. I really felt like, as her mother, it was my responsibility to protect her from pain, and I worried that my decision wasn't doing that. —*Alessandra*

⌇ I feared that she would suffer not only in the womb but if by some miracle she survived the pregnancy, then in the outside world. —*Shayla*

If you're worried about your baby suffering, ask for a referral to a specialist who has experience with your baby's condition. For many conditions, the mother's body compensates for the functions the baby's body cannot carry out. That's why your baby may continue to survive—even thrive—inside you.

⌇ We worried the baby might suffer, but those fears were eased after an in-depth consultation with a wonderful neonatologist.
—*Jennifer*

⌇ I was very scared that the baby was in pain and kept telling my husband that I wish they would induce me so we could get her out and they could fix the problem. My husband kept reminding me that as long as I was carrying her, she was happy and "healthy" as my body was doing all the work for her. —*Jessie*

Many conditions are not inherently uncomfortable for the baby. If your baby's condition is expected to cause pain or discomfort after birth, you can make specific postbirth care plans for your baby. Ask your baby's doctor about palliative care for your baby's particular condition. Include palliative care in your baby's birth plan as well. (For more about this, see Chapter 5.)

Fear of Childbirth

As worrisome as this pregnancy can be, the thought of your baby's birth can be even more formidable. After all, birth is a turning point. What will labor be like when you know it signifies the beginning of the end? Will you get your wish to look into your baby's eyes? Will you be able to bear the physical and emotional pain?

⌒ I feared giving birth so much. I didn't want to know if my baby died during delivery and then freak out. I knew that everyone says the pain of labor is worth it. But it wasn't really worth it for me. I had to go through all the pain and then hand my baby over and say goodbye forever. —*Annette H.*

⌒ I was worried more about the birth of my daughter than carrying her. What I mean is that as long as she was inside me I knew she was OK. I wanted to stay pregnant with her because then I could keep her. I was so sad about having to say goodbye when she was born. —*Chris*

A practical way of addressing any fears of childbirth is to prepare a birth plan. (For a more detailed discussion, see Chapter 6 and the sample birth plan at the end of the book.)

Fears about Your Baby's Appearance

You also may worry about what your baby will look like. Will you reach out to hold your little one, or will you recoil in fear? Especially if your baby's condition is outwardly visible, you may imagine frightening deformities.

⌒ I had been told that my baby had no kidneys, no stomach, and that he would likely not be born alive. It is hard to be honest and to admit that I was afraid to meet my baby. I was afraid what he or she might look like. —*Missy*

⌒ I was afraid of what Anouk would look like. Anencephaly isn't very pretty to look at, and I was afraid of my reaction once I'd see her. —*Monika*

⌒ I was worried that she wouldn't have a nose—because it didn't show on the ultrasound—and that she wouldn't be able to breathe. I was scared to find out what she was going to look like. —*Rebecca J.*

Unfortunately, some doctors feed these fears, perhaps in a misguided effort to encourage families to terminate the pregnancy, or perhaps simply out of insensitivity.

⟶ I worried that my daughter was going to be a monster. That is how they described her to me on the day we were diagnosed.

—*Chris*

⟶ Our doctor showed us an ugly scientific picture of what our baby would look like. He told us all of this so we would be "well informed" about what we were dealing with. —*Elizabeth B. P.*

Even if your doctor tries to reassure you, it is normal to worry about your baby's appearance and how it will affect you. To cope, try to separate your imagination from reality. Instead of dwelling on what you're imagining—which is likely much worse than the actual reality—go ahead and research the facts. By learning more during the pregnancy, your baby's appearance may be less shocking or distressing to you after birth.

If you decide to look at pictures, there are websites created by and for parents that feature personal photos, which can be far preferable to the cold, clinical photos studied by medical practitioners. Even so, medical photos can be informative as well, because you can see that the baby is still a baby.

⟶ I was terrified that I would have haunting memories of my baby if I looked at her. Sometimes when there is a lack of amniotic fluid, the babies can develop clubbed limbs and facial features can be smashed. After looking at pictures of the babies with Gianna's condition in medical books, I felt comforted. They are still beautiful babies. —*Jennifer*

⟶ After looking at pictures of other babies with anencephaly, I worried how my baby would look. I knew that I would love him or her no matter what, but how was the baby going to look? After looking at many pictures over time, they got easier, and I knew that he or she would be beautiful. —*Annette H.*

Worries about your baby's appearance can be a natural consequence of being given information that focuses solely on your baby's abnormalities, ignoring your baby's many normal features. If you have easy access to ultrasound images of your baby, ask the technician to point out familiar and normal body parts to you. Also remember that when you meet your baby you will be looking through eyes of love, and like most parents, you will see something in your child that is beautiful. (For reassurance and evidence of this, see Chapter 7.)

Fears about Death

Finally, you may be fearful of meeting death. What will it be like to hold your dying baby? Will your decisions about medical intervention still feel right? Will she or he die peacefully? These fears are natural and common.

I was concerned about watching my baby die since I had never witnessed a death before. I also wasn't sure if I would be able to help myself from feeling like I wanted to do more to "save" him or her (like life support) when the time came. —*Katharine*

If you are afraid of the dying process, ask your doctor to describe the details and what to expect. Talk to other parents or read about others' experiences. (For more discussion about the dying process and for parents' stories, see Chapter 8). Hearing from other parents might clear up any misconceptions and reassure you that it can be a peaceful and loving experience.

While fears are a natural part of this journey, you needn't be ruled by them. Accept that your worries for your baby's comfort are a natural expression of your parental devotion. Even in the face of reassurances, you may remain worried—and that's OK too.

TECHNIQUES FOR COPING

If you find yourself unable to move past despair even fleetingly, if you feel stuck in a rut of grief, if you feel overwhelmed by the wild swings, or if you simply wish you could feel better so that you can open yourself up to your baby's presence, there are a number of techniques you could try.

A particularly effective way of dealing with stressful situations is to practice cognitive techniques, such as reframing and mindful acceptance, that are based on the idea that how we think about a situation affects how we feel about it.

You've probably noticed that when all you think about is how terrible this pregnancy is, all you can feel is terrible. But whenever you can think about how continuing your pregnancy also gives you the opportunity to nurture your baby, you can feel some joyful anticipation too. Likewise, if you chastise yourself for feeling terrible—or get down on yourself for feeling OK when your baby isn't—you're only adding to your distress. Whenever you can accept the ebb and flow of all your feelings, you can move with your experience instead of struggling against it. Focusing on the positives and going with the flow are two ways of reducing distress.

Reframing involves countering distressing thoughts with positive ones. To give this a try, purposefully counter a distressing thought with a positive one. For instance, if you are dwelling on what a tragic hand you've been dealt, try considering how much love and appreciation you have for this child or imagining nurturing, life-affirming activities such as bathing and dressing your little one after birth. This doesn't mean becoming a Pollyanna. But if you are feeling overrun by distressing thoughts and incapacitated by misery, you deserve some respite. You aren't trying to banish your painful thoughts; you're just trying to find a balance that is less agonizing for you. Whenever you can focus on the positive aspects of this gift of time, you can find some relief.

Mindful acceptance involves paying attention to what's going on inside you and around you, in the moment, nonjudgmentally. You can observe your thoughts and feelings, however positive or negative, and accept them as a natural part of your experience with this child. Practicing mindful acceptance enables you to let your feelings flow through you without fighting or avoiding them. This can give you compassion for yourself and your family and a sense of peace about your journey.

Both techniques can help you be more psychologically flexible and therefore resilient in the face of stress. Becoming proficient in these cognitive techniques requires practice, particularly if you are changing deeply ingrained habits, but you may see results quickly. Many suggestions throughout this book will have cognitive aspects to them. You can also practice these techniques in other areas of your life.[1]

The power of either reframing or mindful acceptance is that even though the situation and your grief won't change, you can change the way you behold this landscape and feel less overwhelmed and better balanced.

Here are more suggestions for coping:

Dare to let yourself imagine meeting your baby. Such thoughts can help you focus on life rather than death and on embracing rather than letting go.

Plan special experiences with your baby during this pregnancy. By including your baby in positive experiences, you build positive memories. (See Chapter 4 for ideas.)

Ask your doctor for extended or repeated ultrasounds. Seeing your baby may help you feel a connection, make your baby more real to you and your partner, or let you feel like you're getting to know him or her as a unique and special individual.

Take good care of yourself physically. Exercise, healthy eating, and adequate sleep can contribute to positive mood and energy and to your ability to tolerate distress.

Commune with nature. The great outdoors and sunshine are natural mood boosters.

Give yourself permission to go to the depths of your despair. After hitting bottom, you can find yourself naturally rising up again.

Pray. If you believe in a higher power, you can grab onto the lifeline of a faith community and familiar rituals—or simply cry out in surrender, asking God to carry you when you cannot walk yourself.

Look for a network of bereaved parents. Go online, contact a pregnancy and infant loss support group, or ask your doctors if there is another family in your area who has been through this and would be willing to meet with you.

Talk more with your partner, or reach out to others in your circle. Having even just one person who can listen to you talk about what you're going through can be immensely helpful for getting in touch with your feelings and moving through them.

The Emotional Journey

Seek professional counseling. Even one or two sessions with a thera-pist, perhaps one who has experience with grieving parents, can help you find solid footing.

Write in a journal or blog. Keeping a diary can be an effective balm, giving you a nonjudgmental forum to identify and express your feelings.

Engage in art therapy. Artistic self-expression, individually or in a group with the support of an art therapist, can help you identify and process your feelings as well as provide a creative outlet for recording your experiences during this special pregnancy.[2]

Other coping ideas include relaxation techniques such as medita-tion, yoga, or deep breathing; immersing yourself in a favorite hobby or sports; or listening to music. You deserve to ease your distress so that you can make the most of the time you have with your baby.

YOU AND YOUR GRIEVING PARTNER

We thought we were drifting apart when really we weren't. We had already started our grieving for our baby and the speeds were different. We were in the same awful car but in different gears.

—Elle

If you are married or in a relationship, you will share this journey and this grief with your partner. At times you may feel in sync with each other, but at times you may feel far apart, each of you caught up in your own unique experience and emotions. Navigating this experi-ence together can test your communication and relationship skills as never before.

This is going to be the greatest challenge we've faced yet as a couple. It's so easy to get concerned with helping my wife so much that I have this gaping hole inside that I'm letting fester all because I thought I was being there for her. In the end I'm not helping her at all; I'm running from my own fear. *—James*

Too many emotions were surging though us. When my wife was at her low, I was at my high, and vice-versa. *—David W.*

Parents often have different outlooks. It is normal for a father to focus more on the pregnant mother than on the baby, while the mother can't help but focus on the baby as she has a direct, physical connection. A father may worry about the woman's physical and emotional health and her ability to carry a difficult pregnancy. A mother may worry about her partner's ability to handle this crisis. Each of you may be more afraid for the other than for yourself.

> My husband worried that something would happen to me, too—that he would lose his daughter and his wife at the same time.
> —*Shellie*

> I was worried about my husband, who kept hoping that this baby would be born without problems and that the doctors were wrong. He couldn't face the reality of all this. I knew that when the reality hit, it would hit him hard. —*Sue*

Along with different worries and different paths, you may also have different coping styles. It is common for one partner, typically the father, to have an "instrumental" coping style, which focuses on jumping into action and problem solving. He may express his grief by working hard and playing hard.

> My husband deals with grief by ignoring it and hoping that it will go away (moving on, focusing on the practical). He does things, rather than discuss his emotions, and it was really hard for us to come together. He kept himself busy doing things. —*Samantha*

> I think the biggest emotion I struggled with was the common compulsion every man has: to *fix it!* —*Scott*

The other partner, typically the mother, may have an "intuitive" style, which focuses on processing thoughts and feelings by talking and writing and generally experiencing the emotions. She may express her grief by crying and ruminating and sharing with others. It can be a challenge to accommodate your differing outlooks and coping styles. You may also experience different needs regarding sexual intimacy.

The Emotional Journey

⟳ I didn't understand how we could possibly be intimate when we faced such a crisis. I longed to feel close and connected to my husband, but the kind of intimacy he needed from me was frustrating. This compounded the feelings and thoughts of wanting to be able to speed up this process. There were many days I wished our life could be back like it was. I did not want to think about anything else but me and this baby. Everything else, especially intimacy, seemed so unimportant! —*Kristin*

Finally, you may experience different social support. Typically people focus on the mother and how she is feeling, because she's the one carrying the baby and because she is more likely to exhibit or talk about her emotions. If you're the dad, you may feel isolated at a time when you need support too. On the other hand, you may feel this is a private matter and are content to keep it to yourself. You can discern your own emotional needs and speak up about them if you wish.

⟳ I don't think the fathers get enough support. I don't think anyone at my husband's office ever really talked to him about what was going on. Everyone seemed to ask about me and how I was doing first, even our friends and families. They would inquire about my husband almost as an afterthought. —*Kathleen*

⟳ I think my husband was a bit forgotten in the whole process. People would frequently ask me how he was doing with everything, but that was about the extent of it. I think a lot of people were well-meaning and had good intentions of being supportive, but they just didn't know what to say or do, so they didn't say or do anything. He eventually confronted his parents and his sister about this, saying that when they neglect to say or do anything, he perceived it as them not caring. I think it gave him relief to confront them this way. —*Heidi*

⟳ My husband wanted to be pretty private. He wanted to keep everything to himself; he didn't want to share with anyone. I said, "I can't do that. Once you're pregnant, that's all people talk about." He finally understood where I was coming from. —*Bridget*

If you observe differences between you, remember that there is no single way to grieve. There's your way—and your partner's way. Accepting your differences can help you empathize and support each other as you each find your own way. Understanding that you're both normal can help you worry less that your partner will crash and burn or that your differences are a sign of irremediable distance. Communicating openly can help both of you feel more united, even as you grieve separately.

We were very honest with each other about how we felt. We respected each other's feelings and did our best to be good and patient with each other during such a hurtful time. *—Missy*

His openness and willingness to listen to my concerns was crucial to my making it through many tough days. He did not judge or discount my feelings, but he tenderly proved his love for me through words and actions. He was definitely in this with me, and it made loving him, even when I did not feel like it, easier to do. *—Kristin*

It took some time to realize what was happening, and it was only when I read an article about grief differences between men and women that it made sense. Once I accepted that my husband was always going to react differently from me, we allowed ourselves to just be ourselves, without any pressure to be anything else. And it worked. *—Elle*

YOUR OTHER CHILDREN

If you have other children, your journey is both complicated and blessed by their presence. On one hand, you have the additional responsibility of figuring out what to tell them about the new baby and how to support them. On the other hand, your life can retain some semblance of normal parenting as you tend to their daily needs. You may also feel some respite from despair as you acknowledge your gratitude for already having one or more healthy children.

Luckily our son was very young and had no idea what was going on, so he just continued being his cute and funny self, and that got us through many days. *—Christine*

The Emotional Journey

Explaining Your Baby's Condition

You may be concerned about how this experience will affect your older children. How much should you tell them—if anything? Will they be scarred for life at having to face death so early? Should they see the baby after birth? Will it be harder on them if they see the baby—or harder if they don't?

There is much you can do to share age-appropriate explanations and to prepare siblings for this significant event in their lives. For a very young child who isn't aware of your swelling belly, you may not feel the need to explain. However, even young toddlers can pick up the emotional stress and changes in their parents. Your job is to go the extra mile to offer reassurance and loving attention, so that your little one doesn't suffer from the natural turning inward that is common for a grieving parent.

It's also important to be aware that even if your toddler has few words, she or he understands many more. While it can be tempting to shield your young children from the terrible reality, you run the risk of confusing them by withholding the truth. Instead, include them by offering simple explanations such as, "There is a baby in mommy's tummy, but this baby's body does not work quite right, so this baby won't be able to live for very long." By being open to talking about it, you can draw your children into what's going on, letting them experience the comfort of enduring this as a family, rather than estrangement in a cloud of secrecy.

> Upon getting our bad news, we had decided to try to shield our older son from this loss. After a while, he let us know that he was way too smart and intuitive to be deceived when out of the blue, he told me that he knew the baby was still inside of my body. Then we told him that Gianna is in Mommy's body and is living but is sick and won't be able to come home with us after she is delivered. —*Jennifer*

Also keep in mind that your young children probably would not understand nor do they need to know all the implications of your baby's condition or your decisions about continuing your pregnancy, so it's unlikely they will be as traumatized as you are by the situation. With your gentle, straightforward explanation, they can translate it into a framework that makes sense to them. Many parents enlist reassuring spiritual imagery, evoking comforting ideas about heaven, souls, or love.

⌒ Our other children were 6, 5, and 2 when I had Rose. We did not try to hide anything from them. We told them that baby Rose would be very sick and that if the doctors could not take care of her that God would take care of her in heaven. They asked a lot of questions, and we tried to keep it simple—she would be very small, she had a bad heart. They wanted to help her, and my 5-year-old said when she was born he wanted her to sleep in his room so he could take of her. My 6-year-old wanted to help feed her. —*Debbie*

Another good strategy for talking to a child of any age is to let their questions be your guide. Many children will express a natural curiosity about what's happening and why. They also will likely have worries about it. Answer their questions simply and honestly along with reassurance that everyone else in the family is healthy and that there is a difference between a tiny, very sick baby whose body isn't working right and big healthy kids like them. Older children may have more in-depth questions about the baby's condition and prognosis. That can be a chance to have important, thoughtful conversations about life and death, medicine, and religion. If there are no answers, you can explain that it is a mystery to you too.

⌒ It was as if my heart was broken once again when my husband and I had to explain to our daughter how very sick our baby was. It was hard enough for us to understand; how could we expect her to? We tried our best to put it into words that she could understand. We simply told her that our baby is not healthy and very sick. She asked a few questions and seemed to accept what we told her. I also had to explain to her that it makes us sad to have a sick baby and that she may see Mommy crying. I told her that we're going to be all right. —*Greta*

⌐ I tried to be as honest as possible about what was happening and my feelings and emotions. My older kids were afraid of me dying too and needed a lot of reassurance. —*Sue*

⌐ Every night before bedtime, we would have "questions." During that time our 4-year-old asked us anything he wanted about his baby sister Molly and what was going to happen with her when she died. I think it was a good ongoing discussion for the three of us to have, and we believe it was helping him to deal with what had happened with Molly so far and to prepare for what was to come. —*Kath*

If your child has pointed questions about the medical aspects of your baby's condition or wants to know what your baby looks like, consider sharing photographs or sketches from websites or medical books that you feel are appropriate. Children take their cues from their parents. If you are respectful and calm and share your child's curiosity, even vivid photographs can yield information that can help you both feel better prepared.

⌐ I was a little worried about my first daughter. We tried to prepare her as much as possible. We showed her pictures of children with cleft lips and palates. —*Holly*

If you try to withhold information from a curious child, you merely engage his or her imagination, which may conjure up images that are scarier than any you'll find in a medical textbook.

Sibling Grief

Just like their parents, children will grieve in unique ways. Very young children may not understand that your baby's impending death is a permanent loss, and even older children will vary in how invested they are in the idea of having a new baby in the family. Some children will seemingly shrug off the news and run off to play, while others will grieve deeply and openly. And over the course of your pregnancy, your baby's upcoming death can also acquire different meaning. Your children may begin to grieve near the end of your baby's life or perhaps not until after your baby's death. The impact of your baby's death will also change over time as they grow and perhaps realize what will be or has been lost. However your children react, let them know that you will answer their questions and support them through this experience.

Sibling Support

⌐ When we told our other four children, they started grieving as well. That was the hardest part of all, taking emotional care of our other children. This was not just happening to mom and dad, but our children were going to lose another brother. —*Bekha*

Supporting your children through their own grief can feel daunting when you are struggling to cope with your own. For many children, what affects them most is the grief that their parents are demonstrating and the disruption to the normal family rhythms. Even very young children will notice that you aren't as cheerful or attentive as before. Children commonly assume that they have done something wrong or disappointed you. That's why it is so important to explain that when you are sad, it's because you're thinking about the baby. This will reassure them that your sadness is not their fault. Also reassure them that although you'll be especially sad for a while, this won't last forever, and you can return to feeling happy most of the time. You can also reassure them that while you'll always miss this baby, you are so grateful that you have them to enjoy and love.

Some children feel ambivalent or angry about the prospect of having a new sibling, and they might feel guilty, wondering if their thoughts caused the baby's condition. You can reassure your children that thoughts are not powerful enough to affect your baby's health and that no one is to blame.

Finally, if your children attend school, talk to their teachers, so that they can look after your children with sensitivity. Contact school administrators to find out what kinds of support can be offered by staff or special programs. For children of any age, contact your doctor, local hospital, or regional children's hospital for referrals to grief programs for siblings. Some hospitals have child life specialists, who are pediatric health care professionals trained to support hospitalized children as well as their siblings in developmentally appropriate ways.[3] Even if you feel you and your other children are coping well, it can still help to ask for some literature or schedule a meeting at the hospital where you plan to deliver. A child life specialist can also guide you in how to talk with your children about meeting the baby and how to include them in your baby's birth and care.

↬ The child life specialist was very nice and helpful. She definitely recommended that our older son meet and hold Joseph when he is born, no matter what the outcome. She said that we needed to keep him updated on what is going on, because he can sense that something is happening. But she also suggested to not make it complicated and not give him future possibilities, such as "if this happens, then this happens" kind of scenarios. —*Janel*

Knowing that your children are getting expert assistance can ease your mind. You needn't be your children's only source of support.

↬ We have four other kids who were 10, 8, 6, and 4 at the time. I was more worried about their dealing with all this than anything else. I made our baby's diagnosis well-known throughout their school and our church so they could get all the support they needed. Our parish school and church didn't let us down and were great supports. —*Sue*

↬ We explained Maggie's diagnosis to our boys with complete honesty. Like us, they tried to make sense of it all. They began working with an incredibly skilled and sensitive children's bereavement counselor. Because our three children wouldn't have the opportunity to make traditional memories, she helped them to make memories while they could. There are wonderful letters from our boys to their sister and beautiful photographs of them lovingly talking to Maggie in my tummy. —*Alessandra*

↬ We started noticing behavior patterns not typical for our kids, so I called their elementary school counselor. I learned more about grieving in that ten-minute conversation than I had learned after the death of our other son. She gave me some very helpful tips, mostly questions to ask our children to open the door for them to share what they were feeling emotionally. We are a very close family and we talk openly and honestly, but the language she taught me was different. For example, "I am so happy that we are having another baby in our family! But today, I am feeling sad that our baby is going to be sick and die. How do you feel today?" Also, acknowledging that I am sad, then stating what I am going to do about it. "I am sad that our baby is going to be sick, but I am going to keep spending time with our family because that makes me happy." Validating emotions: "You are looking a little sad today. Do you know why you are upset?" The best thing we did was have them take a class through this counselor. We had them teach the rest of the family for Family Night. It was fabulous. —*Behka*

You can tailor your words to fit your situation, your children, and their questions and concerns. For expert guidance, you can also consult books about talking with children about death and grief.[4] (For more ideas and support regarding siblings, see Chapters 4 and 9.)

SPIRITUAL AND PHILOSOPHICAL ASPECTS

As you try to comprehend your baby's fate, you may have a whirlwind of questions, not just about your baby's condition but larger questions: spiritual questions about God, fate, the universe, the meaning of life. Pondering and questioning your beliefs is a normal part of coming to terms with your situation. Asking "why?" can be poignant and frustrating. You may feel angry that your prayers aren't being answered.

I remember screaming in the bathroom one night. When my husband came in to see what was going on, I punched his chest repeatedly while he held me. I was so angry and terrified. I kept asking God if this is what I deserved for being such a terrible person. I figured that God was punishing me and I hated him for it. —*Brooke*

I was wondering in the back of my mind: *why?* I struggled with that a lot, yet at the same time I knew God was in control of it all. —*Scott*

Many parents search for spiritual and philosophical comfort. You may find solace in the thought that there are ways of being that have a purpose that you can't yet understand. You may have faith that this path is your destiny or leads to the higher good. You may come to accept that whatever happens is ultimately in the best interests of you and your baby. Perhaps you give up what you cannot control to a higher power. You may also reclaim some of your personal power and decide that you will get through this.

I coped by praying and hanging onto my faith like a life raft. I also realized I had to figure this out for myself and that no one could do this for me. —*Chris*

What helped me the most was faith in God and saying, "We're not in control of everything, and if this is what is meant to be, we'll take whatever happens." —*Greg*

I think that when I finally surrendered and began to pray for God to do what is best for my baby, things were tolerable. It was when I asked God to have this baby be born *now*, or to give him a miracle, that I just couldn't cope. I had to admit that it was out of my control and plead that God take care of my child, because I just couldn't. —*Jo*

Several people have told us we are the perfect parents for Gianna. That is the best compliment I have ever been given. It is a great honor and privilege to be her father. I love her so much my heart often aches. She has taught me to live and love more deeply. I am more deliberate in the choices I make. I want to live a purposeful life and be reunited with her in heaven. Knowing we will most likely lose her has forced me to focus on what is truly important in life. I hate to think of how much of my life I have wasted on unimportant and insignificant troubles. —*John*

I felt that others didn't really "get it." I felt that ultimately their prayers had nothing to do with Frankie or with me; it was between the person praying and God. And so I was alone in my understanding. But not lonely! I felt strong, empowered, and eventually, as I practiced being present with my baby, and, as I realized how tentative incipient life can be, I felt increasingly grateful that I had him growing in my belly at all. —*Susan E.*

For so many weeks, I struggled because I had been looking at my baby through the lens of the diagnosis and not as a creation of God. It was during an ultrasound that I fully realized that no matter the diagnosis, no matter the cause, Elliot's malformations were no accident, no mistake. My child was beautiful and loved since before his beginning. —*Karla*

If you are plagued by asking, "why me?" or troubled by thinking that this ordeal is punishment from a higher power or payback because of earlier wrongdoing, you may find it helpful to explore spiritual beliefs and philosophies that embrace gentle or forgiving ideas about twists of fate. Ask your spiritual advisor to offer reassurance, answer your questions, or help you release hurtful interpretations.[5]

LIVING IN THE TWILIGHT OF DEATH

I prayed for a miracle and at the same time planned his funeral.
—*Kelly G.*

One of the most challenging aspects of continuing your pregnancy is the fact that you are essentially living in the shadow of death. As one mother recalls, "Sometimes I felt a little bit like a coffin, carrying this baby that was doomed." How can you make plans when you don't even know which day is your baby's last? How can you enjoy this time when you're consumed with grief? How can you proceed, when moving through time brings you closer to your baby's final hour?

But over time, your grief can soften and allow you to embrace this foreknowledge. Then you can shift your focus toward using this awareness to your—and your baby's—advantage. Even though knowing ahead is painful, it can be a blessing because it informs how you can use the time remaining. You can use it wisely and lovingly.

As you adjust to living in this twilight, you can attain a sense of acceptance too. You don't like it or succumb to it, but you go with the flow of it. When your baby's survival is out of the question, there is no struggle for finding the magic cure. Instead, there can be a sense of surrender to something bigger than oneself. Death lurking in the shadows may feel horrific at first. But as you adjust to your baby's reality, your shock and horror begin to fade, and you can begin to focus on how precious every day is. Preparing for death can mean appreciating your baby's life to the fullest.

RECLAIMING HOPE

While others may view your situation as hopeless, your hopes don't disappear—they can evolve from hoping your baby will live to hoping your baby will die peacefully, surrounded by love. You may hope that your baby will feel loved, that your baby will be acknowledged, that your baby will be remembered. Those are profound kinds of hope.

At first, you may cling to your hopes for the best outcome possible or envision what could be right or go well. It is natural to hope for a miracle, a diagnostic error, or a baby who beats the odds.

I wanted God to perform a miracle for Emmanuel. I wanted the doctors to be wrong. —*Jana*

There was always a bit of hope that our next ultrasound might show that his prognosis was not as serious as they first thought. There was denial and a secret hope that this might be the first-ever incorrect amniocentesis diagnosis and that he'd be born perfectly fine. —*Heidi*

I hoped that he would be born crying and peeing; I was so ready to fall to the ground and praise God for healing my son. I hoped for him to be a true miracle baby. I hoped for myself that I, as well as my family, would be able to move forward from this.
—*Stephanie*

Even as you hold onto hopes for a miracle, your hopes can shift toward making the best of what is more likely to unfold. Your dreams can be as simple—and powerful—as hoping for a live birth, a few minutes to whisper some loving words, or a comfortable life.

⌐ I hoped that the baby would live and beat the odds! I did, however, realize that this was a fantasy, and in reality I wanted this baby to live for even a short time so that we could see her before she died. I wanted us to celebrate her life no matter how short it was. —*Sherry*

⌐ I hoped that my child would be born alive, that I could see him breathe, hold him, and tell him I loved him. —*Donna*

⌐ After reading a story about a baby with Trisomy 18 who lived four months, I thought, *four months would be nice.* I imagined that as long as possible would be nice. —*Jill K.*

⌐ I asked for ten seconds. I had my conversation with God. I just wanted ten seconds, just to have her be born alive. I didn't want to get greedy. I just asked to see her eyes. I said, "I don't care if this is selfish. I don't care if this is not in your plan. I want ten seconds." —*James*

Hopes can help allay your fears. Whatever you're afraid of, you can hold onto the hope that this experience will unfold in the best ways possible. You may figure out what is most important to you and fervently wish for that particular outcome.

⌐ I hoped she wouldn't feel pain. I hoped I would be able to look at her and not be disgusted or afraid of her. I hoped she would look beautiful to me. I hoped she would cry, that I could hold her alive. I hoped it would bring my family closer together. —*Erin*

⌐ Our dreams were that he would at least be born alive and that we would not go to a prenatal checkup and have no heartbeat. It seemed to me that having him born alive would validate the experience that we went through, the fact that we bothered to carry him. It felt like in other people's eyes it would make him more real. We could say he lived, he has a name, he deserves a funeral. —*Greg*

The Emotional Journey

I wanted Joseph to make it to 20 weeks. That would make the birth a stillbirth instead of a miscarriage. My state gives you a type of birth certificate for a stillbirth, but a miscarriage doesn't get any official recognition. I wanted the government to recognize that Joseph existed. —*Janel*

My hopes for Lily were for her to live and breathe. I wanted her to experience life. My hopes for myself were to have some time with her. I especially wanted her to be well enough for us to bring her home for a few days. I wanted my family to meet her so that they could know who she was. —*Katharine*

My hope for Anouk was that she will have eternal life in heaven. —*Monika*

Hopes also can help you focus your energy on doing everything in your power to have positive experiences. You can make concrete plans to protect your baby, support your children and partner, and make the most of the time you have with your little one.

My hopes were very practical. From the reading I had done, I was expecting a day or two tops. My hope was to hold her and look her in the eyes for five minutes. My hope was that she would be born alive and not suffer. My hopes for my family were that we could accept this fragile baby into our family for as long as we could and that we could love her and make many memories. —*Chris*

I had two major goals throughout the whole thing. One was to be there for my wife, obviously. The other was to try to bond with the baby as much as I could while he was inside. For me, emotionally, I really didn't try to think about the end results during the pregnancy, because I wanted to put those other two goals first. —*Brad*

Our hope was that we could celebrate Gianna's short life, and even though we felt pain and heartache, celebrate her life joyfully and gracefully. —*Jennifer*

Over time, your hopes may become more general and all-encompassing. These overarching hopes can form the foundation of your vision for your time together.

⟶ I hoped that when I met her, I'd have the opportunity to show her how deeply she was loved. I hoped that in meeting her, we'd feel certain that she was comfortable and that her life was her own. I hoped that we would all feel peaceful when the uncertainty was finally over—and that I would feel that I had cared for her in the very best way. —*Alessandra*

⟶ I hoped that Frankie would feel all of the love I felt for him. I hoped that he would be cozy and warm and that his life would really pack a punch for himself. —*Susan E.*

As you settle into your pregnancy, you'll be able to do everything in your power to see your hopes come to fruition. You can also benefit from accepting that you don't have total control over what happens, and that being flexible will make you more resilient. There are many ways you can express your love and devotion throughout your baby's life and beyond, and not even death can break your bond. Even if some of your wishes don't come true, your baby's journey will be no less amazing.

YOUR REORIENTATION AND ADJUSTMENT

⟶ Eventually I just surrendered to love and to the situation. —*Elle*

Central to your adjustment is reorienting yourself to a different process and a different outcome. Instead of viewing this pregnancy as a means to delivering a healthy baby, your pregnancy becomes purposeful in itself. After all, it's during the pregnancy that this baby can live, safely inside your womb. There can be a sense of peace and wonder when you realize that your pregnancy may be the healthiest period of your baby's life, and most likely it will hold the vast majority of his or her life span. Even if your baby has a chance of dying before birth, you can start to see this pregnancy as a shelter for your baby's life, and it becomes a time to cherish for as long as it can last.

The Emotional Journey

Your growing appreciation can also coax you toward accepting your baby's situation as "normal" for this child. You may consider the idea that even though your child has a fatal condition, she or he is actually perfect just the way he or she is. Perhaps "untimely death" is quite timely, an indication of a unique destiny.

When you begin to experience the intensity and richness of this time, another shift can happen. You can stop comparing your pregnancy to other more typical pregnancies. Instead of the common impatience of wishing the pregnancy away in order to reach the goal of birth, you can live in the here and now. While there is tremendous sadness, you can feel gratitude for the gift of knowing what you know, so that you can make the most of this time. And you can come to see this as truly an extraordinary pregnancy.

Indeed, this is fitting, as you are carrying an extraordinary child.

four

Waiting with Your Baby

Settling in for the Rest of Your Pregnancy

⁓ We both desired that Nathaniel complete his journey with dignity and love. I knew I would carry this child and mother him the best I could as long as he lived and grew within me. But I still had to walk the road between the decision and the delivery. I was determined to honor his life and prepare to say goodbye and release him the best way I knew how. —*Annette G.*

When you decide to continue your pregnancy, the idea of spending months pregnant with a baby who is expected to die may seem overwhelming. But as your pregnancy continues to unfold, you can feel a renewed sense of purpose. You can hold on to the realization that continuing your pregnancy is a way for you to nurture this child, and you can set about doing so consciously and with conviction.

⁓ We spent the next several months living in our state of "new normal." —*Alessandra*

As you settle into your pregnancy, you may come to understand more deeply that parenting doesn't start at birth; it starts at conception. Your focus can turn to mothering or fathering your baby now. With this new awareness, you begin to envision this pregnancy as full of opportunities to nurture and appreciate this child. Particularly if you're the mother, you become keenly aware that everywhere you go, your baby goes with you. Even though your baby's life will be far too short, you know that you can infuse it with love.

Settling into your pregnancy will present new challenges along the way. How do you explain your situation? How can you deal with others' reactions—positive and negative? How can you find support and enlist your relatives and friends? How can you include your baby's siblings? How do you find prenatal care tailored to your special needs? How can you make the most of this precious time? This chapter explores specific strategies for navigating the remainder of your pregnancy, embracing this time of parenting, and creating a journey of intentional love with your baby.

INTERACTING WITH OTHERS

Because you are embarking on a journey that many people have never even imagined, you will need to figure out how and with whom to share your news. You may have to deal with those who might worry about you, question your decision, or try to talk you out of it. You may have to figure out what to do with people who avoid you out of a sense of disapproval or simply not knowing what to say. If your doctor scorns your decision, a friend dismisses your baby, or relatives don't rally around, this only compounds your grief.

Most parents experience a mix of reactions from others. You can simply take note of whom you can lean on, whom you can't, and whom to avoid while you carry on. You can learn not to take judgments personally and forgive anyone who cannot understand. You can also decide that you do not owe anyone an explanation, and your competence and growing confidence will prevail. This is your journey, with your baby, and no one can take that away from you.

Explaining Your Situation

At first, you might be overwhelmed by the thought of talking to others. Especially when you're in shock and not ready to face the full reality, it's hard to find the words. And when you're in the thick of grief, whether it's a passing moment or a steady state, you may not feel comfortable opening up your emotional floodgates. But over time, your explanations will mirror your adjustment. As you face the reality, you'll be better able to tell people what's going on. As your grief softens, you can talk without sobbing or raking up intense feelings. As you gain confidence about your decisions, you can explain more openly and matter-of-factly. Delivering tragic or controversial news also takes practice. By trial and error, you learn what goes over well—and what doesn't. You learn who to confide in and who can't handle it.

Some parents break the news to family and friends by e-mail or letters.

The letter was one of the most helpful things we did during our pregnancy because it let friends and family know that we wanted and needed to be open about our situation. We asked for their prayers, and asked for their help in learning about other resources to help us prepare for Gianna's death. Through this e-mail, which was sent to many acquaintances, strangers learned about our situation and embraced us. Many people who had experienced infant loss, or had a close relative go through infant loss, reached out to us to help us prepare emotionally and spiritually. Those who didn't know what to do or say at least knew we were open to talking about our anticipated loss. —*Jennifer*

I decided to be completely open about it. So I sent an e-mail to all my co-workers. I was really glad I did that, because I got so much support. My husband got support too, but it was primarily for me. And then people were able to talk to me about the pregnancy without wondering if they were making me feel bad or anything like that. I made it clear that I was still open to talking about it, that even though it may be a sad situation, I was still pregnant. It was nice because we talked about my swollen legs and the things that I was experiencing in pregnancy, or else it might have just been that elephant-in-the-room kind of thing. For me, that was really helpful. —*Bridget*

One mother wrote:

> It is with a very heavy, sad heart that I am sitting down to write this letter to all of you. Please forgive this e-mail, but I just don't have the energy to call all of you. . . . In the last weeks we had begun to share the happy news of our upcoming baby with you.

Yesterday an ultrasound confirmed that our baby has a disorder called anencephaly. This means that parts of the skull and brain do not develop normally. Although the rest of the baby seems to be developing and functioning normally, babies outside of their mothers do not survive very long or at all with this disorder. . . .

I feel strongly that this is not bad news; it is sad news. This may sound crazy, but this is what this baby is. . . . This baby isn't bad. We are incredibly sad. Then, in some way, it also doesn't feel right to feel sad about what this child has to offer. . . .

Mark and I are united in our wish to continue the pregnancy, as depressing as that may seem. The health professionals have said that our baby may live for a short time. We really want to be able to see and touch our baby. When I imagine having the moments after birth when I can hold him or her, I feel an unbelievable surge of love and sadness. . . . You may be wondering what else I'm feeling. I'm not feeling mad; I'm very sad. I'm not feeling envious of my other pregnant friends (or other pregnant people); I'm very sad. I am feeling uncertain about what will happen and how I will feel over the next few months. I am unsure about how to react to innocent people who ask me how I am doing. I do feel that I know how to take care of myself. As I go through the next 4½ months, I will be needing an unbelievable amount of strength and courage. Having never experienced this before, I don't know if I have enough of either of these qualities. If you can, please pray or at least hope for these qualities for me; I am going to need it.

It rained all day yesterday; I was comforted by that. Today the sun is trying to shine; I am comforted by that too.

Love to all of you,
Katharine

Some parents describe their journey and provide updates on websites, some of which are free and are password-protected for privacy.[1] A Web journal or blog allows parents to go into as much detail as they like and to provide the same information to everyone who has access to their site, avoiding the telephone tree of misinformation that can develop when a situation is complex and emotions are running high. In turn, visitors can sign a guestbook and leave messages of love and support that parents can read in the middle of the night or whenever they need extra encouragement and consolation.

⟶ The website made it much easier for us to relay information about Ashley and even to share personal issues and decisions with everyone. Many people were surprised—and appreciative—about how open we were about everything on the website and in conversation. I wanted people to see Ashley as a real person, a member of our family that we loved whether she lived for one minute or one hundred. I think reading the website helped a lot of people understand why we did what we did. —*Shellie*

You will also be interacting with acquaintances and strangers in the outside world, where an obvious pregnancy is often a friendly and casual topic of conversation. How much detail to divulge to people often depends on your relationship to them.

⟶ You get asked in the grocery store when your baby is due and if it's a boy or a girl. And you sort of have to pick who you're going to tell and who you're not. If it was someone I was never going to see again, it was a "not." —*Jessica*

⟶ At first I wasn't showing that much, and I found myself even denying being pregnant. Someone would ask, "Do you have kids?" And I'd say, "Nope." Normally before the diagnosis I'd say, "One on the way." But after the diagnosis I'd say, "Nope, not yet," because I didn't want to get into it. Then I realized I'd leave the office in tears because I'd been bottling it up all day and denying it. Ultimately what ended up working was, if someone asked me a simple question like, "When is your baby due?" or "Is it a boy or girl?" I'd answer it the way I normally would. But if they directly asked, "Is everything going OK?" then I usually told them. That worked for me. —*Bridget*

⟶ I was congratulated by many strangers who didn't know how my heart wept at their words. Others, seeing me with my four kids, said, "Not another one! How are you going to manage another one?" Oh, please God, I wish! —*Sue*

Waiting with Your Baby

97

⌐ It was like a ton of bricks you'd have to drop on people sooner or later in a conversation. And you'd hesitate doing it, because you just knew even though that conversation wasn't going to impact you too much emotionally, you were going to devastate this other person, and they were going to feel like they had stuck their foot in their mouth. I was the new guy at work then. Talking to secretaries, they'd say things like, "Oh, are you guys gonna have a baby?" And I'd be like, yeah—but here comes the bricks. —*David D.*

⌐ Some people would see my growing belly and congratulate me, ask me all kinds of questions. I was grateful for those questions at times, because I desperately didn't want to ignore my baby just because she was sick. It was inevitable that the sickness would come up, if the right questions were asked. You see, they weren't able to tell us if she was a boy or a girl, also I was very small, so that was a topic of conversation which led to the fact that my baby was sick. Some very caring people I barely knew would hug me and cry with me, while others would try to change the subject and pretend they didn't hear this horrible news. It really helped when they just listened and didn't make me feel bad for telling my story. —*Chelsea*

⌐ We came up with, "Yes, we're pregnant, but the baby has a birth defect and will not make it to be born." That explains the whole thing and doesn't leave any gray areas but also leaves us open to talk about it more, if we feel comfortable. —*Janel*

Reactions from Family and Friends

If you are fortunate, family and friends will rally around you, supporting your decision even if they don't understand it. Others may be able to support you even though they themselves are in pain over your baby's plight and what you must endure. You may have some special people in your life who are willing to ask you how you're *really* doing, and they really listen when you tell them. They may be able to handle your expression of intense emotions and understand that talking about the situation helps you, even when you are brought to tears. Some people are not intimidated by terminal illness and death and can bravely face your reality with you. Those who can simply empathize and walk with you may offer the best comfort of all.

⟳ My mother was always there for me. She was hurting just as much as we were and did everything she could to help us.

—*Brooke*

⟳ Most of my friends were so supportive. One friend in particular just called me every night and listened. She knew that I needed her. —*Annette H.*

⟳ Most of all I needed to cry to someone besides myself alone at my computer every day or in the shower. There were some friends and family who knew I needed to talk about it. They knew that if they talked to me it would lead to sadness, anger, frustration, and a crying fit, but they still called. —*Rachel*

⟳ My co-workers (I am an RN) were very supportive and always asked how I was and how was the baby. I think they thought we were very brave to face this. It really helped when people were concerned and asked about me and the baby. —*Debbie*

⟳ Those who just sat with us and were quiet while we talked or cried with us were the greatest blessings to us. There were eternal friendships created during that time. —*April*

⟳ My family was 100 percent supportive of continuing the pregnancy. They "got it." My mother and father in particular were an unwavering foundation of love and support. If I got stressed or uncertain, they were always there with gentle encouragement and guidance. We did this as a family. —*Chris*

⟳ I allowed others who were willing to walk this journey with me to carry me when I didn't think that I could go on and to pray for me when I had no words to pray for myself. —*Karla*

Typically, some friends and family will be supportive, and others won't. Consider that you can set the tone. If you can talk openly and honestly about your situation, those around you will likely follow suit by acknowledging your baby, expressing their concern and empathy, and offering support. Your openness can serve you well as it invites others to walk with you.

Unfortunately, even in the face of your openness, some people will remain closed. Most parents run into at least a few barriers of silence, doubt, or criticism. How you respond can be determined by your relationship to this person and whether you think it's worth it to build bridges of understanding—or whether it's best to walk away. The following sections hold insights and practical tips that can help you figure out how to handle any uncomfortable exchanges you might experience.

When People Are Silent

⌒ There was one reaction from people that truly stung: when folks didn't say anything about our baby at all. At one point toward the end of the pregnancy I felt bigger than a house—it was very clear that I was very pregnant—and people I knew, who knew our and Frankie's story, would talk about anything but my big belly sitting there between us. To this day, there are people that have not said one thing to me about the life and loss of our baby, and that hurts profoundly. —*Susan E.*

Unsure or unaware of how to be there for you, some friends and family may remain silent on the topic. They may believe that silence is the best way to help you avoid your pain, but the effect on you is isolation, not protection.

⌒ What some of my friends didn't realize is that my whole world had become David. Every day from morning until night, I was trying to discover what my son's life would be like. People told me to "cheer up" and to "get out." They only had best intentions. They wanted to see me think about something else and thought that bringing up David was what I needed least. But what I really needed was to talk about him and what was going on and what I'd found out. —*Rachel*

⌒ Friends and family seemed supportive of us carrying Nathaniel to term, although no one came out and said it in so many words. I think they did not really know how to treat me. They did what they could in terms of bringing meals, sending cards, buying us a memorial tree for our yard. So the tangible kinds of things were done. But on the other hand, people did not seem to want to talk much about the pregnancy. Sometimes it was as though Nathaniel did not exist, even though I had this huge round belly. I felt lonely and isolated on my journey. —*Annette G.*

None of our family or friends made judgments or told us what we should do. That was a help. They all said they would support our decision. But they were afraid. They were afraid to talk to me. I think they thought I would fall apart if they even made general conversation. I hate pity, and I know there was a lot directed at us.

—*Sue*

Most painful are those who withdraw completely. Most likely, they are disappearing in fear or discomfort. Sometimes, people may withdraw if you are putting up some barriers of your own, such as not wanting to impose your needs on others or harboring a sense of shame for not bearing a healthy child. If your friends and relatives seem to avoid you or the topic, you may believe this confirms your need for barriers, when they simply may be uncomfortable and don't know how to help. This can be a vicious cycle, but when you're in turmoil and pain, it can be difficult to be the one who steps up to breaking it.

I struggled with those who completely ignored us, waiting for this to be over so that they could resume our friendship. —*Jane G.*

The rational side of me understands that people probably don't say anything not out of lack of concern but because they are afraid to say the wrong thing that hurts me. Anyway, I suppose I could have had the strength of character to gently bring the topic up myself. But do I always have to be the rational and reasonable one? —*Susan E.*

So many of our family and friends didn't even know what to do or how to help, so they chose to do nothing at all. From the time of diagnosis to the time of delivery I felt as if I were living in a bubble—too afraid to step out into the world for fear of rejection for not being able to create a "normal" child. —*Shayla*

It was a lot different for me than for my wife. She was talking with her friends, reading, and doing all this other stuff. Maybe it's different with guys, or just with the friends I have, but you don't really talk about your wife's pregnancy or things like that a whole lot. Pretty much everyone knew what was going on, but it's the kind of thing that people aren't going to bring up in conversation. People are probably afraid to. It was a little harder for me to talk with people about it. I guess I wouldn't have minded if other people brought it up, but I didn't feel like I wanted to bring it up either, to say, hey, feel sorry for me, my wife's carrying a baby that's not going to make it. That's a hard thing to do. —*Greg*

When people withdraw from you or avoid the topic of your pregnancy or baby, it can help to remind yourself that most people mean well. Your relatives and friends likely care about you and want you to feel better, but they don't understand how supported you could feel if they simply would acknowledge your journey or listen to you share your experiences and feelings. Try explaining this to them. Also consider that those closest to you may be too burdened by their own grief or fear to provide much emotional support. So look outside your inner circle for support. There may be others—perhaps even people you hardly know or would least suspect—who will rise to the occasion.

Our family had difficulty understanding how to relate to us, what to say, how to act. I know now that much of that reaction was due to their love and concern for us and our other children, rather than indifference to our situation. Our friends enveloped us in a blanket of love, prayers, and support. Although none of them could understand what we were facing, they were more readily available to talk, laugh, cry, and pray with us. I think much of that is because they were less invested in us emotionally than our family (especially our parents) and could just step in to do what was necessary. —*Pam M.*

A Gift of Time

‿ Family members who didn't acknowledge our loss hurt us the most. We expected more out of our family and closest friends, yet we learned that it was casual friends and acquaintances who had gone through losses similar to ours who really reached out the most. Despite the insensitivity and lack of support we expected from some, the overwhelming majority of people in our life were really terrific. —*Jennifer*

When People Question Your Decision

‿ I often got the comments in the beginning like "Why are you putting yourself through this?" "Isn't your baby going to suffer?" "Aren't you going to suffer?" "Why don't you get this over with and try again?" They didn't understand me. I often replied that they didn't have to get it—only I did, because I had to live with the consequence of my choice. —*Chris*

Many people, knowing that abortion is an option, may question why you would draw this out. They might think it would be better to not become so "attached," to seek "closure," and move on. They don't realize that your love for your baby started blooming when you found out you were pregnant and did not simply cease with the terminal diagnosis. Ending your pregnancy would not end your feelings of devotion—or your grief.

‿ Many people questioned our choice to carry the baby to term. They did not understand how much we needed our child in our lives and how we wanted to hold on to every second given to us. I will never forget being asked the question, "What do you really want to come out of this?" What I really want is for my baby to be healthy. I want him to have a long and happy life on Earth. I want him to stay with me forever. But I can't have that, so I am willing to accept what God gives me. —*Donna*

‿ My aunt wondered why we would willingly choose to endure pain, suffering, depression, and eventually our son's death. My husband's parents questioned whether our church had "forced" us to make the decision we had. Obviously, this kind of reaction from close family members hurt a lot. —*Heidi*

A member of my family asked me, "Can't you just take care of it?" When I asked him to clarify what he meant, he asked, "Can't you just have a D&C?" I was horrified. I couldn't just "take care of it." This wasn't some situation like removing a mole. —*Stacy*

Some friends did support our decision to carry to term, but they could not figure out why we would want to have a funeral and burial for that malformed baby. Carrying to term was an act of obedience in their eyes, but once we'd have done that, there would be nothing more to do, thus no need for a funeral. They thought that we would be glad to get rid of her as soon as we'd have done what we had to do according to God's commandments. It hurt to see that they just understood the "you must not murder" but not the love we had for our unborn baby. —*Monika*

There were some people in our lives who tried to encourage us to end the pregnancy sooner, because after all I was just supplying life support. That really hurt. I knew my baby wasn't expected to live and that I was her source of life, but I didn't want to end her life any sooner than it was going to end. I wanted her to live for as long as she could inside of me. I didn't want to let go. —*Chelsea*

Most painful are the comments from people who question your decision by dismissing your baby's value.

One acquaintance said, "Nature has a way of fixing mistakes," and I thought, *my baby isn't a mistake; nature made a mistake.* Don't consider my baby to be a mistake, something that never should have existed! —*Jennifer*

One co-worker, a doctor, asked why I was upset because, "No brain, not human." —*Sue*

If people dismiss you as merely providing "life support," you can remind them that every human being needs a mother's support before birth. Your baby's existence is normal and natural for this stage of his or her life. If someone questions why you'd put yourself through a "death watch," you can say that that's what people do when a loved one is terminally ill—they wait, they care, and they love.

While some people who question your decision may be judgmental, it may help to keep in mind that others may be expressing sincere concern for you and your baby because they can only see the suffering involved.

My parents thought this was too hard for us to go through. They asked, what was the point in having us and our baby suffer when she was going to die; wouldn't it be better just to end it? I felt hurt by my parents' reaction even though they just didn't want us to be in this situation. *—Debbie*

It seemed as though many felt I should not continue the pregnancy, but not because they didn't care about the child. They thought being induced would be easier on my husband and me. At times I resented them for thinking that way. It was as if I had to defend my child's life. *—Deanna*

Some might question your decision because they don't understand what's involved. Many people have little to no knowledge of palliative and end-of-life care, and some in your circle may not be able to comprehend your desire to nurture and protect your baby in this way. They may not realize the many ways in which continuing your pregnancy benefits you and your baby. With your patient explanations, they may be able to come around and stop focusing on suffering and death, and—like you—begin to focus on nurturing and life and the special relationship between you and your baby.

Especially early on, when you're feeling overwhelmed, explanations can take more energy than you can muster. You need time to process your own thinking before you can clearly state your mind. And you need to give your confidence a chance to grow. It may help you to avoid these people until you're ready to tackle the issues with them, or ask family and friends who *do* understand to have these conversations for you in the meantime. For the people who are expressing concern for you or your baby's suffering, you have a chance to explain your perspective and gain their support. For the ones who misunderstand, offer them clarification. For the unwavering doubters, forgive them and move on.

⌐ I had somebody ask me while I was pregnant, why would I go to the trouble of bonding with a baby who was just going to die anyway? At first I was indignant. I had three emotions in the space of a second: I was indignant, I was angry, and then I realized he just didn't know any better. I said to him, "I'm his mother. It's not up to me to number his days. It's up to me to provide the best home I can for as long as he's here." And that became my pretty standard response to people. —*Jessica*

When People Deny or Dismiss the Diagnosis

⌐ It didn't help when our families or friends either thought we were lying (why would one lie about something like this?), thought we were exaggerating, or just ignored that there was a problem. I guess I was more realistic—this was life or death; we heard this from the doctors and knew the odds. —*Elizabeth D. P.*

It's challenging enough to face your baby's life-limiting condition without the added burden of trying to convince your friends and family of the facts and likely outcome. It can be frustrating when people deny that your baby has a fatal condition, call on their faith in God to spare you, or simply want to console you with platitudes so that they don't have to face any painful feelings—yours or their own. It can be bewildering when friends or family dismiss what you're telling them, as if you're creating unnecessary drama or refusing to believe in the miracles of modern medicine.

⌐ One of the things that was very difficult for us was that many people did not believe us: that without a truly supernatural miracle, Lucy was going to die. Because of extensive prenatal probability-based testing for genetic disorders, there are many, many stories of babies that were believed to have something wrong with them that have turned out fine, and we kept hearing these stories over and over again. However, anencephaly is easy to diagnose and always fatal. It was actually not helpful to have many people tell us stories of miracle babies. —*Jane G.*

Some were optimistic, probably just to keep our hopes up, but it made me angry at times because it was like they couldn't believe it or process it. So during this extremely devastating time in our lives, they were saying things like "I just know the baby will be fine." Looking back I understand why someone would say that, and I would rather someone say something "wrong" than nothing at all, but it was hard for me to hear such positive thoughts at times, because I was trying to grasp the odds of what the doctors had told us.

—*Jessie*

My mother-in-law was in disbelief. She asked me over and over again if Anouk would really die. It was hard as I felt that I had to support her in moments where she should have supported me.

—*Monika*

In the beginning, we felt that some of our family members and friends underestimated Anya's condition. Sometimes, this made us feel as though they underestimated our assertiveness and optimism. We were not giving up on our baby. We heard comments such as "They can do so much with medicine now," "I know someone whose baby had a heart condition; now the baby is just fine," and "Have you talked to someone about this?" It was hard to get the point across: Our baby is not just sick, our baby is *really* sick. —*Delsa*

If your religious faith is strong, it's especially insulting if people doubt your faith when you're merely facing reality.

I struggled with those who assumed that if we had enough faith our daughter would be healed. One person said that it was good that it was not a genetic abnormality because it would be "easier" for God to heal. —*Jane G.*

Our family never questioned our decisions, but we did have several people look at our decisions and think that we never had any faith in God to heal our son. —*Scott*

Waiting with Your Baby

When People Judge You

You may even encounter people who judge you for your decision. They may question your motives or treat you with disdain. Others may hold ideas that are false. This can be infuriating and hurtful.

⟜ I lost one friend because of our decision. She told me that I was going to make my baby suffer, and I should just realize what has happened to me and move on. We didn't expect people to judge our decision to carry to term, and it hurt so bad that a friend would be so harsh. —*Annette H.*

⟜ One person at work said I was a coward for not terminating. Some people acted like she was a tumor waiting to be removed. It helped when family members would greet my belly when they came over and would say, "Hello, Charlotte girl!" It helped so much to have her validated. —*Erin*

People have every right to imagine what they themselves might do in this situation, but they have no right to tell you what to do or to criticize you. It was not their decision to make, and it's not theirs to judge.

Sadly, it may be close family members who voice the strongest opposition. If your baby has a genetic or hereditary condition, grandparents may worry about their unwitting contribution to your baby's condition. They may try to distance themselves from their own feelings of responsibility by vehemently disagreeing with you. Others may feel angry and deprived of a beloved grandchild, and you become their target of blame.

Sometimes, not responding is a valid option. But if destructive comments come from someone with whom you have an ongoing relationship, it may serve you best to stand up to them. A blanket statement may be effective, such as, "I really need your support, not your judgment." If you can share your grief and love for your baby, that may help them understand your perspective.

If judgmental people are hurtful to you, you can remind them that you are the parent of this baby, not them. If they disappear in a huff, let them go. Also consider that as you grow more peaceful and confident about your decision, it'll be easier to shrug off judgment.

A Gift of Time

There were individuals who disagreed with our decision to carry to term, and even if they didn't verbally express this directly to us, their disapproval of our plan was clear by their body language. While this hurt some, because we did have so much support from others and we felt such peace about our decision, I didn't really care that much. —*Susan E.*

When People's Responses Are Unhelpful

In contrast to silence or withdrawal, some people take up all the space between you and them by expressing their own thoughts and feelings to the exclusion of yours. Instead of listening and offering support to you, they may be so overcome with ideas or emotion that you feel compelled to listen and provide support to *them*. Of course, this is unfair and you may feel quite resentful or very much alone.

Because death is often a taboo subject, others may try to ignore or downplay your grief in an attempt to fix it, perhaps by talking about future babies or by comparing your tragedy to someone else's.

Some people said I could have other babies; they would go into their story of some friend who had a miscarriage and then a subsequent healthy pregnancy. I didn't get it. They do not know if I will ever have a healthy baby, plus I wanted *this* baby, not another. One co-worker told me what his mother used to tell him as a little boy: "There are other people worse off than you." I thought this is true but insensitive. I know others are worse off; it doesn't make me feel better. I was so sad over my baby, why can't they let me be sad, instead of making me feel guilty for doing so? —*Chelsea*

Again, it may help to remember that friends and family generally mean well and want to be helpful, but they may not know how. Insensitive comments often come from awkwardness, not cruelty.

Many parents experience offers of prayers. If people are offering to pray for you and your baby, and this is in line with your own religious beliefs, you may find this immensely comforting. But if others are expecting a miracle and you're a realist about your baby's condition, or if they are imposing their religious views on you, you may find their attempts at support unwelcome.

⟜ Some people were praying that Frankie would grow kidneys. (I asked if they could ask God to throw in some lungs while they were at it. I don't think the humor helped.) At first I resented this prayer for Frankie. Wasn't Frankie perfect as he was? Eventually I realized that those praying for a miracle needed to pray for Frankie for themselves, as they hadn't yet come to the same conclusions about the meaning of his short life like I had. And so my resentment faded. —*Susan E.*

In the past, you too may have offered platitudes, but now you know how hurtful this can feel. Forgive your friends' and relatives' awkwardness, just as those who have faced death and grief before you have forgiven yours. Educate the people you trust and lean on most about what you need. Tell them, write them a note, or give them this book to read. After all, they likely *want* to know how they can support you.

Facing Others' Pregnancies and New Babies

Inevitably, most parents have acquaintances, neighbors, friends, or relatives who are pregnant or who are parenting newborns. Everywhere you turn, you may notice blissfully expectant parents or proud parents with babes in arms.

⟜ My sister-in-law was pregnant with her third baby at the same time as I was pregnant with Elliot. Her baby was perfect and healthy. It was the hardest thing, watching our bodies changing, knowing her baby would live and mine would die. —*Karla*

⟜ I particularly disliked people who invited me to baby showers (and called to find out why I hadn't responded) and tried to put me in contact with other people who were having normal pregnancies. I didn't want anything to do with normal pregnancy. —*Jane G.*

⟜ I worried about my sister who was pregnant with her first baby. We were due the same week. She suffered from the guilt of having a healthy baby knowing that mine would be born dying. I felt awful that her joy was being taken from her. She should have enjoyed being pregnant more than she did. —*April*

I continued working for three months after the diagnosis, and it was difficult because three co-workers were pregnant at the same time as I was. It was hard to see them every day. They were so happy and excited about their babies that it was hard for me to hear them talking. I felt badly for them as well, though. I was this constant reminder for them of what could go wrong. They were always very supportive, but I'm sure I was hard to look at. One of them wrote me the most beautiful note. She knew how worried I was about my impact on her. She said that I taught her the depth of a mother's love. I really cherished those words. —*Kathleen*

If you find it difficult to be around other babies and pregnant women, you can gracefully decline certain social engagements for now. When interactions are unavoidable, it may help to mindfully acknowledge your painful feelings, to share them if you feel up to it, and to recognize the miracle of pregnancy, whether it results in a healthy baby or a baby whose life is expected to be brief.

FINDING SUPPORT

Family members and friends are often eager to support you in tangible as well as intangible ways, even if sometimes they may not know how. Parents have found much comfort in simple but heartfelt gestures of phone calls, letters, e-mails; practical help such as meals, housecleaning, and lawn-mowing; and meaningful gifts that acknowledge the baby.

Physical things that we received were picture frames, angel ornaments, flowers and many meals. We were really touched by *anything* that acknowledged our baby girl and our loss. Things with her name on them were especially meaningful. Letters, cards, and e-mails also lifted us up at moments that were too hard to bear alone. —*Courtney*

My friend showed up right after the diagnosis and brought a hydrangea to plant in my yard. She did not say anything, she just sobbed with me. —*Annette G.*

Waiting with Your Baby

⌐ Our family and friends were good to us, especially when you consider that with our frame of mind, they never knew whether they were saying or doing the right thing, and really neither did I! They called and checked on us often. —*Alaina*

⌐ We had immediate and thoughtful support most all the way around. I have friends and family who carry quite differing beliefs and worldviews, from "conservative, evangelical Christian" to "spiritual-but-not-religious" to "materialist-worldview/atheistic." All of our loved ones were available to listen or help out however we needed. We were very blessed with this. —*Susan E.*

⌐ Our community support was phenomenal! They gave us a "prayer baby shower" attended by more than two hundred people. The peaceful church was lit by candles, with soft music in the background. Not only were prayers offered for Austin, but for the grandmas, grandpas, his sisters, and for his doctors and nursing staff. A calm surrounded me and comfort was all I could feel. I could hear sniffles in the background. I peeked behind me and saw the church filled—standing room only! I saw lots of people with lots of tears. People genuinely cared. The most joy I felt was knowing that Austin's life was of value, not just to me and my husband but to others too. The shower gave us the only gift Austin was in dire need of—prayer. It was that night that we both felt strength and honor. It opened up the door for me to be open and honest with others and to share him with the world. —*Jo*

In addition to seeking support from friends, family, and faith communities, you can also seek support from parent networks and a professional counselor or therapist.

Support from Other Bereaved Parents

⌐ My friend who had also lost a daughter due to severe anomalies was a great support. She told me, "This is the only time that you will have with Gianna. This is the only time you will have to know and love her." Her words helped fortify me. —*Doreen*

I talked to my aunt, who lost her firstborn daughter, Christiana, due to a heart defect. She was alive for about ten hours. My aunt shared some things that I desperately needed to hear. She said I needed to love that baby right now. I had already realized that I was starting to distance myself from my son still in my womb. I was afraid to allow myself to form that bond for fear of the pain that would come from losing him. My aunt reminded me that my baby was not dead yet and to think about the regret I might have from not enjoying all aspects of being pregnant. This was still my baby, created by love, and I made the choice that I could not deny my feelings of love for my sweet baby boy. —*Kristin*

There's nothing like sharing common ground with other parents. You don't have to explain the unexplainable. You don't have to defend yourself or apologize for your reactions. They can understand what you're going through because they've been there, or are there, themselves.

I remember asking everyone at the hospital if we could speak to someone who'd been in our circumstance to try to get a sense of our options and the impact of any choices that we might make. I think I was also desperate to find someone who'd experienced what we had and survived, because in those early days, I remember thinking I might not be able to get through it all. —*Alessandra*

Because pregnancies like yours are relatively rare, chances are slim that there is a local parent group tailored for you. However, in this age of the Internet, you can tap into online support networks of other parents who are currently continuing a pregnancy or who've done so in the past. (See the parent resources at www.perinatalhospice.org for places to start.)

I was lucky to have found some very supportive Internet sites and some remarkable people who had or were living our reality. I connected with one woman in particular. We traded e-mails daily, each of us sharing thoughts, worries, joys and sorrows with the other. To this day, we've never met (I don't even know what

Waiting with Your Baby

she looks like!). But she knows me better than just about anyone, and her tender care has been a salvation on some of my darkest days. —*Alessandra*

You may have more luck finding a general pregnancy and infant loss support group. Many hospitals offer them. Although the other parents' experiences may vary, from early miscarriage to unexpected stillbirth and infant death, you may find comfort and solidarity around what you do share: love and grief for your babies.

⁓ I began to attend an Empty Arms support group. I felt so bad walking in pregnant, but after I told my story, I felt welcomed.
—*Brooke*

Even connecting with one other family can be helpful.

⁓ It was hard for me when we met with another couple whose baby had died. It was like looking into my future. I was like, "Crap, I don't want to be him." But we appreciated their honesty. Their honesty made it doable—they're alive, they're functioning, they're here, they're having dinner. —*James*

Connecting with other bereaved parents can help you feel less isolated, assure you that your feelings and experiences are normal, give you opportunities to develop supportive friendships, and offer hope for the future as you observe how others have managed. And when you are further along your journey, if you wish, you can be one of those parents who turns around and offers support to parents who are coming up behind you.

Professional Counseling

Just like you would see a doctor whenever you need help with physical issues, it makes sense to see a professional counselor when you need help with emotional issues. A clinical social worker, psychotherapist, licensed counselor, or a member of the clergy can give you the extra support you need to get through this crisis.

A counselor who is knowledgeable and sensitive to your situation can help you sort through challenges and figure out how to cope. You can air your feelings at greater length than you can in a support group and work through personal issues that may be affecting your adjustment. Family therapy can benefit your other children and your relationship with your partner.

Even if you know that your feelings are normal, professional support can help you move through it all. This kind of crisis can push anyone to the brink. Your baby's impending death may awaken old pain from previous losses or challenge vulnerabilities you've managed well until now. You may need to examine coping techniques that have worked adequately in the past but that may now be causing you additional pain and getting in the way of your ability to grieve and adjust. This crisis is too big for you to blunder, muscle, or sidestep your way through it. Your baby's life and death can act as a catalyst for growth by compelling you to adopt healthier ways of dealing with crises and emotions. A skilled therapist can support you through this process of change and adaptation.

You may feel the need for sporadic counseling at different points along your journey or for ongoing counseling throughout. Even if you go intermittently, it can be a comfort to know you have access to additional support when you encounter bumps in the road.

Be aware that not all counselors are trained or skilled in the area of perinatal death. The last thing you need is a therapist who doesn't understand your decision to continue your pregnancy or minimizes your feelings of grief and love for this baby. Try asking your doctor or a local pregnancy and infant loss support group for recommendations.

GETTING APPROPRIATE MEDICAL CARE

Perinatal Hospice and Palliative Care

Ideally, there is a perinatal hospice or perinatal palliative care program near you. If so, you can plug into their support. Programs differ: Some are integrated seamlessly into existing prenatal care provided by an OB clinic or by a midwife. Others are hospice-based or independent and don't provide prenatal medical care, although they may help coordinate it; their main focus is providing hospice support for you and your baby. (See Chapters 2, 5, and 6 for more about perinatal hospice and palliative care and visit www.perinatalhospice.org for an up-to-date list of programs and support.)

Contacting someone to ask for support may seem intimidating, even draining. But you may be surprised by how reassured you will feel once you've had the courage to make that phone call.

⟶ We were putting it off and putting it off, and when we finally called, we thought, "This is amazing." —*James*

⟶ It was great. From the beginning, our nurse said, "I will be so honored to be part of your baby's birth. We'll make it the best day ever." —*Jill N.*

⟶ I thought the day our son would be born was going to be the worst day of my life. Perinatal hospice helped me think, "Maybe this doesn't have to be so bad after all." —*Greg*

The options and care that may be offered to you may be more thorough, practical, and sensitive than you expected.

⟶ When I called the perinatal hospice, they said, "Here's the laundry list of things we offer. You pick what you want. Some people use one of these things, and some people use all of them. It's totally up to you." And that made me a lot more interested, because we just didn't want a ton of people in our faces and taking up our time. In the end we probably used almost every service they had. —*Jill K.*

⟶ We didn't want to go to a regular birth class with all these happy people, but we needed to go to a birth class. As a dad, I didn't want to be just standing there. I wanted to be as much a part of it as possible. Perinatal hospice was awesome. They did a one-on-one class for us. We felt special and taken care of, in a way that we really needed to feel. —*James*

Coordinating Your Own Care

What if there's no perinatal hospice near you? You don't need a program to take a perinatal hospice approach to your pregnancy. All you need to do is commit to creating a loving experience for yourself and your baby. You will need to make some decisions and advocate for your needs, which can be challenging when you are overwhelmed with sadness. But you can coordinate your own care by creating a plan in the spirit of perinatal hospice with your regular caregivers— even if you're the first family they have ever cared for in this situation. Having even one health care practitioner who is willing to support you can be immeasurably helpful. Even without their explicit support, you can be energized and inspired by knowing that you are parenting your baby in ways that will honor this child as well as your role as parents. Perinatal hospice isn't so much a program as a frame of mind.

When your caregivers take your care in stride, this validates your path—and your baby's life.

⌒ I can't describe how comforting the midwives were. Throughout the pregnancy, they never treated me shoddily just because my baby had a fatal anomaly. I received top-notch care and generous understanding. Never was I criticized for carrying my baby to term. They were more than happy to give a little extra hand-holding when I fretted about the fundal height or too-frequent Braxton-Hicks contractions. I was very, very impressed. —*Jane T.*

⌒ The doctors and nurses that I met were some of the most caring medical personnel that I have ever encountered. The nurses would all come in and tell me that they were praying for me.
—*Jane G.*

⌒ The care provided at our hospital was outstanding. I felt well taken care of and well-informed about what to expect during delivery and after delivery. They answered all of my medical questions and were available to provide support even after hours. The nurses, ultrasound techs, counselors, social workers, and physicians were top-notch. —*Jenny A.*

⌒ My obstetrician was outstanding from an emotional support perspective, even to the point of turning our grief around. He put his hands on my shoulders, looked me square in the eye, and told me what a beautiful pregnancy I had and what a beautiful baby I had. —*Melanie*

⟶ Our perinatologist said, and these words stuck with me: Of the parents she knew who had made this choice of continuing, none of them regretted it. Here was somebody who had seen families go through it and was telling me that this was an OK thing to do. Especially when my regular doctor wasn't at all supportive, it helped to have her words. Those words stuck with me. They still resonate in my head often. I think that was one of the biggest gifts anyone gave us the whole time. That one little sentence. —*Kathleen*

Overcoming Negative Reactions from Health Care Practitioners

Unfortunately, after deciding to continue the pregnancy, some parents are admonished or rejected by their health care practitioners. A negative reaction from someone who is supposed to be your caregiver can feel shocking.

⟶ Our OB reiterated her position about our baby. She said, "This pregnancy is pointless. It is just going to die anyway." She said that she was not willing to have her staff put in so much work for a pregnancy that should have been terminated weeks ago. My husband and I left that appointment in shock. We had no idea which way to turn. What do you do when your own doctor refuses to help you? —*Jenny D.*

⟶ My regular ob-gyn practice seemed to be annoyed with me that I was carrying this baby to term and how it would inconvenience them. I actually had an OB tell me that I was "foolish for continuing this pregnancy." That was the last time I saw him! —*Pam M.*

⟶ When we went for her fetal echocardiogram, the doctor, after drawing us a picture of a normal heart and then Emma's poor broken one, told us most people have an abortion with this diagnosis. It knocked us both back, and we said we weren't doing that. He asked basically why, if it was due to our religious faith. I felt like we had to justify what we were doing and explain that we weren't in denial about our daughter. —*Kristi R.*

⌐ The OB wasn't very nice. That's all I can say about her character. I think she was mad that we'd taken the choice out of her hands
about whether to terminate. She tried to scare us. She said things
like, "These babies are pretty hideous" (you're not Miss America
yourself, honey) and "If we don't induce, you could carry her for 55
weeks" (gee, I always wanted to be in the Guinness Book of World
Records). —*Jane T.*

You may even continue to be pressured to reconsider your decision. If you to have to keep defending yourself, you may feel deeply
misunderstood.

⌐ I felt so abandoned. They did the bare bones of what they had
to, but never once did they do anything more than that. No one ever
said, "I am so sorry for your situation." No one ever said, "How are
you really doing?" No one ever said, "Would it help to find a professional to talk to?" The only thing I was repeatedly asked was, "There
is still time—would you like to terminate your pregnancy now?" We
were walking blindly, one step at a time. —*Alaina*

⌐ Our perinatologist would say things like, "The outcome will
be the same" (even if we didn't induce) and "Unfortunately, some
people feel like you do" (believing they should carry to term rather
than inducing right away). —*Jennifer*

⌐ The doctor said that he understood the social aspects of my
carrying this baby, and if I wanted to be induced, he would be willing to do that. He then said, "Once the novelty of all this wears off,
then you just let me know, and we can get you scheduled." I was
so shocked I don't even think his words sank in until later. Did he
think I was happy about the way this pregnancy would end? I was
making the most I could out of carrying my son for as long as possible, and there had been many blessings! Did he realize it wasn't
my fault or my choice for that matter to have a baby that would not
survive? How could he say that to me—a novelty! —*Kristin*

⌐ For the third time, the doctor spoke with us about terminating. He firmly believed it was best for us. We told him again we

were not going to terminate—we were going to give our baby girl all the chances she needed to continue to fight and to live. He told us that he would see us again in a month—there was no reason to see us more frequently than that because there was nothing more he could do for us. I asked him what would happen next. We had a trip planned, and I didn't know if we should go or not, since I had no idea how long my pregnancy would last. He said, "Oh sure, go. What will happen is your baby will die, and you will not know it. A few days or weeks after that, your body will go into labor. Wherever you are, you can go to any hospital and they will handle you the same way—it really doesn't matter." Can you feel the abandonment we felt by our doctors and the medical community? How I hated that doctor for his treatment of us. —*Alaina*

We met with our perinatologist a second time and told him our plan, which was that we were going to proceed as though we were the hospice for the baby. He wanted to know why we were making this decision. I said that my dad is sick and is in a hospice program, and we feel that we can be a hospice for this baby. He kind of got choked up. He told us our decision was courageous and unusual, and he said we should be prepared for resistance by members of the medical team. He said, "I need to warn you that you will find that many of your health care providers won't be terribly receptive to that idea, essentially because they're scientists, and they see this as science, and this situation can be ended, so why would you take it to term?" Interestingly, I did face some of the opposition that he had warned us about. For the most part, the doctors seemed to not understand why I would continue a pregnancy that was terminal. They continued to ask me if I was sure of our decision and to remind me that the window for termination was closing. —*Missy*

As perinatal hospice becomes more widespread, parents will experience different points along the learning curve. Your first post-diagnosis appointments will tell you a lot about how much experience and sensitivity your practitioners have with situations like yours. Although many physicians have never had a patient like you, they may be able to support you without missing a beat. Unfortunately, some physicians balk. Your doctor may be concerned about the wisdom of such a path, misunderstand your motives, or say something insensitive. Some shut down emotionally, not knowing how to handle painful feelings or the situation.

⌐ I remember he said that Trisomy 13 babies are "miscarriages that should have happened, even if the child lives for ten years." That struck me as absolutely absurd. I had been feeling this "miscarriage" flip around inside me for weeks. *—Alessandra*

⌐ My doctor had always been friendly and easygoing. After we found out that our baby had acrania, things changed. He acted like he did not have time to waste on me anymore. When we arrived at the appointment, he was very rude and short with us. He kept repeating the fact that the baby would die, as though we did not understand this. He acted as though only an ignorant person would want to carry a baby to term only to have it die. There was no warmth, no sympathy, and no care. I had written down a list of questions because I knew that with the emotions I was facing I would not be able to remember or speak them on my own. Questions like, how long will we be able to keep him in the room with us after he has passed? Most of these questions were brushed off with rude comments like, "What difference does it make? It will not be alive. You need to understand that this baby is incompatible with life." During the visit, my husband asked me to get up and walk out. He insisted that we did not need to deal with someone like this.

—Donna

It can be supremely challenging to cope with a lack of support from your medical practitioners. It may help to know that you and your baby are on a medical frontier—not just with regard to diagnostic prenatal testing but also with regard to relationship-based, emotionally attuned, holistic medical care. Caregivers are mostly trained to take action: to "manage" pregnancies and their outcome, and to actively ward off death, rather than waiting for it to happen. Perinatal hospice requires a different mind-set, one in which the caregiver doesn't feel overwhelmed by a sense of failure, helplessness, anxiety, or sadness when death is the prognosis. So if you feel dismissed or avoided, it may be because your physicians and nurses are not getting the training or support they need to provide the care you need. As diagnostic prenatal testing becomes more widespread, more caregivers will realize that this technology demands new skills from them and will insist on the necessary training and assistance. For now, be aware that some are more skilled and trained than others in working with grieving parents, and you can seek them out. When you make appointments, ask for a practitioner who is known for being sensitive to the needs of parents who are facing the death of a baby. You can also share this book with your caregivers, to give them insight into the emotional experience and needs of parents like you.

Particularly if you already have a good relationship with your regular medical practice or if your options are limited, you might try working with them. See if your physician is open to forging a perinatal hospice plan together. Try stating your case calmly, so your doctor can see that you are capable of a collaborative relationship. You might try saying something like: "I know you may never have had any parents do this before, and I also imagine that you would like to provide us with the best care. I want you to understand that we've thought this through, and we are confident of our decision being right for us and our baby. A lot of hospitals and clinics are providing perinatal hospice already. Please consider working with us. Here is some more information, and let's meet again after you've had time to think about it." Even if you end up not staying with a particular physician, you may still spark a change in that practitioner's way of practice or thinking.

I did go to a perinatologist once, and he applied subtle, steady pressure for me to end the pregnancy since the "baby would die anyway." I assured him that I did not want to take that road and wanted all the time with my baby that I could get. I desired that my child have a natural, peaceful existence for as long as he was nestled in my womb. He seemed really puzzled by my decision, but told his nurse that I was his "hero" as I was leaving his office, so something I said must have resonated with him. —*Annette G.*

Switching Doctors

You and your baby deserve care that is attentive to your unique needs for medical and emotional support. If you are dissatisfied with the attitude or care you're receiving, do not hesitate to search for practitioners who are willing to assist you in your mission. If your OB practice has more than one doctor, you can ask to meet with the other doctors to see which one is the best fit for you. If this doesn't work, interview other medical practices in your area to find someone who is a good fit. You might be fortunate to have a medical professional who can advocate within the health care system for you or who can offer advice on how to advocate for yourself.

My perinatologist was very concerned about me and about making sure that my ob-gyn practice was going to take care of me. He gave me a lecture on what I should insist on, and I say "lecture" with affection; he was very supportive of our decision and of me. —*Pam M.*

If you've been referred to a specialist, you might assume that you'll get better care from that high-risk practice. But some parents find that it's the specialist who is unsupportive, and when they switch back to their regular caregiver, they get all the support they need.

We were pressured by our perinatologist over and over again. She said things like "induce and be done with it." We made it very clear we wanted to continue, but at every visit she reminded us that our baby had a terminal diagnosis and made us feel like we were wasting her time. She said she would not monitor our baby in any way. My doctor back home and the entire staff were made aware of my situation and were very understanding and supportive. —*Laurie*

If your caregiver's reaction is so negative that you feel you must change doctors, you may feel abandoned. You may worry you'll be unable to find anyone, and the idea of striking out on your own to cobble together the kind of care you and your baby need may seem daunting. Your search may take time and energy, but perinatal hospice is becoming more commonplace, and more caregivers are realizing that this is a new standard of care they can offer to parents like you.

⟶ It was very difficult to find a new doctor who would take me. Every doctor I called said they could not help me because I was too far along with such high-risk needs. I finally found a high-risk clinic that accepted me. The doctors were wonderful. They were trained in dealing with these difficult situations. The best thing about my new doctors is that they did not talk about a specimen or statistic. They talked about my child, a real live human who was still growing inside of me. They were genuine and answered my questions with kind words and love in their voices. *—Donna*

⟶ We weren't given any support, nowhere to turn. When I told the doctor I wanted to continue the pregnancy, he said to come back in two months. I switched clinics and doctors, and it was so different! The doctor understood and supported my decision; the nurses were so caring and informative. They treated my baby the same as any other baby. *—Sherry*

⟶ When we called for an appointment with a different doctor, the receptionist was able to get us in the very next day. I went into that appointment ready to fight for my son. I had a list of demands all written out on paper:

- No one in this office will refer to my son as nonviable or as a fetus; he is my son, he is Jordan, he is my baby.
- We want monthly ultrasounds to track his progress.
- No one in the office will ever bring up termination to me.

I must have sounded like a drill sergeant that day as I presented my demands. I was an angry mama bear daring this doctor to attack my young. Very sweetly, he bowed his head for a moment, then told us about his baby who had been born and spent a few weeks in the NICU before going to heaven. He suggested an ultrasound later that week! We were overjoyed. The appointment was the first really good thing that had happened in weeks and weeks. My husband and

I cried that day. Honestly, we cried every day, but those tears were tears of joy and relief. —*Jenny D.*

You needn't look only into obstetrical practices. For instance, family practitioners might be more open-minded about your situation, as they treat people at all stages of life and are more used to handling death. A nurse-midwife can be an excellent choice, as midwifery honors the natural process of pregnancy and birth. You might also consider working with a doula, a trained nonmedical support person who provides physical, emotional, and informational support before and after a baby's birth. Some doulas specialize in families experiencing the death of a baby.[2]

Your Prenatal Care

Regardless of your baby's diagnosis, your pregnancy requires prenatal care. You still need regular appointments to monitor your blood pressure, weight gain, and other typical pregnancy issues.

Prenatal Checkups Tailored to Your Needs

Prenatal care usually focuses on the physical condition of mother and baby. Your prenatal care has a much broader focus. Maintaining a healthy pregnancy is still important for you and your baby, but each prenatal checkup should also attend to your emotional coping, your special needs for encouragement and reassurance, and the kinds of baby monitoring *you* want.

Prenatal checkups can cause emotions to resurface, so you may want to ask for special consideration. Something as simple as being taken to an exam room immediately or scheduling appointments at the beginning of the day before the waiting room starts to fill can help. Or you might prefer to blend in.

There weren't many visits that I didn't leave the office in tears. I always brought my sunglasses with me so I wouldn't have to walk through the waiting room with teary, swollen eyes. —*Amy*

One of the things that showed they cared was allowing me to skip the waiting room and go directly into the examination room.

There is nothing worse than being stuck in a room full of mothers who are expecting healthy babies and knowing that your baby is not one of them. —*Donna*

⌒ My ob-gyn treated me like a normal pregnant woman, and I was grateful for that. My daughter's condition didn't make a freak out of me, and I need to be treated as a normal woman. —*Monika*

You may want more appointments, especially if you find monitoring reassuring or if you would like to be able to see your baby more frequently on ultrasound. Perhaps hearing the sound of your baby's heartbeat is music to your ears—even if it brings tears to your eyes. You can also switch from routine care to special care near the end of your pregnancy.

⌒ Because of his condition, I could feel very little movement, so the only reassurance I had that he was alive and as OK as he could be was through the ultrasounds performed at my monthly doctor appointments. I lived for those appointments, when I could see my precious baby and know that, at least for now, he was still alive and not being harmed. —*Kelly G.*

⌒ Our obstetrician was good. Every appointment we had, he did an ultrasound so we could see her. He let me bring the kids in. I wanted the kids to be able to see her. —*Bianca*

⌒ I continued the pregnancy in my hometown with my regular OB. He had never handled a case like this before, but he was extremely supportive. I got regular sonograms and lots of sono pictures. He would schedule me in the beginning or end of his day so I wasn't around a lot of pregnant women. He monitored me very frequently at the end to maximize the chances for a live birth. —*Chris*

⌒ My ob-gyn was phenomenal. She allowed me to come in as often as I wanted. —*Shayla*

For some parents, ultrasound exams can be therapeutic for processing the baby's condition and trying to look past the defects to see the pure essence of their child.

⌐ At 31 weeks, I had my final ultrasound to simply check on his progress. It was at this ultrasound that my husband and I really got to see Elliot for what he was. We saw the extent of the damage, but we were also able to watch him move around, put his hand up to his mouth as if he were sucking his thumb, and just be our baby. The tech allowed us a good forty-five minutes with him, watching him and loving him. It was then that for the first time I truly saw him as my baby. This moment was pivotal for me. —*Karla*

It is possible that you are the first perinatal hospice family that your caregivers have ever attended to. That, and the fact that every family is unique, means that you need to figure out and tell them what will help you cope and make this journey most meaningful to you. By becoming a full participant in your care, you forge a partnership with your caregivers that will strengthen their ability to support you.

Nutrition and Exercise for Your Special Situation

Knowing that your baby is not going to live, you might question the typical pregnancy-related advice about diet and alcohol use. You might wonder, *If my baby is not going to be healthy anyway, what's the point of abstaining from junk food and beer?*

Remember that you are still a pregnant mom and your baby is still alive, so the nutrition you provide is a direct way of helping your child—and you—be as healthy as possible. Eating nourishing foods and continuing your regular exercise routine—or starting one, with the advice of your doctor—will also help you to feel well physically during this demanding time of your life.

⌐ I was carrying her to term because I wanted her to have the fullest and best possible life she could have. I had to give her whatever I'd give my other children, just out of fairness. To me, that meant continuing to eat healthy, not taking any medications, taking the prenatal vitamins, and so on. I found my disposition was much improved when I continued to "act pregnant" and be on my best behavior. There wasn't much I could give Emily during her time with us. But maybe I could give her good nutrition and make sure her birth wouldn't be accompanied by a caffeine-withdrawal head-ache. —*Jane T.*

At the same time, if an occasional sip of red wine or a latte helps you feel pampered, no need to feel guilty. Nurturing yourself is an essential part of nurturing your baby.

Complications

Some women experience complications with pregnancy, sometimes related to the baby's condition, sometimes not. For example, polyhydramnios, or excess amniotic fluid, is a possibility if your baby has a condition such as anencephaly.

⌐ I was becoming so uncomfortable, especially at night. I no longer could lie on my back to sleep; because of the baby's pressure, I would feel sick. It was really wearing on me. I took naps when I could but then found it better to be extra tired at night to get some sound sleep. I really tried not to complain, yet I couldn't even pretend to be comfortable. My belly was so hard and full of fluid. It seemed worth it for the life of a baby, but why all this when I'm losing my baby? —*Greta*

⌐ I had polyhydramnios, and it looked like I was pregnant with twins. They offered several times to tap the amniotic fluid, but I said nope, I don't want to spark labor. I was just uncomfortable. I slept sitting up. But I was so happy to still be pregnant, so happy he was still with us. —*Jessica*

In a typical pregnancy, complications are nerve-wracking because of the risk to the baby's health or life. Because your baby already has a life-limiting condition, your reaction to any complications may be different. You may feel especially vulnerable because you already know that tragedy can come your way. You may feel doubly cursed—or you may accept it as another unexpected twist along your journey.

You'll also need to make unique decisions about how to proceed. If treatment is invasive, uncomfortable, or risky and wouldn't change your baby's outcome anyway, you can refuse it. Or if you want treatment to make you more comfortable, even if it wouldn't be indicated for a regular pregnancy, it may be appropriate given your special circumstances.

Some pregnancies involve bed rest to allow the baby to mature as much as possible and to avoid complications of prematurity on top of the baby's other problems or simply to maximize the chances of a live birth. If bed rest is recommended for you, you might view it not as being confined to bed but as a time to simply be with your baby.

⌐ I got put on bed rest at just over 35 weeks. That was actually a really special time for me. I was really thankful. There's always so much to do, you're so busy, especially those last few weeks of pregnancy. I was forced to just sit there and be in the present moment with her. We'd read, and I'd talk to her a lot, listen to music. It was actually a very cherished time. —*Bridget*

Prenatal Monitoring

Especially if there is a possibility that your baby may die before birth, you might want to be closely monitored toward the end of your pregnancy. If your baby becomes measurably stressed, perhaps you can be induced or wheeled into surgery. If your baby does die in utero, monitoring can spare you a C-section if your only aim was to have a live birth.

Taking Care of Yourself

⌐ We continued to take care of ourselves and one another. We did so by doing things we normally enjoyed. It was our way of taking care of the baby and being the parents our baby deserved.
—*Delsa*

⌐ Our family beach trips were planned and I was looking forward to going. I wanted to get away and enjoy a vacation. I couldn't let my pregnancy interfere with other plans anymore. It felt as though I was putting my life on hold and I just couldn't any longer. —*Greta*

During this time of waiting, there are many ways to take care of yourself in addition to getting appropriate medical attention. You can continue to do what you enjoy. Maintaining your favored routines, spending time with loved ones, and keeping special plans already scheduled—or making new plans—can do wonders for your mental *and* physical health.

Being attentive to your spiritual life can also help sustain you. Maybe regular prayer or meditation is already part of your life, or maybe it's something you'd like to try to see if it helps during this time. Reaching out to something larger than yourself can help steady you for this larger-than-life experience. There are many ways to pray: alone or with others, in silence, crying out in anguish, whispering in gratitude. If you are part of a faith community, you can request formal prayers or rituals, which can be deeply meaningful. If you don't consider faith a part of your life, you can nurture your spiritual side in other meditative ways, such as spending quiet time outdoors, listening to music, or simply lighting a candle at home and being present with your baby.

EMBRACING THE TIME REMAINING

I had only one chance to love Emily while she was still in the world. Only twenty more weeks. We tried to take advantage of all of them. —*Jane T.*

I tried to enjoy this as a pregnancy, not just as a tragedy. These will be our memories with Joseph. Sometimes I forgot that there was a baby in there, not just a bad outcome. —*Janel*

As you settle in to your pregnancy, you can view this time not as waiting *for* your baby, but waiting *with* your baby. You can actively embrace this time and affirm the existence of your baby in many ways, such as by naming your child if you wish and if it fits with your tradition, and planning activities or projects that hold meaning or honor your baby's place in your family. You also can simply enjoy quiet moments with your little one.

Every day that we had felt like a bonus. Every day that we were still pregnant felt like a gift. He was happy inside me, he was fine

A Gift of Time

inside me, he was healthy inside me, because he didn't need those things to function well inside me. He didn't need lungs. —*Jessica*

⌐ We decided early on not to complain about our situation. We knew this little life deserved to be treated with dignity and respect no matter how short in duration it may be. We chose to make the most of our time with Gianna. —*John*

Learning Your Baby's Gender

With the advent of routine ultrasounds, parents no longer need to wait for the traditional delivery-room proclamation from a doctor: "It's a boy!" or "It's a girl!" Many parents choose to learn their baby's gender during pregnancy, while others prefer to save it for a natural and happy surprise after birth.

In a pregnancy where you already know some crucial—and devastating—information about your baby, your decision about learning gender might be different from what you had originally planned. You might decide to wait to preserve some sense of normalcy and excitement about the baby. Or maybe you'd like to know whether your baby is a boy or girl because you want a fuller picture—not just of his or her problems but more about your baby as an individual.

⌐ We had decided that under the circumstances we would like to know the sex of our baby. We didn't need anything more left unknown. The doctor confirmed that it was a girl. Wow, another daughter. It made it seem so much more real for both of us to know that our baby was a girl. —*Greta*

⌐ The radiologist hadn't taken any pictures from the scan. She hadn't found out the gender. I guess she thought it wasn't important. It left me feeling that much more desolate: not only was I not going to have a baby, but now I didn't even have something to hold onto or a way to know about this baby I was going to lose. When I cried about not having ultrasound pictures, my husband called the clinic and asked for copies. The radiologist said we could come back and take more pictures for free. It took five minutes of the woman's lunch hour, but I'm sure she's going to heaven for that simple kindness. She showed us the anencephaly in more detail, how the top of the head had simply failed to form above the eyebrows. She took three pictures. And she determined that our baby was a girl. —*Jane T.*

Naming Your Baby

Given the circumstances, many parents decide to name their babies before birth. In some religious and cultural traditions, naming happens only after birth or just before burial; many of these parents bestow a nickname in the meantime. Whether you use a name or nickname, it can feel tender and personal to refer to your baby by a chosen name. A name invites others to use it, to understand the uniqueness of your little one, and to talk more easily about your baby. Hearing your baby's name spoken by others can be gratifying and affirming.

We decided to name our little girl and break our family rule of not naming our child before birth. We wanted to be able to refer to her by name and bond as much with her as we could while she was alive. —*Courtney*

After knowing that he was a boy, I wanted to name him. I wanted to give him a name so that the doctors would know he was a person, not just a fetus. —*Amber*

For parents who may still be trying to keep their distance, a name can make the baby too real. You may need more time to grieve and adjust before you feel ready to pick a name.

I wanted to name the twins. My husband was very resistant to naming our sick baby. He still would like to simply pretend that it didn't exist. —*Samantha*

Choosing a name takes on added significance when you know your baby will die. You want the name to be meaningful and a name that you love, but you know that all too soon it will be printed on a death certificate. Eventually, it will become a name that you will not get to hear very often. Do you choose a treasured name, maybe the one you had already planned to use before your baby's diagnosis? Or do you save that name in case you're able to have another baby in the future?

⸺ It is so strange to name a child that you know will die. Do you give that child your favorite name? It came to "yes." And luckily we had two favorite names (for our twin girls) and got to use them both. It was hard to give up hearing "Nora" as often as I would hear "Anika." I love to hear Nora's name, and I don't get to hear it that often really. But I am so happy with the names we picked. —*Kristi F.*

⸺ When we picked out his name, we decided that he would be named after his grandpas. We thought and thought about which name would go first. I was saying different orders to put the three names in and I said it, "David Michael Joseph," and I realized that was a perfect scolding name. That was it: "David Michael Joseph! You get your butt down here and pick up these toys you left lying on the living room floor!" That was how we picked out his name.

—Rachel

⸺ Picking a name for this baby was harder than I thought it would be. It was especially hard after finding out that she was unhealthy. I wanted this baby's name to have a meaning. A name that has a story of its own. Just any name wouldn't do. —*Greta*

Whatever you decide, there is power and love in bestowing a name on your baby.

Finding Ways to Feel Close to Your Baby

⸺ I began the deliberate process of falling in love with my baby. I began to talk to him, telling him that I loved him. —*Karla*

Sadly, unless things turn out much differently from what your doctors have predicted, you will not have years to enjoy your child. But even though you aren't going to get to keep this baby, this is your time with your child. You still have a profound opportunity to parent your little one and create memories together. *This* is the time to enjoy—and cherish.

Waiting with Your Baby

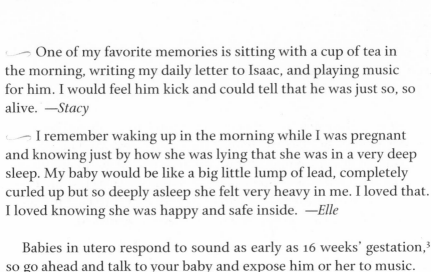

One of my favorite memories is sitting with a cup of tea in the morning, writing my daily letter to Isaac, and playing music for him. I would feel him kick and could tell that he was just so, so alive. *—Stacy*

I remember waking up in the morning while I was pregnant and knowing just by how she was lying that she was in a very deep sleep. My baby would be like a big little lump of lead, completely curled up but so deeply asleep she felt very heavy in me. I loved that. I loved knowing she was happy and safe inside. *—Elle*

Babies in utero respond to sound as early as 16 weeks' gestation,[3] so go ahead and talk to your baby and expose him or her to music.

We made it a point to talk to our child as much as possible. We never missed a chance to tell him we loved him. One of my favorite memories of pregnancy is having my husband kiss my belly every night and tell the baby goodnight and "I love you." A lot of love came from having this child. He showed us the true meaning of love. *—Donna*

Anytime I yelled or was nervous or cried, I was afraid that Frankie was receiving that negative energy. If he were to live for many years to come, at least he could make up for that with lots of joy and laughter. But he wouldn't be, so I made an attempt to do that prenatally by playing the piano for him every day and by playing a recording of my husband reciting nursery rhymes against my belly. I sang to Frankie a bit and talked to him sometimes, too. I tried to celebrate his life the best I could. I certainly sent waves of appreciation to him often. I felt so lucky to have him living inside of me! *—Susan E.*

I began to play music for Carter through headphones around my belly. I also talked to him a lot. I even sat in the rocking chair and rubbed my belly while sobbing lullabies. *—Brooke*

We spoke to her often, telling her how much we loved her, and I told her daily her father was a very handsome man. I believe every little girl should know her father is strong and handsome. *—John*

I talked to him about his big brother. I sat and spent time with just him, telling him about how special he was to God. Elliot responded to my voice by moving around all the time. He seemed to sense that it was important for him to just be my baby. I loved him for that. —*Karla*

My husband would lie in bed and put his mouth up to my stomach and say, "Hey, Noah Sam, it's your Daddy. I love you and I cannot wait to see you and kiss you. Mommy and Daddy are going to love you every second of every day." —*Jenny A.*

Being attuned to your baby's behavior can give you a glimpse of your baby's personality and preferences.

Emily had her own personality. How much was imagination and how much fact, I can't tell. But she seemed stubborn. Although the medical professionals asserted she would be both blind and deaf, Emily reacted to sound. More than that, she could react in specific ways to specific words I said! She disliked noise, and she jabbed furiously when I turned over at night. She kept my husband awake by kicking him when we cuddled, and yet she held totally still whenever her brother touched my tummy. She put us in mind of Mary in *The Secret Garden*, solemnly telling Colin, "If everyone thought I was going to die, I wouldn't do it." And we hoped not—we sincerely hoped not. —*Jane T.*

Revel in the experiences you can have with this baby. You'll have special memories and associations that you can always cherish.

We started to imagine that Alaina was with us at that moment. We took her to a Fourth of July parade, swimming, to a comedy show so she'd hear laughter. We took her to the orchestra. —*James*

My husband did neat things like suggest we take Eli to the zoo. I was seven and a half months pregnant, looking very much nine months pregnant, waddling around the zoo, talking to Eli about everything we were seeing. We did things with Eli, things we could do to make memories together. —*Jessica*

Waiting with Your Baby

We went skiing; we go every year. I had not been planning on skiing; I was 20 weeks, and I wasn't going to take any chances. I changed my mind. I thought, "She needs to go skiing." It was bitter-sweet. But I was glad that I got to take her skiing. I tried to get on the chairlift myself without anyone else so I could talk with her. I just talked to her about what I was seeing and how pretty it was. I was telling her about the sun shining and the sounds and the sights and how beautiful it was. —*Bridget*

Do whatever is meaningful to you. This is your time with your baby.

Pregnancy Photographs and Ultrasound Pictures

Just like you might take a snapshot of a first tooth, you can make visual keepsakes of this time with your baby. You can record the sur-roundings and events of your baby's prebirth life with photographs and videos of family outings, vacations, the seasons, your home, ev-eryday life, and your loved ones.

Some parents schedule a sitting with a professional photographer who specializes in pregnancy photography. If you have a knack for camera work, you can make some artistic images yourself. You could be bare-bellied or fully clothed; alone, with your spouse, or also with your baby's siblings. These images can be tender and artistic depic-tions of the miracle and beauty of a belly swelling with life.

You can also ask for more time in your regularly scheduled ultra-sounds and request snapshots to take home with you. Parents who are expecting a healthy baby proudly display grainy black-and-white ultrasound photos on their refrigerators at home or on their desks at work. You can be just as proud of your baby.

I asked the doctor if he could take a 3-D photo for us to keep. It was amazing to see her in 3-D. She truly looked like a sleeping baby on the picture. I loved it and I was excited to show it to our fam-ily and friends. My mom said it was hard for her to see a photo of our baby that she may never get to meet. As for me, I couldn't have had enough of pictures to look at. I wanted to see her as much as possible. —*Greta*

Including Siblings

If you have other children who are old enough to be experiencing the sadness of your baby's diagnosis, let them also experience the joy of being a sibling. Just as this is your time with your baby, this is their time with their baby brother or sister. To make the baby more real to them, share ultrasound photos, let them feel the little kicks, and if you've chosen your baby's name, use it regularly. Watching the baby grow, preparing for the birth, making mementos of this time are all ways to help your children process this experience and move through the emotions.

Even if your other children are too young to understand what's going on, any memories you can create now are memories they can cherish later. You can record these experiences in a journal or with photography. Over the years, they can return to the story of their baby sibling, and these tangible keepsakes can allow them to continue to process their experiences with a maturing perspective. If your baby has a healthy twin, for example, these keepsakes can be concrete evidence and affirmation of that special relationship for the surviving child.

We tried to include the children in the pregnancy as much as possible. One thing that we do each pregnancy, which may sound bizarre, is allow the children to color on my big belly with washable Magic Markers. The boys enjoyed participating in this as much as their big sister, and by doing this I felt that we were sharing the joy of a new life with them. Gemma loved her "pictures" and would usually kick up a storm! —*Courtney*

I explained to our 4-year-old son that Molly could now hear us and that he could talk to her if he wanted. He asked if he could get his toy kazoo and then proceeded to lean into my belly with his kazoo, singing to his baby sister! Then he asked if he could sing her a lullaby. He sang a song I have sung to him since he was a baby and that my father used to sing to me. After he finished, he leaned in again and said, "Goodnight, Molly. I love you. Sweet dreams!" My husband and I told him what a great big brother he was already and how lucky his baby sister was to have him, even before she was born. We were so amazed by the wisdom, kindness, and thoughtfulness of a 4-year-old. The more I observed him wanting to connect with Molly that night, the more it made sense to me that no matter what the outcome, and even if it might make things a little harder for him if and when Molly died, that being able to have a relationship with her at that time, even in utero, would be special and important for both of them. —*Kath*

While you may worry that fostering their sibling bond will intensify the grief of your other children after the baby dies, this bond can actually help them cope. Just as you are reaping the rewards of purposefully parenting before birth, your children can reap the rewards of being brotherly and sisterly. You'll all benefit from having shared this experience as a family, and you'll all find comfort in your memories.

Other Keepsakes and Creative Activities

If it appeals to you, journaling, putting together a scrapbook, creating a photo album, burning a CD of images and sounds, or producing a home video can be therapeutic ways to process your experiences, engage in creative expression, and create keepsakes. If you have the skills, you could sew your baby something to wear, build a keepsake box, or create a piece of art or music that illustrates this time in your life.

Holding on to This Gift of Time

As you travel through the remainder of your pregnancy, your thinking can grow along with your belly and your baby. You may have wondered at first: What's the point when this baby is going to die anyway? Why draw it out? Why not just get it over with and move on with our lives? As you continue to adjust and reorient, your thinking can evolve to: If this baby is going to die soon, then why *not* embrace the time remaining? Why *not* protect this baby? Why *not* use this time to create some memories and welcome this baby and allow this baby to have a peaceful, natural goodbye? This experience and this baby *are* part of our lives.

As your thinking evolves, the possibilities expand for finding meaning and treasuring this time. Even though you aren't going to be able to keep this baby, you still have a profound opportunity to embrace the time you do have. You can still parent this child. You can wait with your baby, protect your baby, and love your baby for as long as your baby is able to live.

— Time takes on a different meaning, and therein lies the gift.

—Susan E.

five

Making Medical Decisions

Choosing Care for Your Baby

Sometimes you need to advocate for more medical care, and sometimes you need to advocate for less medical care. —*David D.*

Even with a terminal condition, many babies will survive for a time after birth. You may need to make significant decisions about how much medical intervention to provide for your baby during this time.

Like your first decision about whether to continue your pregnancy, deciding about medical intervention can raise difficult questions about ethics and what is truly in the best interest of your child. Just because doctors can intervene medically doesn't necessarily mean that you *should* or *must* ask them to do it. Interventions aren't necessarily appropriate, humane, or beneficial to a dying baby. There are varying levels of care, from the basics of providing nutrition, hydration, and comfort all the way to experimental surgeries that may not even offer the hope of making your baby's life better.

It can also help to remember that your baby's life-limiting condition is beyond your control. But you can exercise a great deal of control over what your baby's quality of life will be like between birth and whenever death finally comes.

Your decision to continue your pregnancy was a significant milestone in parenting this baby. The decisions you will make about medical care after birth are another profound way of caring for your child.

You probably already began researching your baby's condition when it was diagnosed. This information may have confirmed your decision to continue your pregnancy or helped you decide. Now your research may take a different turn. You may be hungry for more details about your baby's condition and anything that may give you a glimpse of what your baby's life and your time together might be like.

⌐ I read as much as I could about anencephaly along with books that were about other mothers losing their babies. I read and read and read. My husband heard the facts, knew what was going to happen, and that was all he needed. He didn't want to learn much more, but for me I had to. The fear of the unknown was less and less after research. —*Annette H.*

⌐ I was too distraught to even talk about it. I poured myself into researching everything that I possibly could about anencephaly in twin pregnancies. As a scientist, it was easier for me to face the medical questions rather than the emotional fallout of what the experience would be like. I just sat in front of the computer and stared. —*Jane G.*

⌐ I spent a majority of my time researching the heart defect and any other possible syndromes our baby might have. My husband worried about me; he didn't like me spending so much time on the computer researching so much. I couldn't stop and still have not been able to stop researching. —*Chelsea*

Even if you're spending hours gathering information, this is a reasonable quest. Your acquired knowledge helps you make informed decisions and identify what's in your baby's best interests. Being informed can also restore feelings of control and mastery during this uncertain time.

We were just trying to get as much information in every possible way that we could. Show me odds, stats, numbers. The thing was, they didn't have much. But we didn't want only half the information. We're adults. Don't treat us like kids. We wanted as much information as possible so we could make the best and most informed decision. —*James*

To make informed decisions about your baby's medical care, you may need more specifics about what kinds of life-prolonging interventions are possible, what they would entail, what their risks and benefits are, and whether they would improve your baby's life and comfort or whether they would cause your baby unnecessary pain.

Keep in mind also that deciding to turn away from life-prolonging intervention does not mean turning away from medical care or doing nothing. There are palliative, comfort care options that actively keep your baby comfortable and respond to his or her special needs. (You can find more on palliative care later in this chapter.)

My husband did a lot of research on the Internet. I had experience working with the adult heart failure and heart transplant population; seeing what adults had to go through, I knew surgery would not be my choice. My husband and I tried to keep an open mind and kept strong opinions from one another until it was time to make the decision. Thankfully, we felt the same way. Every now and then, we'd read a story about a child who lived to be 8, 9, or older. It would give us a glimmer of hope, but then we knew the surgery would be more for us, not the baby. Speaking to a reputable pediatric cardiothoracic surgeon helped in making our decision. He was very upfront and did not sugarcoat the facts. We sometimes toggled back and forth, but it would always come back to the same reason: "Compassionate care would be for the baby, surgery would be for us." —*Delsa*

Many parents turn to specialists to try to make sense of their options. If you are considering life-prolonging intervention, specialists can help explain the feasibility and projected outcome, given the particulars or severity of your baby's condition. This information can help you make decisions about intervention or simply provide the details you need.

⌐ We ended up talking with neonatologists from three hospitals in the state. After these conversations and subsequent distressing appointments with the perinatologists, it became pretty clear to us that Gemma's numerous medical conditions were beyond repair. After months of going back and forth between the options of aggressive treatment and compassionate care, we decided to deliver locally and hold and love our little girl for as long as she was able to live. —*Courtney*

⌐ I knew all about the diagnosis, but I didn't know the concrete practical reality of what life was like. Our doctor told us some of the practical, ethical questions we were going to be dealing with. He explained to us that these kids just have a weak constitution, a weak inherent ability to thrive, to breathe. So, do you have a sleep monitor in their room? There are very difficult considerations for how aggressively do you want to treat that. Do you do intravenous treatments? An IV in a newborn, especially a little one, is not trivial. He got us off to a good start in terms of deciding how aggressive we were going to be with her. —*David D.*

⌐ We went back to have another ultrasound to try to get a better look at her heart. Several doctors had recommended that we do that because it would be nice to know what we could expect. But at the later ultrasound, the doctor asked, "Why do you want to know? What are you looking to know here?" I think he was thinking, *if I give you information, then you're going to go do some crazy fix*. We said we would just like to know, just to know how long she might have after birth. Because two weeks is a lot different from six months. Or ten seconds. —*Jill K.*

If you aren't given the information you seek, this can make you feel as though the doctors are deciding for you. If you are leaning toward aggressive intervention and doctors are dismissive, you may feel they are giving up on your baby too quickly or that they are making recommendations based solely on a diagnostic label, not on your baby's unique characteristics.[1]

⟶ We were told that heart surgery for a baby with Trisomy 13 would be "a huge waste of resources." —*Courtney*

⟶ There was pressure on us to sign a "do not resuscitate" order on Grace before she was born. That bothered me. I didn't sign it until afterward. I was convinced that they needed to hear that we wouldn't sue them. I also felt that they needed to hear from us that we truly understood her condition (fatal) and that we weren't expecting any miracles. —*Chris*

⟶ My new doctor was wonderful in every way. And I hated him from the start. Now I am so glad he was there, but when I first met him I wanted him to look at my record and say that he would try and save David's life. Instead he told me the same thing: David could not survive. So I bargained with him, which was more like a plea from me, by asking him if they would do everything possible to save his life if he was born alive and if he was born after 24 weeks. He said that if that were the case, there would be no question they would try if that were my wish. —*Rachel*

It is natural for you to want interventions that will help your baby thrive even for a short time or at least to explore these options. Being told your baby is not worth the cost is deeply offensive, and it can spur you to dig in to defend your baby against what feels like eugenics or rationing. A far more constructive process is to be given the facts and the time to make your own decisions.

In contrast, some parents feel pressured to opt for what seems excessive, such as when the intervention would be considerable and the outcome uncertain or likely to be poor. You may feel that your baby isn't being viewed as a whole, just as a collection of parts that perhaps could be worked on individually. You may feel some specialists are missing the forest for the trees. Would intervention prolong life or merely prolong dying? Or you may be told that a late-term abortion is your only other alternative to extensive treatment.

One thing that made me mad was when one of the perinatologists said to me, "Many of these babies do well after the surgery." I wondered, did he actually read our medical file? While it's true that babies who only suffer from congenital diaphragmatic hernia have a chance at surgery and survival, Ashley had many more things wrong with her. The prognosis is very grim when CDH is combined with other defects. I sat there knowing that I was going to let Ashley peacefully die, and he was talking about medical intervention and saving her. I felt like he just didn't get it. —*Shellie*

When I talked about compassionate care, the doctor told us that we would have to go in front of a committee at the hospital to prove that not pursuing the surgeries was in the best interest for our son. I couldn't believe what I was hearing. One doctor even informed us that they would pursue legal custody if we chose not to allow surgery. We didn't understand why we couldn't deliver Kevin and love him for as long as it was intended to be on this earth. At one point in our conversation with the doctor, a late-term abortion was offered. He said that my husband and I could fly out-of-state at our expense and terminate the pregnancy. This doesn't make sense. We were told we couldn't love Kevin for as long as it was meant to be without repercussions, but we could fly to another state and have an abortion without repercussions? —*Amy*

If the doctors have a "do everything possible" mind-set, they simply may be doing what they always do. If there is no existing palliative or hospice support at your hospital, they may not know how else to think about your baby's care or where else to refer you. If you can state your case clearly, they may be open to doing things differently. And you may have the option of inquiring at other hospitals, as practices can vary.

We asked that nothing would be done on Anouk after birth; we just wanted to have her in our arms. The medical team didn't understand at first. The neonatologist told us that after birth, the baby would be placed in an incubator in the NICU so they can check her vitals, control her temperature, etc. It was not about aggressive medical care but about control. We told him that we did not want that, but his first reaction was: "But we always do it like that. It's best for everybody." We then told him that we did not want that control; we knew that she would die shortly after birth, and we did not want a "beep" telling us that she was dying. We wanted to hold her in our arms all her life, should she be born alive. Then we asked him to imagine it was his own child. What would he want to do? To have strangers care for her, spending her only time outside of the womb in an incubator far away from her parents, or would he want to have the baby with him and his wife? There was nothing the doctors would be able to do anyway. He gave it a thought and then told us: "You are right, I never considered things that way." —*Monika*

It wasn't until I called my regular doctor that a door was opened for us. I explained to him that my husband and I felt at peace with our decision to provide compassionate care for Kevin and the turmoil we were in with the other doctors and hospital who opposed our choice. He informed me he respected our decision and would talk to some authorities at his hospital. Twenty-four hours later, he called. We were authorized to deliver Kevin and provide compassionate care to him, and my case was being transferred back to his office. When I hung up the phone, I looked at my husband with tears in my eyes and said, "We got it—we got compassionate care." He and I stood in the kitchen in each other's arms and cried. It was a bittersweet moment. We got the call that our son would be able to die with peace, respect, and dignity. —*Amy*

Considerations Regarding Medical Intervention

When we hear about medical intervention for a life-limiting condition, we usually hear about the "miracles." Hospital press releases and superficial media coverage can sometimes paint a too-rosy picture. As a result you might have hoped desperately that medical science could provide a cure for your baby too. It can be crushing to learn about survival statistics and the suffering that this path can entail. But this is exactly the kind of information you need to know, so you can realistically weigh the risks and benefits for your baby.

For many terminal conditions, even aggressive intervention cannot save lives. But for certain life-limiting conditions, aggressive interventions may offer some chance of extended life. However, they may be lengthy, complicated, experimental, and have low success rates. Treatment doesn't offer a total cure, and the condition requires ongoing intervention and may remain life-limiting.

If your baby has a condition for which there are treatment options that could extend life, specialists can help assess whether your baby is likely to survive more than a few hours or months or years. Even if your baby might survive for a time, you need to have a true picture of the risks, course, complications, burdens, and resulting quality of life for your child. Ultimately, you'll have to decide if these possibilities present a path that you want to embark on with your baby.[2]

Initiating and Discontinuing Life Support

Because Asher had very little brain tissue, he could live on a ventilator, but we would eventually have to decide when to take him off. We thought it would be better to not ever have to make that decision. —*Kristy*

For some babies there is the option of temporarily using mechanical life support to extend the baby's life. Technologies available might include a ventilator to push air into the baby's lungs or ECMO (extracorporeal membrane oxygenation), using a heart-lung bypass machine.

But extending life does not necessarily extend *living*. In some cases, these technologies merely extend a baby's life by prolonging the dying process. However, using these measures to extend life for a day or so may be appropriate if, for instance, doctors are uncertain about the extent of your baby's condition, and life support would allow time for them to evaluate your baby and recommend treatment and for you to make informed decisions.

If you are considering employing mechanical life support, be aware of the burdens and challenges. Resuscitation and invasive medical technology can be very hard on babies, forcing the body to function in ways for which it wasn't built. It can also be very painful. Depending on your baby's problems, she or he may very soon become clinically brain dead, and the lungs and heart continue functioning only because of the machines. When this happens, artificial life support isn't really supporting life, only imitating it.

Another challenge of initiating life support is deciding when to remove it. "Pulling the plug" can be emotionally wrenching. You may want to avoid that scenario, or you may dread the thought of having your baby tethered to invasive tubes and noisy machines. Many families decide that opting for hospice and palliative care is the kinder, gentler path.

AMBIVALENCE ABOUT MEDICAL DECISIONS

There seems to be so much against this baby—too many challenges. Would she be up for them? Maybe. Should we let nature take its course? Not every living being is meant to survive. This baby is naturally not meant to make it. Would interfering with this natural process be selfish on our part? What does our baby think? She probably wants a chance to live in this beautiful world. Will we ever be at peace with our decision? —*Christine*

As you gather information about your baby's condition and possible treatment options, you are faced with the gravity of the life-and-death decisions you are making. It's normal to feel ambivalent and unsure. It is also normal for you and your partner to be on different timetables.

We went back and forth about giving her comfort care or aggressive care. It was really hard to choose because we did not want her to suffer, and we did not want to feel as if we were holding on selfishly. —*Lizabeth*

I was really scared that I wouldn't feel right about the decision. I think my husband knew right away he didn't want to do the surgery. I didn't want to do the surgery either, but I didn't know. I couldn't imagine watching our child die and I just didn't know. —*Kristi F.*

～ One minute we'd ask ourselves, "How can we not do anything (medically) for her?" The next minute we'd think, "How could we put her through the suffering that medical intervention would bring?" I started to think early on that comfort care might be the best thing for Ashley. It took my husband a little longer to be at peace with that—he didn't want to feel like we were giving up hope or not fighting to save Ashley. I think he knew in his head that medical intervention would not save her life, but the heart is a different story. A part of me felt that way too. But if Ashley would only survive a very short time, I wanted her to know us and to feel our presence. I wanted her life to be peaceful, not filled with tubes and machines, suffering and pain. —*Shellie*

Just like you may have wished for a miscarriage to take the decision about continuing your pregnancy out of your hands, you may also wish for your baby's prognosis to be clearly grim at birth so you won't have to bear the responsibility of making decisions about intervention. You might wish that a doctor would just tell you what to do. Or you may secretly hope that if you do consent to intervene, your baby will die anyway—but at least you could tell yourself (and everybody else) that you tried.

～ If we did do the surgery, I already sort of wished that she wouldn't make it. I can't believe that I write that now, but that is what my gut felt. I wished that she would save herself from further suffering, that she and God would take it out of our hands. I realized that meant that if we decided to do the surgery, I would be doing it to take the responsibility off my shoulders. I would do it just to feel like I had done everything possible. I would do it to keep myself from feeling guilty. I would put my daughter through open-heart surgery and keep her from feeling our love just to make myself feel better. I couldn't make her do that for me. —*Kristi F.*

～ I sometimes wished someone else could make the decisions for me. I didn't want to make life-and-death decisions for our child. —*Shellie*

Even though you may wish you didn't have to make these decisions, you are, in fact, the best person for the job. As the mother or father, you are closest to your baby in body and spirit. Also remember that you are not choosing death or the timing of it; you are choosing to allow nature to take its course and choosing to give your baby a good life.

SEEKING OUTSIDE ADVICE

You may find it helpful to seek input into your decisions about medical intervention. Close family, trusted friends, health care practitioners, other bereaved parents, or clergy may be able to offer helpful perspectives. Or you may simply seek reassurance that you have their support.

⌒ I still felt so alone. I wanted to talk to someone who made the same decision we had. Luckily one of the doctors had a friend who had gone through the exact same experience and made the same decision we had. That connection helped me so much. She gave us really good advice: to give our daughter a name, to make her part of the family even though she was still in the womb, to give her all the love that we had. She said that we were making a humane decision in forgoing heart surgery—this is the way Sarina's life was meant to be. It was natural and her path in life was not long. Everyone has a path, a journey, a reason for being. She told me we were doing something "selfless," as hard of a decision it was, because it was the least amount of suffering for Sarina. —*Christine*

⌒ I really needed to find a way to come to peace with not doing anything surgically. Our pastor came over and talked with us for three hours. He told us that there were different levels of technology that were appropriate for different people. Basically, he helped make it OK to not do the surgery. He also told us that we needed to bring in the people that we loved and needed help from to be part of the decision. We realized that he was completely right on that one. Although I didn't want others to tell us what we needed to do, we needed more than just support from our families who would do whatever we wanted. We needed them to really believe in our decision. —*Kristi F.*

Affirmation of your decision from your doctors can be reassuring as well, in light of their medical expertise. When you have agreement, you also have assurance that your plans will be honored.

⟶ We told the doctor our plans for interventions that we hoped would be available to Jordan and about the interventions that we thought were too extreme and too painful to perform on a very sick infant. The doctor agreed with all of our plans and was glad to see how informed we were about our son's diagnosis. —*Jenny D.*

⟶ Some of the staff at the clinic discussed comfort care with us. Probably the most helpful conversation was when we spoke to the neonatologist. She began the discussion by asking us where we were at and if we had made any decisions. Once we told her we were thinking about comfort care, she seemed to validate that decision in some way; we felt like she agreed with us that it would be the best thing. —*Shellie*

For parents who consider themselves pro-life, sometimes there is uncertainty about how that translates into medical decisions. Some confuse being pro-life with being "pro-every-possible-medical-intervention." One perspective to consider is that many religions that passionately defend the sanctity of life also teach that one is not obligated to undertake disproportionate medical means in order to sustain life. A sharp ethical line is drawn between forgoing extraordinary treatment, thus allowing death to come naturally, and taking direct actions intended to end a life. Many religious traditions do not insist on artificially maintaining life at all costs, but they do insist on *reverence* for life. This is a helpful guiding principle for many parents.

Bioethicists are another source of insight for parents. You may find sage advice from your hospital's bioethics committee or professional ethicists at a nearby medical school or university. They could assure you that a medical procedure isn't judged to be a good or bad idea based on the procedure itself. Instead, the benefits and burdens are weighed by how it would affect an individual patient in his or her specific circumstances. A feeding tube, for example, would be appropriate in some situations and inappropriate in others. (You can find more on nutrition and hydration later in this chapter.) It isn't the technology itself that drives your decisions; you can use your judgment or use the insight of your advisors to see your baby holistically and take the entirety of your baby's condition into account. Seeing the whole picture avoids falling into the trap of what is called the "technological imperative," the assumption that just because a technology exists that you are obligated to use it.

Religious parents can take the view that declining extraordinary medical intervention isn't playing God; it's stepping out of the way to let God's will be done—whether that be an earthly miracle or welcoming their baby to heaven.

⌐ We wanted just comfort care for Asher. We knew if God was going to perform a miracle he would not need chest tubes and ventilators to do it. —*Kristy*

⌐ Although we ended up choosing comfort care, we never stopped praying for a miracle. They do come, just not always in the way we would have chosen. —*Courtney*

DECIDING TO WAIT AND SEE

Decisions are even more complicated when no one is sure how the baby will be after birth. If your baby's prognosis or diagnosis is uncertain, you don't need to decide before birth what to do afterward. You can continue to research what the options might entail and come to some tentative conclusions about what you might do depending on how your baby responds after birth.

⌐ While they presented several options and helped us weigh the pros and cons of life support, it was clear that we wouldn't really know much until he was born—and that's if he were born alive. —*Heidi*

A Gift of Time

⌐ Since we were still unsure of the extent of her deformities, much was going to be decided after her birth. We decided that if her deformities were too severe (seizures, severe heart problems) we would sign a "do not resuscitate" order. We knew that we'd be keeping her alive for us, and we thought it selfish. If she was born alive, we were going to get her immediately so that we could hold her as much as possible. If the doctors determined that her abnormalities were not too severe, then we were going to do as much medical intervention as possible. —*Jamie*

⌐ My husband and I decided, after much thought and prayer, that we would have her intubated immediately after birth so that the doctors could observe and evaluate her, and we would go from there. —*Jessie*

It's also important to keep in mind that babies can surprise everyone. Some conditions are so rare that the few cases on record may not accurately predict how your baby will do. Even babies with conditions generally considered terminal, such as Trisomy 13 and 18, can have significant differences. Some babies are born without the major heart defects that often are a hallmark of those conditions, for example, and may be able to live longer with minimal intervention.[3]

⌐ We looked for a doctor who would be willing to assess her at birth, and who was willing to give her oxygen, or a feeding tube if she lived that long (the neonatologists we talked to were not even willing to discuss either option). The doctor we found knew that chances were slim but was willing to make choices based on the realities of Sidney's life, not based on statistics. —*Laura W.*

This wait-and-see approach can also be appropriate for parents who can't imagine doing anything less than "everything." If you are still hoping beyond hope for a miracle for your baby, it can be a relief to hear that your baby can be evaluated after birth, and decisions can be made then. If you wish to pursue extensive intervention, or at least want to keep your options open, this is a way to give your child a chance, if there's one to be had.

Making Medical Decisions

⟋ I was in complete denial and wouldn't stop until I found a doctor who at least said he would do something, anything to try and save my so wanted and loved little boy. In my mind the only thing I could think of was how I would feel like a murderer if I didn't believe I'd done everything I could do to give David a chance that he deserves if he wants to fight. —*Rachel*

If you decide to wait and see, living with uncertainty can be very stressful. Here are a few coping strategies that might work for you:

- *Take one day at a time*. Is today the day that you need to make a medical decision? No? Then let it go for now.
- *Trust the process*. Hold onto the idea that events will unfold as they should, toward a higher purpose.
- *Adopt a wondering attitude*. Instead of pinning your hopes on a certain outcome, say, "I wonder what my baby's evaluation will be after birth." And hold onto the idea that this is your child's sacred journey.
- *Let your baby—not your baby's diagnosis—lead you*.

OPTING FOR HOSPICE AND PALLIATIVE CARE

⟋ To a parent, the options are sometimes perceived as "the black door of death" versus "a chance or hope that a treatment might be beneficial." I love the perinatal hospice idea because it opens that "black door" and eliminates the fear that may result in a family making a treatment choice that they will regret. The hospice removes the fear of death and indeed reveals or creates beauty in the process. —*Barbara*

It may seem that the decision before you is framed as "doing everything" versus "doing nothing." What kind of parent wants to do nothing? This has overtones of abandoning a less-than-perfect child or willingly letting a baby die. Even if you are opting against certain medical interventions, perinatal hospice and palliative care is not "nothing." It is an intense, active, holistic way of caring for your baby as well as you and the rest of your baby's family.

A Gift of Time

Palliative care can be an alternative to surgeries or other major intervention and in its fullest form encompasses "comfort care" and much more. As defined by the World Health Organization, palliative care provides relief from pain and other distressing symptoms, affirms life and regards dying as a normal process, and intends neither to hasten nor postpone death. Specifically regarding children, palliative care is the "active total care of the child's body, mind and spirit, and also involves giving support to the family."[4] Palliative care can also be provided along with medical intervention that might extend your baby's life.

So what would palliative care mean for your baby? It depends greatly on your baby's condition and how long he or she might live. It could be as simple as providing a warm blanket, a quiet room, a loving touch, and hushed respect. If your baby lives long enough to go home, it could mean home visits by a hospice nurse, feeding tubes or supplemental oxygen if needed, and guidance and support for you as your baby's condition progresses. But the principles are the same: relieving pain, affirming life, and neither hastening nor postponing death.

While opting for palliative care can ensure your baby's comfort, deciding against medical intervention can be wrenching because it seems to violate the primal parental instinct of keeping your child alive.

I felt guilt, because I knew that there were many people out there who would have thought very differently from us. They would do all that they could to keep their child alive. What parent wouldn't? It seemed so unfair that we were put in a position to make such a decision. How could a parent decide to let their child die? —*Christine*

We decided after talking to our pediatrician, my ob-gyn, and the NICU staff that we would provide comfort measures to Riley when he was born but that we would not take extensive action to sustain his life unless his prognosis at birth showed signs of hope. Making a decision like that goes against everything that makes sense to a parent. —*Christie*

Making Medical Decisions

It was a hard decision to make. You are supposed to protect your child and preserve his or her life. I feel in a way that we did protect him. We protected him from painful procedures and treatments that would have not really changed his outcome. I think the prevailing opinion in this country is to always do everything medically possible when people are sick or dying. I think our culture is so afraid of death that it thinks of it as something to avoid at all costs. I think if we had a better understanding of death as a normal, natural, although emotionally painful, part of life, things would be different. —*Kathleen*

For many parents, the decision not to intervene is relatively clearcut because their baby's condition is so severe and life outside the womb is expected to be very short regardless of any attempts to extend it. There can be an element of peace in choosing palliative care when medical intervention offers no good outcome.

Because every doctor told us he could not live longer than five minutes outside of the womb, we chose to hold him and love him without being interrupted by doctors or nurses. —*Donna*

The doctors had said that if we wanted, they would try to keep him breathing. We decided that, if there weren't any kidneys and there was no way of him surviving, we didn't want them to prolong his life by machines. I wanted him to be in peace. —*Deanna*

A perinatologist and former hospice nurse explained the types of medical interventions that our baby might require. They helped us understand the benefits versus the outcome and explained what "comfort care" is. We wanted Jonah to know our voices, our touch, and our love for him regardless of how long he lived. Not wanting him to endure the needless pain of a ventilator or other machines, we chose to hold, love, and cradle our son instead of attempting heroic medical efforts. —*Heidi*

We just thought, we're going to let her do what she would do.
—*Bridget*

For other babies, intervention might buy a short amount of time, but you may decide that the extra time does not outweigh the burdens that the interventions would impose on your baby. You may also want to avoid opening the door to a spiral of other complications and decisions.

⟶ We basically decided that if there was a 50 percent chance she wasn't going to make it past five days anyway, there was no sense in spending those five days on a ventilator in a NICU. —*David D.*

⟶ It was definitely an instinct from the very beginning. We still went ahead and researched the medical intervention to make sure we were making the right choice, but it was clear that there was no cure. We knew that medical intervention might increase the length of her life, but we didn't see an increase in quality. We put ourselves in her shoes and thought she would prefer to spend a short life in her parents' loving arms over a slightly longer life in a hospital having painful procedures. We picked a good life over a long life. —*Jill K.*

⟶ I couldn't see putting him on a ventilator. Being a nurse, maybe I see it from a different perspective. I just couldn't do it. Our perinatologist also said, once you start doing things, you're sort of on a slippery slope. At some point, you're going to have to decide to stop it—and that's a really hard decision to make. So she said they always recommend comfort care and that's it. —*Kathleen*

⟶ If you operated, you might get two weeks extra, but she would be in the hospital in pain, on drugs, recovering from major surgery. Then all of a sudden the liver fails. Then what? You could do that, but there's no question that the baby would be in pain. So we chose hospice care. I wanted her to have the best, most amazing life she could have. —*James*

A significant advantage of knowing before birth that you will not be pursuing extensive intervention is that you can stay with your regular doctor or midwife and give birth at your local hospital rather than traveling to a specialized medical center. This can make the birth experience less stressful for you and can make it easier for family and friends to offer support. Even if you'll be in a large hospital, your advance decisions can still make your experience more peaceful.

Making the move to arrange for hospice or palliative care can be difficult. You may feel that picking up the phone requires you to admit that your baby will die. But enlisting their help can actually ease your fears.

It took me well over a month to finally pull my head out of the sand of denial and give hospice a call. —*Heidi*

I was so mortified by the thought of contacting hospice. I had this idea that if I was even found to be talking with someone from hospice that it would mean that I want to just give up and let my David die. Once I talked with the hospice nurse and shared my fears I learned the error of my ways, but that was not an easy road for me to walk. I wanted so much to hate this woman who lets little children die. I just didn't want it to be my baby that needed her. —*Rachel*

Formal perinatal hospice support is available in some areas but not others. Even if you've been told that there is no perinatal hospice support for you, you can contact a regular adult hospice program and ask if they would be willing to help.

I contacted a children's grief and bereavement specialist from hospice and I asked her if she could help us. We started a relationship that continues today. She and hospice were the exact things I needed to carry this baby to term and plan for what was ahead. She had never had a case like ours before, but she embraced us and walked with us. —*Chris*

Some adult hospice programs have even started formal perinatal hospice programs because of a parent like you, someone who came to them and said, "No one else knows what to do with me. Will you please help?" Having the courage to contact a hospice can help not only you and your baby but other families to come.

If your caregivers have not had formal training in hospice and palliative medicine, much information is available to them in the medical literature.[5] They may be willing to be pioneers with you in providing the best possible palliative care for your baby.

Nutrition and Hydration

Depending on your baby's condition, if your baby is born alive, he or she may have a normal suck reflex and may be able to nurse from the breast or a bottle. You can think ahead: Would you like to attempt the sweet intimacy of nursing your baby? Would you like to try bottle-feeding so the baby's dad and others can share in this tender care? You can also plan to try both.

Keep in mind that some babies begin dying as soon as they are born and will not be able nor want to nurse. Other babies can live for a time but will be too weak to nurse or take a bottle. Others have facial or other physical anomalies that make it impossible to suck or swallow. Also be aware that newborns generally need only small amounts of colostrum until breast milk comes in several days after birth. In addition, a dying body needs little or no food or liquid, and force-feeding someone who is imminently dying could actually cause discomfort.[6] As your baby's system gently shuts down during this natural process, you don't need to worry that your baby is hungry. Still, even if your baby is dying or too weak or tiny to nurse, offering your breast can mean a lot to you. Expressing colostrum or breast milk and placing a drop at a time in your baby's mouth can be a touching symbolic gesture, without presenting a burden to your baby.

If your baby appears strong enough to live more than a day or so but cannot feed by mouth, you may need to consider providing nutrition and hydration through a feeding tube. To nourish a baby in this way, densely nutritious liquids can be provided through a nasogastric (NG) tube, which is a narrow, flexible plastic tube threaded through the baby's nose and into the stomach.

Feeding tube decisions can be difficult, especially when a newborn is involved. What could be more nurturing and instinctive than feeding a baby? Nutrition and hydration are basic and necessary forms of care. But when a baby is dying, or when a feeding tube offers no reasonable benefit, extends the dying process, or would be burdensome to the baby, you are not obligated to take this step.[7]

Still, feeding issues are intensely emotional, and some families face criticism and may need to defend their decision.

⌐ The neonatologist wanted a feeding tube within six hours of birth. I balked; I wanted to wait a bit and have a good chance to assess his condition first. If he was only going to live a few hours, I didn't want him to have to endure having a tube shoved up his nose and down his throat. The neonatologist's reaction was that I was a bad mother; I wanted to starve my child to death. I was so angry. I wish I would have said, "You know, I've been told many times to terminate this pregnancy, and I haven't. If I was interested in killing this child, I could have done it weeks ago and saved myself the agony." I was so stunned I didn't know quite how to respond to his accusations. I think I just sat there. Thankfully, the nurses were completely supportive and came to my rescue, and the perinatologist was like a tiger. She said, no, we were not being unreasonable, and we were not trying to kill our child. Of course I didn't want to starve him or do anything that would intentionally hasten his death. I wanted him to stick around for a long time but not at any cost. I didn't want to selfishly make him endure uncomfortable procedures just so I could have a little more time with him. If he was going to live for only eight hours, I didn't want to stick a feeding tube down his nose. That's one of the things, from my nursing experience, that I never wanted to have. Having put so many of them in—it doesn't last long, and it's not painful, but it's really uncomfortable. I didn't want that to be part of his life if it didn't need to be. —*Kathleen*

Pain Relief for Your Baby

⌐ Once we made the decision to continue the pregnancy, we quickly decided to offer Maggie the highest quality comfort care and refrain from any invasive procedures. We were realistic about her diagnosis and her prognosis and felt the highest priority was keeping her pain-free. —*Alessandra*

For many parents, the desire to protect their baby from pain is paramount. Many conditions are not inherently uncomfortable for the baby. If your baby's condition is expected to cause pain or discomfort, you can make advance plans with your doctors to provide pain relief if needed. (In case of severe pain, which is rare, it is possible to inject medication into the umbilical cord immediately after birth, avoiding a needle stick into the baby.[8]) Most doctors are not routinely faced with providing pain relief to newborns and may not be familiar with medications or proper dosages, so you can explore options with them or to ask for a referral to an anesthesiologist.

A much greater factor in whether your baby experiences pain is what you decide about medical intervention. Some families who have sadly traveled this path in the past decide to do things differently based on what their previous baby had to endure. Or perhaps you have witnessed intensive care in action and know that's not what you want for your baby.

— We decided to deliver the baby, allow tests to confirm his condition (but no more than necessary), spend as much time with him and hold him as much as we could—but to not let him suffer the pain as his sister had. *—Pam F.*

— I had visited a friend's infant son in the PICU, and when I saw infants hooked up to all those tubes, surgeries, etc., I instantly knew that I could not do that to my son. I had this overwhelming feeling that if Colm was only to have a short while with us, I did not want him to be connected to tubes and machines. I wanted him in our arms feeling all of the love we had for him. *—Pam M.*

You can even decline minor routine procedures such as the standard vitamin K shot, a "heel stick" that draws blood for genetic testing, and eye drops given to prevent infection. These are unnecessary discomforts for your baby.

And you can be insistent about advocating for pain relief for your baby. A recent study published in the *Journal of the American Medical Association* emphasized the need to treat pain in newborns aggressively and reiterated some of the possible methods, including using acetaminophen or other medication; anesthetic creams to numb the skin before needle sticks; or even a small dose of sucrose with a pacifier, which can block pain signals in newborns.[9] They also recommended "kangaroo care"—warm skin-to-skin contact between an undressed baby and a bare-chested mom or dad, which comforts the baby as well as offers a tender experience for the parent. You can also speak or sing softly to your baby.

These recommendations are a continuation in the evolution of thinking about pain in newborns. As recently as the 1980s, newborns were believed to be unable to experience pain.[10] Physicians also have been hesitant to medicate tiny babies, for fear of overdosing. But the evidence that newborns can experience pain and need pain relief is now beyond dispute, and leading pediatrics groups in the United States and Canada have issued strong statements advocating pain prevention and management protocols.[11] Pain management in newborns is a hot topic, and your baby's doctors should be prepared to interpret signs of pain and take action if needed to make your baby most comfortable.

Resuscitation

It may be difficult to think about now, but you can also think ahead to resuscitation decisions you might be asked to make at birth or as your baby approaches death. Do you want "heroic measures"? Do you want teams rushing into your hospital room or your home to attempt cardiopulmonary resuscitation or intubation? What about gentler, low-tech measures such as "bagging," suctioning, or supplemental oxygen if your baby simply needs a bit of breathing assistance? Thinking through these difficult questions during your pregnancy, and then putting them in writing, can give you a sense of control.

The biggest thing we had to put in our file and make known was that no heroic measures be done. This was something that I was never able to fully say. Even though my husband and doctor had it in our file, I just couldn't ever say those words. I knew that when the day came there was no way I could say "do nothing," so in our birth plan I specifically said that my husband would make those decisions. I knew those were the right decisions, but I also knew

I wouldn't be in the right mind-set to make them when the time came. —*Camille*

A "do not resuscitate" order, also known as a DNR, is much more commonly associated with an elderly person who is very ill and near death. Like many of the issues you are facing, this is another one that seems horrifically out of place when thinking about a newborn baby. A DNR can seem to be a cold-hearted withholding of treatment, as if someone is dictating who deserves to live and who should die.

What a DNR can do, however, is make clear to your entire health care team what you do or do not want for your baby. The process of signing one can also help you understand what is actually involved in resuscitating someone. It is not as simple—or as successful—as often depicted on TV.

Another way of thinking about making your wishes clear is to consider using a newer term, "AND"—allow natural death.[12] While the medical implications are the same, the phrasing better conveys your protective intent that your baby will not be abandoned and will be cared for with compassion and dignity until death arrives naturally.

If your baby might live long enough to come home, you can also think ahead about what you would do if your baby dies there. If you call 911, first responders may be required to attempt to resuscitate and may initiate medical treatments you do not want. One family who experienced the death of two babies learned from their experience with their first baby about what not to do:

Jacob's death was not peaceful, and we were not prepared. We called 911. Big mistake! It was early in the morning and the police raced over, sirens blaring, and after they determined he was dead, they brought detectives and more police because children aren't supposed to die. They were investigating us. It was awful. Several hours later, they finally reached our pediatrician and he called off the hounds. —*Behka*

Instead of calling 911, work out a plan with your baby's doctor for what to do at the time of death. A hospice worker or other health care practitioner could come to the house to confirm your baby's death and support your next steps. If you want to keep your baby's body with you for a few more hours, even overnight or longer, you can.

Your Baby's Best Interests

I did not want him to suffer in any way. I wanted to be sure that all decisions regarding his medical care had his best interest at heart and not my own. —*Kristy*

Your decision to forgo disproportionate medical intervention is a powerful way to advocate for your baby. You are preserving your child's comfort and dignity and simply accepting the human condition—the reality that death at some point comes to us all. You are not saying "yes" to death; you are saying "yes" to your baby's natural life.

We ended up choosing compassionate care. We chose her life, not her death. —*Christine*

In the same vein of us not terminating her life, we weren't going to do any interventions, no surgeries. We're just going to love. That's all we can do. That's all we're asked to do. —*James*

six

Getting Ready

Preparing for Your Baby's Birth, Life, and Death

⌒ Making the birth plan was such a labor of love. It was an important way to parent Ashley before she was even born. Maybe it was also helpful to have something "planned" since our whole situation felt so uncertain and scary. —*Shellie*

As you continue settling into this pregnancy, getting ready for your baby's birth is your main task. In addition to making medical decisions, you can make plans for giving birth and spending time with your baby afterward. If your baby is born alive, you can learn what to expect when death eventually comes. You can also make preliminary plans for memorializing your baby and selecting a final resting place. You can find comfort and strength in knowing that you are parenting your baby in profound ways—not in ways you had initially expected when you learned you were pregnant, not in ways you had hoped for, but in ways that this baby needs and that you as a loving parent are in the best position to provide.

BIRTH PLANNING

⌒ We were encouraged to make a birth plan. This felt like something positive; such tasks made the pregnancy more bearable. It was something that I could busy myself with. It was in my control. Working on the birth plan brought my husband and me together. It was something we could focus on. —*Christine*

A birth plan is a way of conveying your wishes for your baby's birth and for the care of your baby and you. It can include preferences for labor and delivery, such as pain relief for the mother, and goals for spending time with your baby, such as ways to create memories together and include family and friends. You can also integrate your baby's medical care plan, outlining your advance directives regarding evaluations and testing, aggressive intervention, and palliative care.[1] In addition to the ideas in this chapter, you can get ideas from the sample birth plan in the back of this book, from your caregivers, or online.

⌐ I wrote a birth plan after researching on the Internet. I printed them out, circled the things I liked, and then made my own. —*Chris*

⌐ The birth planning was amazing. All the questions the perinatal hospice staff asked, I thought, *wow, I never thought of that.* They were consummate professionals. It was so tailor-made to what we wanted. —*James*

Birth plans have a negative reputation among some physicians, so it's possible you might run into resistance. Your caregivers may have had experiences with birth plans that were littered with unrealistic demands or had no built-in flexibility or acknowledgement that labor and birth rarely go according to the best-laid plans.

⌐ I told the doctor I'd thought about writing a birth plan for the delivery. He immediately shot me down and said that if I was the type of mom that wanted to have a birth plan, then he probably wasn't the doctor for me. I was shocked and couldn't believe what was coming out of his insensitive mouth. As if I had a choice in the matter! As if I wanted to be in this situation! He believed that a birth plan made the atmosphere more tense. He suggested I just "tell" the nurses what I wanted and that would result in a much more pleasant atmosphere. I got the sense that having a plan really annoyed him. —*Kristin*

But the benefits of having a written birth plan in a situation like yours, in which time will be of the essence, are many and very real—

for you as well as your caregivers. For you, it can provide a format to help you think about the upcoming birth, understand your options, explore what other parents have chosen, and evaluate what will be important to you. A birth plan can decrease your anxiety by ensuring that your wishes are clearly communicated and by giving you a sense of control in a situation where so many things may feel out of your control. It provides a structure so you and your caregivers can work together to make your baby's birth as close to what you are envisioning as possible.

A birth plan can also benefit your caregivers in important ways. It can offer insight into your needs and desires so caregivers don't have to try to read your mind. It ensures that all parties have similar information. It allows for advance planning and offers a format for discussion. Having this information ahead of time decreases *their* anxiety, too. A birth plan gives all of you a road map to follow together.[2]

Overriding Wishes

A good first step in writing a birth plan is to summarize your vision for your baby's birth. Try to come up with a short statement that can help guide you and your caregivers. Perhaps you would like your baby to be held for his or her entire life, or to bring your baby home if possible. Then you and your caregivers can work together to fill in the details to make it happen. Some examples:

⟶ We feel that we have an incredible and unique opportunity to bring Lily into the world and show her only love and comfort for as long as she lives. We hope to offer this to Lily with strength, courage, and grace. —*from the birth plan of Katharine and Mark*

⟶ We may have only seconds or minutes with him (or her) alive, but we may also be blessed with hours. Whatever we are given, we mean to make the most of it, and we ask for your help and support in accomplishing that. Our primary goal is to ensure that Frankie has every chance to meet us and that he is protected from unnecessary pain and suffering. —*from the birth plan of Susan E. and Steven*

We would like to make the most of any time we have with Ashley. Please treat us with extra sensitivity and respect. We hope you will see beyond Ashley's "problems" and provide her with love and tenderness. Please see Ashley for the unique person she is, a beloved child of God and our sweet daughter that will leave us much too soon. —*from the birth plan of Shellie and Mike*

By stating your overriding wishes, you are creating a mission statement that helps guide the myriad details of how you would like your baby's birth and hospital time to be managed. This big picture ensures that your ultimate goals won't have to change, even if you do need to accommodate unexpected detours during labor, in your baby's condition, or even in the mother's condition. A flexible birth plan is a statement of your preferences, not a list of demands. Assuring your caregivers of your flexibility encourages them to be open to your desires as well. Your birth plan is a work in progress—it can always be adapted as new information arises or if your wishes change.

If you can't think of any overriding wishes at first, another approach is to start thinking about specific preferences you might have for your baby's birth and for your time together afterward. Your overriding statement may come more easily at the end of your planning process. You may find that on some level you *did* know the kind of birth experience you hope to have, and you can put it into words then.

Preferences for Labor and Birth

Caesarean Birth or Vaginal Birth

Many mothers can proceed with previous plans to have a spontaneous labor and vaginal birth. Giving birth this way can add a welcome aspect of normalcy and naturalness to the experience, and physical recovery is much faster than for a birth by caesarean section. For most babies, a C-birth offers no benefit and doesn't change the outcome, so a vaginal birth is optimal. But in some cases, birthing decisions are more complicated. You may need to weigh how to give birth in light of your baby's condition or position. If your baby is unlikely to survive a vaginal birth, are the risks and recovery from major abdominal surgery warranted? Or because of your own health reasons or obstetric history, you may need to schedule a C-birth. How do you pick a date? These decisions can be agonizing to make.

⟶ The doctor flat out told us that there would be no way the baby would survive labor. I was overwhelmed by the thought of having to choose between a delivery that would physically be "better" for me versus a C-section wherein we could possibly see our son alive if even for a couple minutes. —*Kristin*

⟶ We wanted to do everything we could to have Gemma born alive and spend as much time with us as possible, so we spent a lot of time researching, asking questions, and praying for God to give us clarity on this issue. For quite some time this was not a clear-cut decision. We didn't know how hard to fight for her to be born alive and we didn't know whether or not we wanted to put me through major surgery to achieve this goal, or whether or not it was even necessary. —*Courtney*

⟶ I was relieved when my doctor said a C-section would be the best. Yet this posed a whole new set of questions: How do I choose when my baby will be born, knowing that it will be the same day he dies? How do I choose, knowing the sooner it is, the greater the chance of him being born alive? How do I sacrifice weeks of life inside the womb for mere minutes of holding him alive? The choices in this pregnancy seemed to get harder the farther along we got.

—*Karla*

If your baby is likely to die during a vaginal birth, the option of a C-birth may or may not be offered to you, depending on whether your doctor thinks that this major surgery is medically justified or wise. If it is important to you to see your baby alive and maximize the amount of time you might have with your baby after birth and before death, discuss this with your doctor as this is a benefit that your doctor may have overlooked. After all, elective caesarean sections are routinely performed for much less serious reasons. You may decide that giving birth to a live baby is a goal that supersedes all else.

If your doctor remains concerned that the physical benefits to your baby and the emotional benefits to you do not outweigh your health risks, talking this out will help you make an informed decision that balances what is best for mother *and* baby.

⌒ I wanted to increase the chances that she was born alive, and I felt a C-section would do that. My doctor didn't agree with me in the beginning. "Why put yourself through all of that?" So I spoke to another doctor and was going to switch. He told me that he knew my doctor and asked me to give him another chance—he would speak to him. When I returned for the next visit, my doctor told me that they had spoken and that he would do what I wanted. He said he "got it . . . You just want to hold your baby for five minutes. Tell me what you want, and I will support you." After that he never looked back. —*Chris*

⌒ The final decision was based on our ultimate goal of a live birth. —*Courtney*

Or you may decide that delivering naturally, once again letting nature take its course, is best. You may want to be alert and able to be with your baby, instead of spending that precious first hour or more being stitched up and monitored in the recovery room. You may feel the health risks and the burdens of recuperating from surgery are too high, or you may have other factors (including needing to care for small children) to consider.

⌒ This was an agonizing decision, because we knew that a C-section would decrease the chances of a stillbirth somewhat. My OB encouraged me to deliver vaginally, and after much soul-searching and spiritual guidance, we decided that I would deliver vaginally. —*Jennifer*

Even if you're certain that you'll have an uncomplicated vaginal birth, it is important to contemplate the possibility of a C-birth so you'll feel better prepared should this issue arise. You'll also be able to discuss with your doctor or midwife your preferences for anesthesia and whether it would interfere with your ability to spend meaningful time with your baby. Becoming informed and evaluating options now might help you avoid disorientation, scary surprises, or having to make snap decisions later.

A Gift of Time

Pain Relief for the Mother

You can use your birth plan to specify your pain relief preferences for labor and birth. Whether you are hoping for a drug-free birth or are hoping to alleviate as much physical pain as possible, ask your doctor or midwife what they recommend.

Your wishes regarding pain relief might be the same as they were before you knew your baby's condition. Perhaps you've always envisioned a certain type of birth and still want to make it happen. Or your pain relief preferences might shift. For mothers experiencing a typical pregnancy and expecting a healthy baby, the hard work of labor is rewarded by a healthy baby at the end. Your baby's diagnosis changes that equation. Knowing that your baby's birth will end very differently can make the idea of physical pain seem profoundly unfair, even unbearable. Some mothers decide to ask for more pain relief than they would have otherwise, choosing to avoid adding unnecessary physical pain to their emotional burden. Others decide to give birth as naturally as possible, choosing to view it as a way of fully entering into the experience or to spare the baby from possible side effects of anesthesia. Either way, talking with your caregivers ahead of time can help ensure that your wishes are followed.

Heart Monitoring during Labor

Many hospitals routinely monitor babies' heartbeats during labor, so if the heart rate drops precipitously or shows other signs of fetal distress, doctors can perform an emergency C-section. Given your baby's diagnosis, you can consider ahead of time whether emergency surgery is something you would even want and if you would like monitoring.

We weren't going to have a crash C-section or anything like that, but we just wanted monitoring to know what her status was. —*David D.*

We decided not to monitor her heart rate. I knew that there was a chance that she would die during labor, and I did not want to hear her heart stop. That would have been too much. I have never regretted that decision. —*Jamie*

Getting Ready

Where to Give Birth

Knowing your baby's diagnosis ahead of time may also factor into your decision about where to deliver. If your baby is likely to need intensive care immediately after birth, or if there are uncertainties about your baby's condition, you may decide to deliver at a larger hospital with a Level 3 neonatal intensive care unit. Or if you are planning to provide palliative care only, you could decide to deliver at a small hospital close to home, with your familiar local doctor.

We were given the option to deliver in the city and stay in a ward especially for families in situations like ours, and at first that is what we wanted. I thought it would be good to be far away from our own hospital, so that we wouldn't have sad memories from there. However, after a while, our decision shifted. We decided to have Sarina where we had our firstborn. She was part of our family and would always be, and we would always have her in our hearts. I wanted to keep her birth in my memory as well. *—Christine*

Perhaps you would like a joyful birthing room filled with people, or perhaps you are envisioning something more peaceful and intimate. Maybe you would like to hear calming music during labor. You can specify these wishes in your birth plan too.

Cutting the Baby's Umbilical Cord

One simple task that takes on added meaning for a baby whose life will be limited is cutting the umbilical cord. In a typical birth, fathers often are invited to participate. Some are eager to finally have the opportunity to take direct action for their new little one; others are a bit squeamish. Likewise, fathers in this situation also may have different perspectives. Some, knowing that their chances to take physical care of their child will be few, are conscious of the moment and grateful for it. They may even feel cheated if a doctor does it without asking. Others, especially if their baby's condition is so severe that cutting the umbilical cord is literally the cutting of a lifeline and signals the beginning of the dying process, may recoil from this task and prefer to delegate it to a doctor. Specifying your wishes ahead of time can prevent a difficult moment in the birthing room.

Medical Care Decisions for Your Baby Following Birth

Your birth plan can include your decisions about medical intervention for your baby (discussed in Chapter 5). Writing out a plan makes it easy for your baby's doctor to review it and discuss it with you. Together you can make improvements or clarifications, add more flexibility, and even get the doctor's signature, which can give these plans more weight in the hospital. Having these medical care decisions laid out in your birth plan also lets your caregivers know ahead of time what your decisions are and prepare for them, which makes them more likely to be honored. And the process also can help clarify for you what to expect.

⁓ Talking to the neonatologist was really helpful for me. It was the first time anyone really explained to us what we could expect on delivery day, as far as what the baby would be like when he came out or how long he might live. How long he lived would depend on how long he could breathe, or if he could breathe. I hadn't really thought about that. I hadn't really pictured what would happen when he was born. —*Greg*

Communicating Your Wishes

Once you have settled on your statement of overriding wishes and some preferences and plans for your baby's birth and time in the hospital, you'll need to convey them in writing to your caregivers. Be concise; brevity makes your birth plan easier for busy caregivers to read—and to follow. If you haven't done so already, it is important to consult with someone at your hospital to confirm that your plan is workable, to revise it if necessary, and to ensure that any special arrangements can be made.

Some hospitals already have a protocol for forwarding written birth plans to the appropriate doctors and departments. Hospitals that use electronic medical records may be able to upload your written birth plan into your chart. In addition, some hold in-person meetings or care conferences, bringing together relevant parties such as your OB or midwife, your baby's pediatrician, a neonatologist, or other specialists. If this kind of meeting isn't typically done, it's a good idea to arrange it anyway. Also pack an extra copy when you go to the hospital to deliver, so that you and others can refer to it easily.

⟿ Those meetings were tough—our circumstance was the antithesis of what pregnancy is supposed to be. But I am glad we held them. It gave us a measure of comfort and control, and it enabled the medical team to see our situation more personally than they may have otherwise. *—Alessandra*

⟿ I found it very helpful to articulate our needs and hopes to the medical staff. It felt good to be listened to. *—Susan E.*

⟿ My husband and I walked out of that meeting feeling so good. I had thought we'd get to the hospital and have to find our own way the day it was happening and maybe have to fight for what we wanted. We both left knowing that all we had to do was get to the hospital. We will be taken care of. They will look out for us. That was a big relief. *—Kathleen*

WISHES FOR AFTER YOUR BABY'S BIRTH

In addition to summarizing the medical care decisions you've made, birth planning also is a way of thinking through experiences you might like to have with your baby, especially opportunities that you might not otherwise have time to seize in the hospital if your baby's life will be brief. Once again, think about your overriding wishes for this time. Do you want your baby to be cradled in peace? Do you want your baby to be welcomed by friends and family?

Imagine the kinds of memories you would like to have: maybe skin-to-skin contact, holding your baby to your chest, rocking your baby, singing to your baby. Consider ordinary baby care that will take on added significance: giving your baby his or her first bath, putting on a diaper, smoothing lotion onto your baby's skin, swaddling your baby in a special blanket. Well-intentioned nurses might do these kinds of tasks for you as part of their normal routine, but if you want to do them yourself, include this in your birth plan and be ready to speak up if necessary.

If your baby is expected to be transferred immediately to the NICU, you can plan who will stay with you and who will go with the baby. If you are expecting a C-birth or are otherwise unable to visit your baby for a time, you can send along a small blanket or another comfort item. If you wish, sleeping with the blanket overnight or expressing a few drops of colostrom onto it will carry some of your scent so your baby can sense your presence. And you can arrange for someone to have the job of keeping you informed of how the baby is doing while you can't be near.

Spiritual Rituals

If you wish to hold spiritual rituals with your baby, a birth plan can help facilitate that. If you have a specific person in your religious or spiritual community whom you would like to have notified, include the name and contact information in your birth plan. If this person cannot be available, many hospitals have chaplains who can step in. You may wish to pack ritual items or things that hold spiritual or religious meaning for you.

If you wish to have your baby baptized, blessed, named, or ritually circumcised and it is possible that your baby will be stillborn or will die soon after birth, talk to your clergyperson or spiritual advisor ahead of time. Some families are deeply distressed to learn that their religion does not allow newborn rituals for a baby who has died before or shortly after birth. If they learn this only after their baby has already died and their urgent request for a ceremony is refused, parents may feel abandoned by their religion, feel that their desires are being judged as "wrong," or feel that their baby is being rejected. It can help to learn the reasoning ahead of time: In many traditions, newborn rituals are reserved for the living, just like medicine is for the living, and administering either one after death would be inappropriate—even malpractice. Most faith traditions believe that even if certain rituals do not take place, a merciful and loving higher power would never abandon an innocent child.

Some clergy are open to adapting rituals in light of new medical situations and increased understanding of bereavement. For instance, if circumcision and a naming ritual are the central newborn rituals in your tradition, you might wonder if babies who die before this ceremony takes place are given names. The fear that your baby might not only be taken from you but also might be deprived of his or her name might make your distress even worse. Talk with your religious advisors to find out how these situations are handled within your religious framework. They likely have had experience guiding parents who have these questions. In some traditions, boys can be circumcised as well as named after death, and babies who have died are given traditional names derived from the words for "comfort."[3]

As another example, if baptism is part of your tradition and you fear your baby will not live long enough to receive this sacrament, you still have some options. Baptism doesn't need to be performed by a clergyperson. In an urgent situation, anyone can baptize a baby, even a nurse using tap water from the hospital sink—or you, using your own tears. Some clergy are willing to perform a baptism even if the baby has just been declared dead, under the reasoning that it is impossible to know the precise moment that the soul leaves the body. Another possibility is baptizing your baby *before* birth. After all, your baby is still alive, veiled from the outside world only by a thin layer of the mother's body.

A few days before my due date, we called our priest and asked him about baptizing our son. The priest did something very special for us and Baby John. He gave our son a conditional baptism using holy water and oils directly on my abdomen. It was a beautiful ceremony with loving and assuring words. —*Elizabeth D. P.*

If your baby is unable to be blessed or recognized by a religious authority and this was important to you, you will have another loss to grieve. If traditions fail to serve you, there are still beautiful and comforting words and rituals that you can use or create, if you wish. A naming ceremony could be held by your family, your baby's body could be blessed and anointed with words and oils of your choosing, or other prayers could be offered.

Whether your spiritual beliefs are faith-based or not, there are many rich cultural traditions you can research and tap into if they resonate with you. Be open to the possibilities that lie outside your religion, culture, hospital protocol, and even your own plans. There are many meaningful actions associated with childbirth and welcoming newborns into the family. Something as simple as bathing and dressing your baby's body in special clothing or wrapping in a handmade blanket can be meaningful. Alternatively, holding your unclothed baby against your bare skin can express your deep bond, feel so precious, and make for treasured photographs. It could be meaningful to take your baby outside—before or after death—to be held in the sun or under the stars. If you do wish to take your baby outside, this is another important reason to create a birth plan and discuss it with your caregivers in advance, because they may need to circumvent standard hospital policy for this.

Meaningful actions can also evolve in the moment or come from a deeply felt need. Leave room for spontaneity, knowing that you cannot predict the circumstances or how you will feel when you're actually spending time with your baby.

Planning for Keepsakes

Keepsakes, including photographs, are priceless for many families. They are tangible proof that your baby existed, objects that you can later touch and admire and smell, things that may make you cry, smile, and swell with pride over your baby. They can trigger vivid, treasured memories. They can also serve as a bridge to help you share your baby with others who didn't have a chance to meet your little one.

Examples of keepsakes you might want to consider include the baby's hospital bracelet, bassinet identification card, hat, blanket, bath soap, or anything else that touches your baby that holds meaning for you. Perhaps you'd like a lock of your baby's hair, ink footprints and handprints, or plaster of Paris molds of your baby's hands and feet.

You can also bring your own special items to the hospital—perhaps a special blanket, a stuffed animal, a soft washcloth and towel, fragrant bath gel or lotion, and baby clothes. Some newborn clothing comes in preemie sizes, if your baby is expected to be small.

⌁ As I looked through the pile of blankets to find the perfect one, it was hard to imagine wrapping my baby girl in it and never bringing her home. This blanket had to be soft and pretty yet something that I didn't mind letting go of. I thought of the special blankets that my mom and grandma made for my older daughter. I cried as I wished I would have a special blanket made for this baby too. The next day, my mom surprised me with a gift bag, saying, "I wasn't sure when to give this to you." I pulled out a beautiful small pink crocheted blanket and a tiny white dress. I instantly started to cry as my mom hugged me. I was so touched that she took the time to make a blanket for my baby. It meant so much as a gift from my mom. —*Greta*

Many hospitals have incorporated collecting keepsakes as part of their protocol when a baby dies. Some still have not. Even if your hospital does help families collect keepsakes, specify the ones you want in your birth plan so nothing will be overlooked.

Photography

Many parents consider photographs to be their most treasured keepsakes. Photographs can offer exquisite affirmation of your baby's existence and importance to you and others. This visual record can also portray your baby's story.

Because photographs can be so important to bereaved parents, you'll probably want to include photography in your birth plan. You can think ahead about what kind of photographs you would like. If your baby is expected to be transferred immediately to the NICU, consider having someone with a camera accompany your baby. Babies in intensive care tend not to have as many photos taken of them, leaving families with fewer photos to treasure later.

Particularly if your baby is expected to be stillborn or die shortly after birth, the idea of photography may seem inappropriate, even morbid. Some parents think, *Taking pictures of a dead baby? Why would I want to remember something so horrific?* Yet many parents who have traveled this path are deeply grateful for the photographs they have, and their only regret is that they don't have even more. Taking photographs after your baby has died is not morbid; it is part of a long tradition of bereavement photography, the act of taking pictures to help remember and make peace with a loved one's life and death.

Below you will find some ideas and tips to consider.

Professional Photographers

Some hospitals have partnerships with for-profit photo companies that provide standard newborn photographs, in which the baby is taken from you briefly for a photo session elsewhere in the hospital. While these photographs are certainly better than nothing, the photographers are accustomed to taking basic headshots of healthy babies, and you might be disappointed with the results. You'll also need to weigh whether it's worth it for you to be separated from your baby for these standard shots. Another option is to hire a professional photographer. Your hospital may already have a relationship with professional photographers who specialize in working with families whose babies are dying or have already died. Many of these photographers volunteer their services or are funded by grants and donations, and their photographs can be stunningly beautiful.[4]

A professional photographer is one possibility. Consider, too, that photographs taken by you or those close to you can be deeply meaningful. Especially with a good digital camera, or even armed with disposable cameras, hundreds of photos can be snapped, documentary style, capturing every nuance. You could also designate as photographers those people who understand what a special time this is or those who have an affinity for capturing emotions and relationships.

Lighting

For softer images, avoid using flash. Also avoid direct sunlight, as this can create harsh or unintentional shadows. Make good use of available light from windows, lamps, overhead fixtures, and sunlight reflecting off walls, so you and your baby are bathed in light from multiple directions.

Black-and-White Images

Make sure that at least some photographs are taken with black-and-white film or can be digitally changed to black and white. Black-and-white images of people allow the depths of emotion and relationships to shine through, while colors divert attention from this overall effect. Black and white renders photographs more aesthetically pleasing by evening out skin tones, hiding the dreariness of sur-roundings, and removing distracting elements such as colorful prints and clashing hues. These images also have a timeless quality.

Documentary and Portrait-Style Photography

Documentary photography unobtrusively captures your baby's story as it unfolds, while portraits are posed with carefully staged lighting, props, and clothing. Most parents opt for using both of these styles to some extent, but you may have a clear preference for one over the other.

The biggest advantage of documentary photography is that it quietly follows you and your baby as you go about spending time together. Photos could show your baby being cradled by you, being cared for by nurses and doctors, being baptized, being bathed, being held by siblings, being introduced to family and friends, and being kissed and loved at the moment of death. Because the time after your baby's birth can be such a blur, this kind of photography also can later help you process the chronology of what happened and evoke the emotions and tenderness of various real moments you experienced with your baby.

An advantage to portrait photography is that you can get certain stylized images that carry special meaning or symbolism. These portraits can also result in images that may seem softer and easier to share with others. Poses could include cradling your baby's feet in your and your partner's hands, holding your baby skin-to-skin on your chest, family portraits with siblings, close-ups of your baby's fingers with yours, or perhaps slipping your wedding ring on your baby's fingers or toes. If you have multiple babies, you may want to nestle them together to represent their special relationship.

Note that a documentary photographer who is attuned to the significance of these portrait-worthy moments also can capture these images as they naturally occur, such as when you are holding and admiring your baby's tiny feet, or when a sibling bends over to kiss your baby, or when you snuggle your twins together on your chest. You can even imagine the moments and details that you think will be significant to you and write them down as a guide to all your photographers.

Particularly Cherished Images

Whether you request documentary or portrait photography or a combination of both, your favorite photographs may be those that show emotion, relationships, and details. The ones that portray your baby being held and gazed upon can be especially affirming, as these images capture the love and wonder that you and others feel for your baby. Photographs of tears and smiles can affirm the emotional intensity of this time. You may also appreciate photographs of your baby naked, cradled in soft blankets or loving arms, so that you have images that capture the identifiable physical details that make your baby both normal and special. Photos can also focus on sweet details of your baby's body, such as wisps of hair, tiny hands on yours, a dimpled chin, or a birthmark. Even if your baby has visible anomalies, you will look at these photographs with eyes of love.

Whatever photographers, styles, or equipment you employ, photographs can help you remember the love and tenderness lavished upon your baby—and upon you. (For more ideas regarding photographs after your baby dies, see Chapter 8.)

INCLUDING YOUR BABY'S SIBLINGS

Your birth plan can specify whether and how you would like siblings to be included. To accommodate the unexpected, state your overriding wishes for your other children, so that they are included in the spirit you intend, whatever happens. For instance, you might state, "I want my children to meet their baby sister (or brother) and to be able to hold and touch the baby and ask questions for as long as they are interested, even after our baby has died." It's also a good idea to designate a support person to accompany each child and meet their needs during this special time.

⌒ The doctor first strongly advised us against letting our older children see Anouk, saying that babies with anencephaly look frightening and that it would be too difficult for young children (ages 3, 5, and 6) to cope with that. We told him that we did not want them to see Anouk without a covered head, but that we felt that it was important to them to see their little sister. Except for the top of her head, Anouk was a normal baby. We asked him what he would do if this was his baby and his children's sibling. After a few minutes he agreed with us. It was a very quiet and friendly discussion, where both parties respected the other. I'm very grateful that we had that discussion. We were able to speak about all our wishes and make the neonatologist not only accept them but understand them.

—*Monika*

In unfamiliar situations, children look to their parents for cues of how to react. If you think you can feel unafraid for them, answer questions simply and honestly, and share your children's curiosity about the baby's condition, they will likely take your baby's appearance in stride.

If you are worried about the long-term impact on your older children, recent research has found that siblings highly value having been able to hold and see the baby and to show concrete expressions of love during the baby's brief life and death. Photographs also were found to be helpful to siblings. For siblings too young to remember or born subsequently, photographs provide a way of learning about the baby who died. Photos also can help preserve memories, maintain a continuing connection with the baby, integrate your baby into family history, and become a way to spark conversation between parents and the surviving siblings as they grow into different developmental stages.[5]

INCLUDING YOUR FAMILY AND FRIENDS

It was really important to me that the family be there. I wanted him to be real for everybody. I wanted them all to be part of the experience because I knew that down the road I wanted to be able to talk about him. And I knew that having them experience it would make it so much easier to talk to them about it. The more real he was for them, the easier it would be—a day, a week, a month, a year, ten years later—to use the name Josh in a sentence and have it not feel strange. —*Jill N.*

Your birth plan can summarize whether and how you would like family and friends to be included. Perhaps you would like as much privacy for the birth as possible, with only your partner and caregivers in the room. Perhaps you have other close support people you want to have around you during the birth. Maybe you would like a private waiting area set up for grandparents and others whom you wish to have in the room as soon as possible after the birth. Specifying your wishes in your birth plan can help your caregivers follow them.

⌒ We had been told that Lucy most likely would have ten minutes to live. We had arranged that all of the grandparents would be in the waiting room to meet her and that my mother would be in the delivery room as my support person, as well as my husband. —*Jane G.*

Especially if you ask friends or family members to accompany you in the hospital, you'll want them to be well-informed about your wishes so they can support and even advocate for you.

⌒ My husband and I established what we called the "Dream Team" of close friends who were designated to certain tasks. One friend was given the title "first runner-up" in case my husband was not able to complete his duties as birth partner. She didn't like this title and wanted to be called "second in command"—we had a lot of fun with that. She went with us to our birthing classes and helped me to prepare the rest of the team. Another friend was assigned to making sure that my teenage sons were well taken care of at the hospital. Her job was to hand them money when they were hungry and offer to take them home if they needed a break. Another was in charge of photography. And a male friend was to be my husband's support when Jordan would be whisked away from me and brought to the NICU. I didn't want Jordan to be without either of his parents, and I didn't want my husband to be alone in such a scary time. —*Jenny D.*

If you're usually hesitant to ask others for help, remember that your family and friends may be at a loss for how to help but eager to jump into action if you ask. Sharing your birth plan with those close to you is a way of inviting them into your experience.

OTHER PRACTICAL PREPARATIONS

You may have additional unique needs to consider, including special childbirth classes and practical preparations if your baby might live long enough to come home.

If you have never given birth or witnessed someone giving birth, one aspect of your preparations will be learning about the childbirth process itself. Countless books, websites, classes, and other resources can help prepare you for the physical aspects of labor and birth. You can sign up for regular birth education classes at your hospital if you are comfortable attending classes with other couples who are expecting a healthy baby. If you would prefer not to put yourself in that situation, some hospitals offer private, one-on-one birth preparation, and some childbirth educators offer private in-home teaching. Your caregiver may be able to make a referral for you.

If it's possible that your baby will be able to come home for a while, you can decide if you'd like to buy a few essentials and have them ready at home. If you'd rather not come home to baby items that you might not need, you could give a shopping list in advance to someone who could run to the store if needed and buy a car seat, diapers, and other items for you. (See Chapter 7 for more about bringing baby home.)

PRELIMINARY FUNERAL AND BURIAL PLANNING

⌐ We met with a funeral director one month before Lily's birth to discuss our situation and details that we needed to settle on. We also decided on a cemetery that was very close to our home. Even though this seemed kind of surreal, it was somehow comforting to have some of this work done before she arrived. —*Katharine*

⌐ Toward the end I started asking my husband to start making funeral plans and that sort of thing. And that's when it became very clear that my husband was not focusing on the end result. Not in denial of it, but just, let's deal with it when we get there, let's deal with it when it's time. —*Jessica*

Whether you do it before or after birth, you will need to make decisions about what to do with your baby's body after death. Is an autopsy necessary? Do you prefer a full funeral, a memorial service, funeral prayers, a private graveside service, or no service at all? Embalming? Burial or cremation? What kind of casket, shroud, or urn? Burial in a cemetery? Scatter the ashes or keep them?

You can even provide after-death care for your baby's body yourself. You will have tended lovingly to your baby until death, and you do not have to stop then. Reclaiming traditions of caring for the dead in the intimacy of home can be another sacred way of caring for your baby. Legal requirements will vary, but it is legal in all U.S. states and many other countries to provide at least some aspect of loved ones' care after death.[6] Embalming—in which bodily fluids are removed through large-bore needles and then replaced by highly toxic chemicals to slow the rate of decomposition—is rarely required by law and is prohibited in some religions.[7] You can transport your baby yourself and keep your baby at home instead of in a mortuary, or you can drive your baby from the hospital to the burial or cremation site. (For more information on transporting your baby's body, see Chapter 8.) You could have a vigil at home, perhaps nestling your baby in a cradle and creating a peaceful space in a bedroom for family and friends to say meaningful goodbyes to your little one. You would need to do some planning and learning ahead of time, such as investigating necessary paperwork and practical matters such as keeping the body cool. Home funeral advocacy groups can help you with details.[8]

We had never really faced death before, but the second we heard the term "home funeral" we knew that whatever that was, it was probably going to be right for us. It was clear that we were not going to have a lot of time with our son in the physical body he was born in. We didn't want to waste even one moment of what we were given! We couldn't imagine letting him spend the time after his death in a mortuary. Plus we felt strongly that our baby belonged with his parents. —*Susan C. and Camilo*

Regarding whether to bury or cremate your baby's body, you may have religious or family traditions to guide you. Perhaps you have a family plot in a cemetery or a special place you can envision keeping or scattering your baby's ashes. You may like the simplicity and dignity of cremation, which is less costly than burial and has environmental advantages as well. Cremation also offers more flexibility for choosing a final resting place, including keeping possession of the ashes. Or you may prefer a "green burial," which returns your baby's body to the earth in a natural way.[9]

It may seem cruel that you must simultaneously create a birth plan and a burial plan. Some parents decide to focus on their baby's life while their baby is still alive, deferring decisions about their baby's funeral and burial until after their baby has died. Others prefer to make as many arrangements as possible ahead of time so they don't have to make decisions in a rush later, especially if the mother will be recovering from a C-birth. If it's simply too much to contemplate, you can make some decisions now and wait on others. For example, you could pick out a burial site but hold off looking at grave markers; decide on cremation but choose an urn when you feel ready (ashes can be returned to you in a temporary container); select a casket but decide later whether to leave it open during visitation or the funeral; or decide to have a funeral but leave planning the details for later.

These preparations can be even more painful if the people assisting you don't know how to handle situations like yours. If you have an unpleasant experience, don't lose hope. You can take your business elsewhere. There may be funeral homes or cremation societies in your area that will serve you for free or at a reduced price in an effort to be sensitive to your special bereavement; ask your hospital's social worker or a home funeral advocacy group for recommendations. It can also give you courage to remember that making these arrangements is a way for you to care for your baby.

⌐ We made an appointment at the local mortuary. They kept referring to us in a very loud voice as "the people with the baby." Forty-five minutes of hearing that! I should have walked out. The man was horrible. In retrospect, I think the funeral director just didn't know what to do. But you would think people at a mortuary would be better at dealing with death, even if it isn't an ordinary death experience. My husband remembers that they didn't even have any tissues. We found a new mortuary. The next funeral director was wonderful. One of his close friends had lost a baby who was stillborn at 39 weeks. He was up-front with us; he said, "You know, we're on uncharted territory here. We have not done this before." When he said that, it made me realize that just because this is my normal, it isn't everybody else's normal. It is not normal to preplan an unborn infant's funeral. —*Kathleen*

If your baby will need an outfit to be buried or cremated in, you may want to shop ahead of time. You may want something special to wear as well, keeping in mind that the mother won't yet be back to her pre-pregnancy shape. It can seem surreal to be doing something as ordinary as shopping for such an extraordinary event.

⌐ I handled everything the best I could, but when it came to buying the outfit for the funeral, I lost it on the cashier. She asked when I was due and said that I must be so excited. I replied, "Not really, because he is going to die!" She immediately lost all her color and finished ringing me up. —*Brooke*

⌐ Never in my worst nightmare did I ever imagine I would have to be shopping for a dress to wear for our daughter's funeral before she was even born, and never did I ever think I would ever have the strength to do such a thing. I had decided that Gemma's funeral would be a celebration of her life and that in celebrating her life I would ask everyone to wear pink. We even found a pink tie for Daddy. —*Courtney*

⌐ We got him a cloth diaper to bury him in. My husband didn't want to bury him without a diaper. And a disposable diaper didn't seem right because eventually he's going to decompose, and then there'll be this disposable diaper left. —*Kathleen*

Buying an urn, shroud, or casket for a baby is another experience that feels surreal. As difficult as it is, taking ownership of these tasks can help you feel empowered and provide meaning and memories

Getting Ready

that you can hold onto later. You could even make these items your-self, if you or someone you know has the skills for it.

⟳ The funeral director brought out the Styrofoam caskets with the pink and the blue gingham. My husband finally said, "Do you have something you wouldn't bury your pet in?" I was picturing a beautiful wood casket, but I didn't realize it would be so hard to find. We got online and found an abbey in Iowa that makes caskets.[10] They were beautiful. The monks build them from oak from their own sustainable forest. We had the casket delivered to our house and we had it for a few weeks, which most people find very bizarre. We had it on our dresser. But this was the one thing we were going to be able to get. And it was going to get buried. We were never going to see it again. It was nice to have, to get to feel it and touch it and spend time with it. —*Kathleen*

Choosing a Burial Plot or a Place to Scatter Ashes

Some parents decide to bury their baby in a different town from where they live. You may want to give your baby a permanent resting place that is familiar or holds meaning for your family. You could also have the benefit of holding two services, one where you live now and one where the baby will be buried.

If you choose cremation, it is legal in many places, including all U.S. states, to keep the ashes at home or scatter them on your own property or on someone else's property, with the permission of the landowner.[11] Some religious traditions require that ashes be interred respectfully in a cemetery or burial vault, to ensure that human remains don't end up desecrated. Perhaps you'd like to keep your baby's ashes in a special urn or keep some in a piece of jewelry. Maybe you'll scatter them in the future, or have them mixed with your own, many years from now. If you are planning to scatter your baby's ashes, returning your baby to a natural spot can be a fitting way to acknowledge the circle of life.

Funeral or Memorial Service

A funeral or memorial service is another factor to consider. Under outdated thinking about miscarriage, stillbirth, and infant death, parents were—and sometimes still are—discouraged from holding a funeral. The death of an infant has been a taboo subject, so to some people a public recognition of the baby is considered unnecessary, even in poor taste. Some hospitals still offer to bury babies in a common plot, under the assumption that this does the families a favor by relieving them from making arrangements or sparing them the expense. However, many parents find meaning and comfort in making these final arrangements on behalf of their baby. It's one of the last acts of parenting you will be able to do for this child. If you want to have a full funeral and burial, complete with announcements and music and family and friends to support you, that is your right. Whatever your heart wants to do to commemorate your baby, don't be cowed by suggestions from others that it is too much. If you prefer something much more private, or a simple graveside service instead, that is your right too. But the choice is yours.

Another option is to have a memorial service at a later date. This is especially common with cremation, as there is no timeline for putting the remains in a final resting place. If you plan to bury your baby, having a funeral service at that time can make sense. But you can also limit this ritual to your immediate family and hold a memorial service another time. Some parents feel they benefit from a lag as it lets them catch their breath and tend to their other children and to themselves in the weeks or months following their baby's birth and death. A delayed memorial service also gives family and friends the opportunity to offer their condolences and support yet again and also gives you the gift of being comforted down the road when you may need reassurance that your baby has not been forgotten.

GETTING CLOSER TO BIRTH

The remaining weeks of the pregnancy went fast, too fast, and I found myself feeling panicky when I would think of the impending birth. I couldn't slow down the clock, even though I tried. I kept doing all the things with Elliot that I had always done, sometimes feeling redundant, sometimes feeling like I couldn't do them enough, all the while knowing that what I did in the remaining weeks would have to last a lifetime for me. —*Karla*

Getting Ready

⟶ As Lily's due date drew near, I was just trying to get through the days without thinking about it too much. Reminders came more and more frequently, though. Lily was quite a kicker, and I could sometimes even see kicks on my wife's tummy. And of course there was planning: making a birth plan, planning a baptism, having an anointing, and planning the funeral. With all this kicking and planning going on, I was only partly successful at forgetting about things. —*Mark*

⟶ I tried to be "normal," doing my hair and makeup each day, getting dressed, putting on a happy face, and inquiring into the well-being of others, but my heart was broken in a million little pieces and I had no idea how I was going to say goodbye to a baby whom I loved so much. I had no idea how I was going to live the rest of my life without this little boy in it. —*Karla*

In the final weeks of your pregnancy, with your overriding wishes carefully considered, medical decisions made, a birth plan discussed with your caregivers, and family and friends lined up to support you, you may feel logistically prepared. You may have attended childbirth classes to help prepare you for the physical aspects of labor. You may feel intellectually prepared, medically prepared, even spiritually prepared. But try as you might, it is normal to feel unprepared emotionally. All you can do is experience your baby's birth and short life *in the moment.* That's also the beauty of it.

You may feel a sense of resolution and peace about decisions and plans you have made, having had weeks or even months to let everything settle in. You may feel like you have all your bases covered and confident that whatever scenario plays out, you'll be able to manage.

⟶ During the last few weeks before Ashley was born I really felt at peace about our decision for comfort care. If we were blessed to have some time with her alive, I just wanted to enjoy every minute with her—to hold her and cuddle her and stroke her hair. —*Shellie*

⟶ We were well-prepared for anything. I was prepared for a stillbirth, and I was prepared to take care of a sick baby for as long as she lived. —*Holly*

A Gift of Time

As the days pass and bring you closer to the day your baby will be born, it can seem that your senses and emotions are heightened. Any remaining fears may seem magnified in anticipation.

⟶ I could visualize the moments leading up to her birth, but for the actual birth and the moments with her in my arms, I couldn't go to that place. It was almost as if my mind and heart were protecting me from the most heart-wrenching time in my life. Maybe I would have run away to a beach and tried to stay pregnant forever if I could have seen how painful leaving her at the hospital would be. I knew the time would be sacred and beautiful. I just couldn't picture myself actually going through it. —*Laura H.*

⟶ I knew that as long as Sarina was inside of me she was fine. So the closer I came to delivering, the more afraid I was for her. I didn't want her to experience pain; I didn't want her to suffer. I wanted her to have a peaceful life, even though it was only going to be very short. I wanted her to feel our love and know that we loved her so very much. I knew that after I delivered, that I would no longer have control of her life. —*Christine*

⟶ The day before her birth, we realized that we had prepared for every possible scenario, except that she might not be born alive. We knew that was very possible, but that was the one scenario that we hadn't been able to reconcile with. —*Jill K.*

⟶ Coming to the end of the pregnancy and knowing my baby would die so soon was incredibly difficult. I became less serene and more frantic, more panicked. I remember going to the supermarket and buying eggs and the date on the eggs was two weeks away, and I knew that my baby wouldn't live that long—that even the *eggs* would last longer. I broke down crying in the dairy aisle of the supermarket. —*Elle*

⟶ Though I had prepared myself all pregnancy long for the fact that I would lose him, no amount of preparation could prepare me for a still and lifeless baby. The loss that I would soon face was so overwhelming to me and I had no idea how to bear it. I missed him so much already, and he wasn't even gone yet! —*Karla*

Getting Ready

As your due date nears, you might want to take action to help calm yourself or provide some distraction. Friends and family may wish to pitch in for you. Although this time of anticipation is intense, it can also be rich.

     ⌒ My friend gave me a relaxation party two nights before I had Aubrielle. They gave me new pajamas and many other things to help me at the hospital. It also helped me to know that they cared for Aubrielle and that she was important to them too. I had a great time spending time with my friends and relaxing. —*Holly*

     ⌒ I had a wonderful evening with friends. I stayed out *way* past my bedtime. We all gathered to enjoy pampering—facials, manicures, foot massages, lots of delicious food and wine. We talked, laughed, and left our troubles behind for a little while. Each woman brought with her a bead that was used to make a necklace for Ashley and me. Each bead was chosen with great care and had special significance. —*Shellie*

     ⌒ My family came to the house for a "Labor Day" picnic. This gathering helped us get through the day, knowing what we were headed for the next day. We had a cookout, hung out in the pool, and talked about old family memories. The time came that I had to start preparing myself for the morning. My sister and I at one point left to get gas for the car. At the gas station a song was playing and we both just starting crying and held each other. This was a moment that meant so much to me. My sister and I had gone through some tough times previously, and to this day I feel as though this was the beginning of our relationship that we have today. Kevin was already working his magic and he wasn't even born yet. —*Amy*

Whether you feel confident or apprehensive, completely ready or wishing you had a bit more time, you will have done what you were able to do to prepare for the big day. That is all that is asked of you. It's time to meet your baby.

seven

Welcoming Baby

Birth Experiences and Meeting Your Baby

As the nurse handed her to me, all I could see was how perfect she was. All anyone had been telling me for weeks was about all of the things that were wrong with her. No one had told me that I would look at her and fall totally in love. —*Alaina*

I remember seeing her in my husband's arms and being consumed with love. I just loved her so much. Even with her cleft lip and palate, she was perfect and gorgeous. So beautiful. I cannot put into words how much love I felt for her. —*Holly*

Everyone told me that Maggie's arrival would be joyous. I couldn't quite believe that. How could it be? The clock on her short life would start ticking when—if—she took her first breath, and I couldn't imagine anything joyous about the ending staring us right in the face. But, then—Maggie was born. And I was never so glad to see anyone in my life. —*Alessandra*

I was sort of in a fog at the hospital as things led up to Lily's birth. Somewhere in the back of my mind, I was hoping that this day would somehow pass without too much pain. But once Lily was born, everything changed. A wonderful thing happened: I found I had no choice but to love Lily! I wanted to know what she was like. I wanted her to know me. I wanted the very best for her. These emotions were very intense, not diluted by time, practicality, worries, or any of the usual things that become part of love between people. And they were not really even wanted in an intellectual sense, because loving Lily definitely meant being very sad and experiencing pain. This was simply the burning desire to know, and to be known, in a very pure form. This experience was very painful because the distance between my desire and reality was so great. And it felt exactly right. —*Mark*

No matter how your labor and delivery unfolds, the birth of your baby is a momentous event. However apprehensive or grief-stricken you might have been during the pregnancy and birth, after your baby is born, your fears can fall away and your focus turns to your little one. Whether your baby is born alive or still, your time together is going to be as extraordinary as your baby is. Whatever happens, this profound time belongs to you and your baby and is yours to cherish in your heart forever.

APPROACHING THE TIME OF BIRTH

As in typical pregnancies, for many mothers labor begins naturally on its own. Other mothers will have their baby's birth scheduled, either by induction of labor or a caesarean birth. If you're waiting for labor to start spontaneously, you may feel the suspense of uncertainty. If you know the specific date and time of your baby's upcoming birth, this date may loom large before you, overwhelming you with its inevitability. Or you may feel a sense of serenity or anticipation.

Preterm Birth

For some mothers, labor begins prematurely and comes as a surprise, even a shock. When labor starts weeks before expected, you may feel especially unprepared.

I felt so unprepared. My thoughts were racing: *What's happening, Lord?! Why are you allowing this to happen now? I'm not ready! How can I get pictures of my baby? I don't have an outfit to dress him in. I don't have his special blanket. I can't believe this is happening!* Yet I was excited to meet this life that had been growing inside me; he seemed to be such a fighter already. What would he look like? Would he survive labor? Would we see him alive? Would he recognize my voice? Would he hear me whisper, "I love you"? Would he open his eyes? Would he cry? How would I react? Would my parents make it in time? It was so surreal. —*Kristin*

⁓ I don't think I will ever forget how I felt the moment I woke up and realized my water had broken, exactly four weeks before my due date. I wasn't panicked, but I was startled—and apprehensive. Not scared, really, just uneasy. In the car on the way to the hospital, I looked at my husband and said, "Here we go." He nodded to me and we both knew that the next hours were sure to be overwhelming and definitive. We'd waited months to meet our daughter and were prepared in every way, but still, we didn't really feel ready. Would we ever be? —*Alessandra*

If you feel logistically unprepared, you may have to improvise and rely even more on family and friends. You may not even have written a birth plan yet. But you can still hold onto your overriding wishes as your guiding light and make your time with your baby just as meaningful.

Scheduled Birth

If you've set a birth date in advance, you have the clarity of knowing the day your baby will be born—and perhaps die. At first, this date may seem far away. And then it's upon you. As it approaches, you may feel overcome by feelings of sorrow or anxiety.

⁓ The night before, I could not sleep. I kept thinking that this was it, the last night I would have with my son. Tomorrow he would die. That night was all I had left. I kept thinking over and over that this is it. I continued to sob the entire time. —*Brooke*

⁓ I couldn't sit still; I cleaned my house top to bottom. Even as the time neared for us to leave for the hospital, I found other things to do and to clean around the house. My family just stood watching me with sad eyes. I was so nervous, on the verge of breakdown, but I held it in and kept together. Eventually they were able to coax me out of my safe home and to the car that would lead to the hospital. —*Chelsea*

⌢ The night before the C-section, my husband and I went to bed and just lay there holding each other like we did when we first received the news that Kevin's heart was sick. We talked about our emotions and our anticipation of the next day. After about an hour of sleep, I decided to get up and take a shower. We had to be at the hospital at 6:30 a.m. As the water fell on my back, I stood with my hands on my stomach and prayed. I prayed that when it was his time to go that he would feel no pain and would be welcomed into the gates of heaven with open arms. —*Amy*

In some cases, an induction is scheduled if labor doesn't appear to be starting on its own near the estimated due date. If this happens, you may take it in stride, or this turn of events may send you reeling.

⌢ I went two weeks over. I ended up being induced. I said I might as well pick a date because I can't be pregnant forever—as much as I would like to. The doctor let me go past the due date, because it's not like the baby was going to be a healthy baby. —*Bianca*

⌢ At 39 weeks, the doctor said he didn't think I would go into labor naturally anytime soon. He said we could wait one more week or he could go ahead and schedule an induction. We decided to wait. I really did not want to be induced; I wanted to keep my baby inside my womb where she was safe and sound. A week later, the doctor said that he scheduled me for an induction and that we needed to be at the hospital the next day. My stomach dropped out of my body, my heart began racing, and my head was spinning. It was hard to wrap my brain around what he was telling me. My doctor patiently listened to my babbling and gently told me he thought we should keep the scheduled induction, that it really is inevitable. I hung up the phone and began to sob at the realization of what was to come. —*Chelsea*

While a scheduled birth may present an unwanted deadline, knowing when to expect your baby's arrival has some advantages. You have a target date for finishing your arrangements. Friends and family can travel to be with you. You're less likely to be caught with loose ends.

Preparing to Deliver a Baby Who Has Died in Utero

⌐ I actually felt rapid kicking for about an hour and then never again. I am almost certain this was the moment she was dying. I was all alone in the middle of the night at home. —*Shayla*

Some parents receive the crushing news that their baby has already died before birth. For some, the baby's condition was so severe that parents and doctors were aware that this was a possibility. The news may even bring a sense of relief. For others who were expecting their baby to be born alive, the news comes as a devastating shock.

⌐ At 2 a.m. I woke up and instantly knew something was wrong. By 5 I had called my OB. She told me to go in to the hospital. It was like a dream, but looking back, I know that I knew Emma was gone. I packed her things and mine, and I was strangely calm. Even when the nurse tried and tried to find her heartbeat, and when my doctor came in and then they did the ultrasounds, I just stared out the window. I may have had some tears, but not like I would have expected. I just knew she was gone. For some reason, the thought came in to my head that Emma was safe, I didn't need to worry about her anymore. —*Kristi R.*

If your baby dies before labor begins, you may think you have to get your baby out right away. In fact, there is usually no danger or rush. Because your baby has been inside you all these months, he or she doesn't carry any microbes that you don't already carry.[1] Talk to your caregivers so you can be monitored. One consideration is that the sooner you deliver, the better condition your baby's body will be. Your baby's skin may show signs of weakening and tearing in certain spots as early as six hours following death in utero and certainly by twenty-four hours, so you'll want to be mindful of this when making plans to deliver.[2]

If you had your heart set on seeing your baby alive, even if for just a moment, you may feel that your chance to say hello has been ripped away. Remember that when your baby is placed in your arms, you can still cradle, kiss, examine, and love your baby. Even death cannot take this precious time away from you.

WHEN BIRTH IS IMMINENT

Whether you're headed to the hospital for a scheduled birth or you're experiencing the onset of spontaneous labor, this is a clear demarcation, an unmistakable signal that something momentous and inexorable has begun. The dramatic climax of meeting your baby is coming. You're not just along for the ride; you are a co-creator of this extraordinary experience in your life.

A wide range of emotions and intensity is possible and perfectly normal. You may feel excited, sad, or filled with anxiety.

When my water broke at 3:30 a.m., I was actually giddy with anticipation. All day I felt happy that she would soon be here.
—*Katharine*

When we got to the hospital, I could see the fear in my husband's eyes; I know he could see mine as well. I whispered, "I'm scared." He said, "I know, so am I." —*Chelsea*

One very vivid memory I have is of my husband and me walking down the hospital hallway to our private room, past the rooms with new moms and crying babies. It was an extremely sad moment for me, because I knew I would be leaving the hospital empty-handed, and that is so not how it was supposed to be. I almost fell to the floor as we walked to our room. —*Christine*

I was avoiding the bed like the plague, choosing instead to sit on the couch on the far side of the room, where it was a sunny happy fall day outside. I could see the little plastic bassinet along the wall with the lights attached to the top, and I knew that is where my dead baby would be lying soon after birth. I knew, and because of that I wanted to burn its image into my head forever. It's something that I can associate with my son, so that makes it important. —*Rachel*

You may feel calm, resigned, or even numb.

⌒ I remember thinking as we were in labor: *It's over, it happened so fast*. There was a realization that we can't extend this life any longer. —*Brad*

⌒ On the way to the hospital, I don't think my husband and I said more than two words to each other. We just listened to songs on our CD of "Kevin songs," and this ride was quicker than I ever remembered. As I went through the admission process, I was wondering if all of the people I was interacting with knew that Kevin was going to die. I wasn't sure who knew and who didn't know. As the elevator doors opened to the third floor, I took a big deep breath and said to my husband, "This is it." The rest of the preparation was a blur. From the monitors to the IVs to the paperwork, all I was wondering again was if all of these nurses knew my baby was going to die.

—*Amy*

⌒ The sun was shining outside; cars were rushing along the road; people were busy and seemingly happy. I entered an unlit labor room; the blinds were closed and there were shadows cast upon the walls and floors. The room looked barren: a bed, a bassinet, in anticipation for what? I was here to have a baby, but there was no excited anticipation, no adrenaline surge. I was here to do a job, give birth and say goodbye. —*Doreen*

⌒ We were pretty matter-of-fact. It was like, all right, it's time to do this today. Up until that point, it was so well-planned, so well thought-out, so it was like, now it's just implementation. I felt like I had to be the rock because my wife was going to be in pain and she was going to be exhausted and her hormones were going to be raging, so I couldn't afford to be sad or down or anything. I almost had to shut off everything and just react. —*James*

Experiences with Caregivers

Like during your pregnancy, having supportive caregivers during your labor and delivery can make a tremendous difference. If you must explain your situation or your birth plan to caregivers you haven't met or who haven't been informed, you might need to gather your strength to advocate for yourself and your baby, just when you feel most vulnerable. Or you may find yourself enveloped in a cocoon of empathy and support.

⟶ When I arrived at the hospital, I discovered that no special arrangements had been made. No one had told the nursing staff about my situation. I had to tell them myself. —*Annette G.*

⟶ When we got to the hospital, the doctor on call was one I'd never seen. He told us there is no medical reason for a C-section since the outcome wouldn't change. I told him that my regular doctor and I had agreed that if Carter was alive at the time of birth, I would have a C-section. So I wouldn't sign any papers and refused to let him touch me. He left the room in a huff. He came back a while later and said he got in touch with my regular doctor, and she agreed to come in on her day off and do the C-section. So she did. —*Laurie*

⟶ The nurses were so wonderful and supportive in the hours that we waited for my C-section. My nurse read through our birth plan and went over it with us to be sure she was completely clear about our wishes. Just before they disconnected me from the monitors to take me into the OR, they let me listen to my son's heart for a few extra minutes. I was very touched that they thought to do that, because my mind was spinning and I hadn't thought to ask. Then as the nurses walked me into the OR, they asked me if I wanted them to say a prayer. If I could pick two or three of the most special moments out of the whole thing, that was definitely one of them. They were standing on either side of me, walking me in, and they were praying aloud as they walked me down the hall and into the OR. —*Kathleen*

⟶ I had the most wonderful OR nurse in the world. As I was getting the epidural in my back, she put her arms around me, buried her face in mine and told me to talk to Frankie, to tell him how much I loved him and that I was there for him. I did just what she said and it did help me. (I hoped it helped Frankie, too, because I was worried that he was feeling my nervousness.) This nurse obviously knew what she was doing and was not afraid to be with my husband and me during this very difficult time. —*Susan E.*

⌐ I'll never forget the look on the anesthesiologist's face as he finished. He looked at me with tears in his eyes before turning away and, patting me on the shoulder, he said, "May God be with you." —*Sonya*

Even if you have specified your medical decisions for your baby in a birth plan or in conversations with your doctor, you may be asked about them again during labor. If so, you may feel like you are being asked to decide again. Instead, you can think of it as your caregivers being conscientious about confirming your wishes, not that you are being second-guessed.

⌐ It was hard when the doctor asked us that dreaded question about whether we wanted them to do all the "lifesaving" measures. My husband and I had already discussed what we wanted to do, and so we said that once he was born we wanted to hold him right away and love him into eternity. —*Kristin*

Emotions during Labor

As labor progresses and your work to give birth becomes increasingly intense, you may find that the physical and emotional pain blocks out nearly everything else. Or you may find that you are able to reach a plateau of determination and acceptance.

⌐ It was long, lonely, excruciating, painful, and difficult. I was in a room near other laboring women, so I could hear the sounds of their labor and delivery. The nurses on that shift were unsympathetic and even a little cold. So I was on my own. It really felt like it was just me and God in this wilderness of contractions and fear of what was to come. But somehow, there was also an assurance that I wasn't really alone. —*Kelly G.*

     ⍺ I didn't talk during that whole time pushing, I had my eyes closed and we had music playing. It was very peaceful and, to me, it was kind of a meditative state. —*Bridget*

Labor is an emotional time for fathers as well.

     ⍺ David Michael had already died before my wife went into labor. She was given pain medications to deal with both physical and mental pains, and when she slipped into sleep, I went for a cigarette (actually about seven, but who's counting?). I called my parents and in-laws, my brother, and my best friend and wept. —*David W.*

You may have family and friends at the hospital keeping vigil for you, ideally in a private room set aside for them. You might consider writing a letter for them to read while at the hospital during this emotional time, thanking them for being there for you and inviting them to meet your baby with open arms and loving hearts. Here are excerpts from a letter that one couple wrote:

> We want to thank you for being here today. We are glad you are here; we need you here. Thank you.
>
> We have tried to plan as much as we possibly could for this day. But, at the time of this letter being read, we are now in an unknown place. We do not know what will happen.
>
> It is our hope and prayer that each of you will be able to visit with Gemma before her spirit leaves her body to go dance with the angels. We know however, that this may not be possible. Be not afraid. We want you to meet, love, and embrace our precious baby girl. Please try to look beyond any physical characteristics she may have. We have been looking forward to seeing our precious Gem for months now, looking forward to rubbing her little cheeks and kissing and wiggling each and every one of her little toes; whether she has ten or twelve, each is as special and amazing as she is. These are precious moments that will not come back and cannot be replaced. Please join us in celebrating the life of our little girl. Feel free to smile with us and to cry with us.
>
> We also want to thank all of you for your prayers, love, and

support over these past several months. . . . We will need you for months to come, to listen to us and to acknowledge and remember the life of our little Gemma Therese. —*Courtney and Terrence*

Pain Relief

Even if your birth plan outlines your goals and preferences for pain relief, you may want to reassess your needs when the time comes. Your contractions may seem more tolerable than you had expected, and you might be able to get by on little or no medication. Or once labor becomes more intense, you might need more than you had planned. If you are unable to manage the pain for whatever reason, medicated relief can improve the quality of your experience during and shortly after birth. But tell your caregivers that you want to remain as mentally present as possible so they can adjust medications and dosage accordingly. Give yourself permission to listen to your body and advocate for yourself—or have your partner advocate for you.

I was still unsure about receiving an epidural. I didn't know if I wanted to experience everything that I could of Noah's birth, or if it would be better not to experience all the pain (and then the memories) and enjoy the delivery without the physical pain. I kept asking my husband, as if I needed his permission and for him to say that it would not mean that I was not strong enough. Of course, he said it was up to me, but he did finally lovingly encourage me to just get it. The anesthesiologist took two tries to get it just where it needed to be, and though I sat there for over thirty minutes through several contractions, I was glad because it worked wonders. As my friends, pastor and his wife, and parents came to the hospital, I was really glad for my choice because I just remember our talking and laughing in joyful expectation of the birth of our son. —*Kristin*

It wasn't too bad except for the back labor. That was torture. I felt that an epidural was the only relief from the excruciating pain, and I was very sad to think that all of the work and pain of labor would not result in a baby we could bring home. —*Shellie*

⌒ I couldn't stand it any more and called the nurse for the pain-killers to be put into my IV. I said my pain was at a five although it felt more like an eight or so. I was thinking that it would only get worse because nothing was going to happen for a long time, and I didn't want to run out of numbers. I welcomed anything that would dope me up at that point. I so wish now that I had just said no. Later I couldn't stay awake because of all the painkillers. That was my time with my son and I couldn't even keep my eyes open. —*Rachel*

⌒ I have always thought that when I had a baby I would have an epidural—no need to be brave, I thought. But with the nurse in front of me asking if I wanted one, I wasn't sure. The last few hours had been brutal and I couldn't imagine someone inserting a needle into my spine on top of it. The nurse reached out and took my hand and said, "Honey, what is coming is going to be hard enough for you. You don't need to suffer through the pain as well." Her words rang in my mind and I knew that I wanted to be in the best shape I could be when my daughter was born. I told her to go ahead with the epidural. —*Alaina*

Whatever your decisions and experience regarding medication and pain, birthing your baby is a triumph.

If Delivery Needs to Be Reevaluated

After a trial of labor, you and your doctor may decide that a cae-sarean section is needed. Perhaps your labor is not progressing well, your baby is too big or in a position that makes vaginal birth risky or difficult, you are experiencing difficulties that endanger your own health, or your baby is in distress. If you are attempting a vaginal birth after caesarean, your doctor or midwife may determine that a C-birth is necessary after all.

⌒ I began to notice Jordan's movements slowing down. My hus-band and I went into the hospital for a non-stress test to find out that Jordan's heart was beginning to fail. We were admitted and told that we could choose to deliver him by caesarean section or allow him to pass away and then deliver him stillborn vaginally. We knew immediately that we wanted the emergency C-section. It was such a flurry of action: doctors and nurses running around to prepare the OR and to get us ready for surgery. During this very chaotic moment, the sweetest nurse we could hope for came to sit with us. She told us about her own baby who had died years earlier. Our doctor also came in to pray with us before surgery. —*Jenny D.*

We had planned to have a home birth because we wanted to have Frankie in our home for at least a little while with our loved ones present. We wanted this inevitably difficult experience to be sprinkled with joy and love. And it was, but not exactly how we had hoped. Eventually my midwife conferred with my doctor on the phone, and it was decided that Frankie was probably doing the splits (he was breech) and that I should get to the hospital to have him delivered by C-section. So we had to give up on the idea of having Frankie in our home. At that point my husband didn't really care, he just wanted me to be safe. —*Susan E.*

If you know in advance that a caesarean section is a distinct possibility, or if you decided as part of your birth plan that you want one should your baby be in distress, then you'll have the advantage of feeling like this unscheduled birth was somewhat planned. But if a C-birth was never indicated during your pregnancy and you hadn't contemplated what to do, you may feel completely caught off-guard. Whether you've prepared yourself or not, decisions are not always clear-cut. Even if a C-birth is clearly needed, the idea of major surgery can still be frightening.

To say that I was very nervous for my unplanned C-section is a huge understatement; I was so afraid I couldn't stop shaking. They told me this was a natural result of the epidural. That information didn't matter to me because the shaking felt like a pretty accurate reflection of how I was feeling inside. When my husband came into the room, he put his face right next to mine and talked to me softly in order to soothe me. This helped because I felt not just nervous but like I was going to pass out from the drugs and the tension. Later my husband confessed that he was scared out of his mind and felt like he was going to pass out too. But we hung on together. —*Susan E.*

⌐ I had not slept nor eaten since Tuesday afternoon, and I was a wreck by Thursday at noon. The doctor came in and said we needed to make a decision. He said I could not continue like this because I was dehydrating, I was exhausted, and the baby was still not coming down. I told him to give me a couple more hours to think about it all. So he left me to ponder. I was scared to do the caesarean. I wanted to be with Gabriel every minute I could and I was afraid of how I would recover. So I asked if we could all get in a circle and pray. My family and friends gathered around my bed and my brother begin to pray. It was one of the most touching and memorable times of my life to look around and feel the love of everyone around me. I didn't feel alone, just scared. As soon as it was over, I looked at my husband and told him if the baby was still alive then we were going to do the caesarean. So the doctor and nurse came in and I asked to hear the heartbeat. As we listened, I heard it again, that galloping sound of his little heart beating. I told the doctor I wanted to do the caesarean. —*Sonya*

MEETING YOUR BABY

After all the waiting and wondering, your baby is finally born! Whether your baby is born alive or still, you may feel like bursting with new-parent emotions: joy, pride, amazement, wonder, exhaustion—and most of all, consuming, intoxicating love. Despite your baby's diagnosis, the pure transcendent truth of this moment is that your baby is here, your baby is yours. Your baby *is*.

Before, during, and after birth, your baby's fate will unfold as it should, beyond your or anyone else's control. Your job is simply to be attentive to your baby, whether your baby has already died, lives for a few precious minutes or hours, or even lives long enough to be discharged from the hospital. Whatever happens, you can take your little one into your loving embrace. You can gather keepsakes and take photographs. You can rest on the support of compassionate caregivers and friends and family. You can trust your baby's path. You can bask in timeless love.

A Gift of Time

Birth Experiences with Babies Who Are Born Still

⁓ During my pregnancy, I longed for the day when I would finally meet my son. So there are no words to describe the profound sorrow and yearning I felt when Nathaniel was stillborn. I did not realize how profoundly it would affect me to give birth to a stillborn baby. His death was beyond my comprehension, but in that moment my aching heart held a whispered hope that one day I would understand, and in that I found peace. —*Annette G.*

The silence in a birthing room when a baby is born still may seem deafening. Where there should be lusty cries from a newborn, there is only hushed murmuring, a quiet clatter of medical instruments, a rustling of towels and sheets.

Hopes for the baby to be born alive are sometimes extinguished at the moment of birth.

⁓ I remember the doctor saying, "It's a girl." I looked up for a second and I saw the longest blue little baby. Then I heard the doctor ask if she was breathing. It took a moment and I heard a "no" from the nurse. The doctor then repeated that to me. I just lost it. I wanted to hold her while alive more than anything. —*Annette H.*

⁓ I knew that she was dead almost immediately. I asked anyway. They told me that there was no pulse and I asked to hold her. I was so calm. I finally had a resolution. It was not what I wanted, but I think a small part of me was relieved that it was finally over. The twenty-six weeks of agony and wondering were over. —*Jamie*

⁓ Suddenly my baby was in my arms. I waited for her to cry. I was in some sort of state of shock. There was my baby; I could feel her warm body in my arms. She felt very heavy to me. I was confused; I looked at my doctor, waiting for him to tell me what to do. I kept saying she needed to be washed off and someone should take a picture. My husband stood beside me, gently looking and touching Caelyn. Time seemed to stand still for me, Caelyn in my arms not moving, the doctor sewing my tear, the nurses moving around the room like busy ants. Then one of the nurses came to me, put the stethoscope on Caelyn's chest and listened. I patiently waited for her to say her heart was still beating; she was just sleeping. She just shook her head and said all she needs is for me to hold her and love her; so I did. I knew then that she was gone, but I held her and loved her. —*Chelsea*

You may have longed for the chance to see your baby alive, even for a moment. Many parents of stillborn babies speak of their sorrow about never seeing their baby's eyes or feeling their baby's grasp. You may grieve that your baby was not alive to feel your kisses or hear the loving words you spoke after birth. But the fact that your baby is no longer physically alive cannot steal the power and meaning of your baby's existence. Nor can it invalidate the nurturing you devoted to your little one before birth. Your baby's entire lifetime was spent cradled safely in your body and in your love. Your baby may not have lived outside the womb, but your baby *lived*.

If you already knew your baby was gone, there can even be a feeling of peace as you labor and give birth.

My midwife explained that with a stillborn baby, she didn't want to be pulling her out at all. It was best for Mariah to come out just with my pushes. It was a very peaceful time as the midwife reminded me that there was no hurry, and I could push when I wanted to. It seems strange that I would describe it to be peaceful but it really was. I had an epidural so I had no pain, and neither did Mariah. —*Greta*

When Emma was born it was so perfect, I could not have planned it any better. All along I felt that when Emma was born I would be overcome with emotion. Seeing her would make all of this real. I was so scared of that moment; I had been dreading it for so long. The hospital was quiet and the lights were dimmed in our room. My nurse was by my side, and my doctor and my husband were going to "catch" Emma. My husband actually held her as she was delivered and laid her on my stomach. I did cry, but then I was so happy to see her it was indescribable. —*Kristi R.*

Being present when a baby is born still can affect your doctors and nurses profoundly too. Caregivers who bravely enter this experience with you and treat your baby tenderly are immensely comforting.

— There was an incredible nurse present. After Caitlyn was born, the nurse picked her up and said, "Oh, come here, sweetie." It was the most beautiful moment I have ever witnessed in a stranger as she treated Caitlyn as the precious child she was, regardless of the fact that she wasn't alive. —*Shayla*

Birth Experiences with Babies Who Are Born Alive

— When she came out, everybody just stood there. It was quiet. Because nobody knew what was going to happen. —*Bianca*

Especially if you're not sure whether your baby will be born alive, it can seem as if everyone in the room is holding their breath to see if your baby shows signs of life. Then if your baby does take a breath, the room is filled with rejoicing.

— Anouk was alive! It was our biggest fear that she wouldn't survive the birth, and once we saw that she was breathing, we were in seventh heaven. We were grateful and so happy for every second she was alive. Although I clearly knew that she was going to die, I was so happy. Joy filled the room around us, joy and peace. Anouk started breathing gently: uncertainly at the beginning, but then in a more and more regular way. —*Monika*

— When Michael was born, he let out one small cry to mark his place in the world. With that, everybody in the room started to cry because they certainly never expected he would be born alive or that he would be able to let out a cry. —*Missy*

— She emerged into the world purplish-gray, still, silent, and not breathing. The nurses slipped a cap on her head and laid her unmoving body in my arms. My husband quickly grabbed the jar of Lourdes water by my bedside and pronounced the words of a conditional baptism: "If you are able to be baptized, I baptize you in the name of the Father, and of the Son, and of the Holy Spirit."

Welcoming Baby

Abruptly she gasped, and I exclaimed, "You're alive!" The nurses sprang into action, suctioning her and doing other things I can't remember. I was so delighted she was alive. I remember seeing with disappointment that all our prayers hadn't healed her, but it didn't matter at that moment. She was here. I was holding her. She was alive. She was Emily Rose, my daughter. It was all I wanted.

—*Jane T.*

~ Lucy Mae slid into this world and let out the most beautiful little noise. She was immediately put on my chest, and I was so glad that she was born *alive!* She was able to grasp my finger in her tiny little hand. —*Jane G.*

~ The doctor placed him on me and said, "It's a boy!" We'd not known until that point what gender he was. I remember whispering to my husband, "Is he alive?" The doctor said, "Very much so." I was so happy. What a special gift. I had steeled myself for him to be stillborn, and here he was, alive! —*Tracy*

Many parents describe overwhelming feelings of joy and love. But how could this be? How could you be joyful, when you've just given birth to a dying baby? Your baby's imminent death may seem irrelevant for the moment, because all you can see is *life*.

~ From across the room I was able to hear the one and only sound I would ever hear my son make. It sounded like the squeak of a tiny kitten. My heart overflowed with joy. —*Jenny D.*

~ They pulled Ramona out of my abdomen and peeked her little head over the curtain, and it was the happiest moment of my life. My husband was so happy; I could see it in his eyes. I was crying immediately. Once they cleaned her up, I got to see how beautiful she was. She did have a cleft lip, her head was smaller than it was supposed to be, but she also had a nose and was able to breathe on her own. She had the longest eyelashes I had ever seen! It was the most beautiful experience ever. —*Rebecca J.*

~ The whole process was as amazing as it gets. The whole process of a life coming, to see Alaina's head, to see my wife working so hard. When Alaina's head came out, I couldn't tell if she was alive or dead. I thought, *I'm not going to react.* When the doctor pulled her completely out, she made this noise, and I thought, *My God, she's alive.* Everything broke down. I didn't have to be stoic anymore, I didn't have to be strong for my wife. Alaina looked at me, and I thought, *this is everything I asked for.* She had huge blue eyes. And the doctor put her on my wife's chest, and I was just like, unbelievable. She's here, and she's looking at me. It was the most powerful, amazing experience. We just took it in, like nothing else mattered. I had two people to love now. —*James*

⌐ It was more than we could have asked for. Every doctor said that he could not survive more than five minutes outside of the womb. As the nurse listened to our son's heartbeat on the stethoscope, she said, "It is impossible. He is too little, he has been given no oxygen, his heart is not formed properly." I just smiled and said, "I know." —*Donna*

If your birth plan and your baby's birth played out the way you'd hoped, you may feel a sense of accomplishment and be especially pleased with the aspects that were normal.

⌐ I remember the nurse coming over and telling me that Maggie had been baptized. That was a relief for me. I was glad something important had been taken care of and had gone the way we'd planned. I also remember the neonatologist laughing because Maggie had peed on her immediately after she had been born—that was so good to hear. It felt so normal and I was grateful that, finally, something in this journey seemed normal. —*Alessandra*

⌐ The nurses put him right up next to me, all gooey (but not a bit gross) from the delivery, and my husband cut the umbilical cord— it all seemed so normal, so right, so beautiful. For a brief moment, our dream had come true—our beautiful son was here—and he was alive! —*Heidi*

Welcoming Baby

First Sight

Seeing your baby for the first time—really seeing—can be a wondrous experience. You've probably seen black-and-white images many times on ultrasound, but those were grainy, otherworldly views. During your pregnancy, it was seeing through a glass darkly; now it is face to face.

It was amazing! When he looked me in the eyes, it was like he knew exactly what was going on. —*Scott*

She was so beautiful, so perfect-looking. For a minute I thought maybe we did get a medical miracle because she just looked so perfect. She opened her eyes and looked right at her Mommy and Daddy, as if to say to us that she knew everything we had been through and we had done a good job! —*Jennifer*

When they brought him to me he was so beautiful. His eyes were looking directly into mine and I said, "Hi, sweetie." After a few seconds Dominic started to cry. I rubbed his tiny, little cheek and I felt so much love for him. —*Tami*

I will never forget her coming out of me. I placed her on my chest and smelled her; she smelled divine. Like damp grass in the shade. She was crying and I remember bringing her to my face and letting my breath just warm her face, and she was so soothed. I loved being able to soothe her, to feel her relax in my arms, knowing she was safe. She knew me immediately—I was her mother and I was able to *be* her mother. —*Elle*

My husband held him up to my face, all swaddled up in the blanket that my mother made for him, and he had his little hand up by his face. I was lying on the operating table and my husband said, "Baby, here is our son, Noah Samuel. Isn't he the most beautiful baby you've ever seen?" I can still remember vividly how I looked at him and kissed him and wondered how I was going to live without him. I loved this little baby boy that my husband and I made together with every stitch of my being. He was so beautiful. So very precious and beautiful, and he was ours. —*Jenny A.*

The first sight can also bring emotions surging to the surface.

⟶ I will never forget how it felt when the doctor put her on my chest. I'd not cried during labor, but as soon as I saw her and felt her against my skin, it all came out. —*Delsa*

⟶ My husband looked absolutely overwhelmed by this wonderful little person. I think he was surprised by the depth of his love for her—actually, I think that made it all harder for him. He looked so very sad. He brought her over to me, so I could see her. She was beautiful. —*Alessandra*

⟶ It was the most bittersweet moment. My heart was just lost to her the second I saw her. It was truly "love at first sight." —*Martina*

Even if your baby has died or is close to death, what you may notice most is this life you created and carried. In spite of your baby's condition, you may see only a beautiful child for whom your devotion knows no bounds.

⟶ I could not take my eyes off of my baby. What a sweet and perfect baby. As a mother, I could not see any imperfections in my child. All I saw was a sweet little one that I loved more than life itself. —*Donna*

⟶ Even though she was dead, I saw *life*. It was wonderful seeing her. I was amazed at what we created. My husband and I have talked about it many times. It was simultaneously the best and worst moment of our lives. —*Jamie*

⟶ He was purple and lifeless and cool. But he was so cute and soft. They laid him on my chest, all wrapped up with just his face exposed. All I could do, while lying there as they stitched me up, was hold him close to my face and kiss his sweet soft skin—and cry.
—*Pam F.*

As you admire your baby, you may notice endearing or normal features, perhaps some family resemblances that affirm your baby as a full-fledged member of your family.

Welcoming Baby

⟑ As the nurse handed Hope Elizabeth to me, all I could see was how perfect she was. She was a deep reddish-purple color, and she was very limp and fragile. But she had my husband's chin and sweet little ears and lips. Her fingers and hands were amazing. —*Alaina*

⟑ I was in awe seeing him for the first time. He looked beautiful to me. He was weighed just over three pounds and was seventeen inches long, but he felt solid and real against my chest. I wanted to remember everything about him and tried to memorize the way his wavy dark hair laid against his forehead. His nose was just like my grandfather's; his tiny perfect mouth was shaped like a bow. His hands were small, but his fingers were incredibly long. I remember wondering if he would have been a musician. His tiny feet and perfect toes were so adorable. —*Annette G.*

⟑ He had a cleft in his chin, which I was so pleased about, because my husband and older son both have chin clefts. I was thinking, *Oh, there it is, you've got it too!* —*Jill N.*

Some parents feel a resurgence of anger, disappointment, or grief over their baby's condition. Or you may feel so overwhelmed that you are simply numb. Whatever you are feeling, you are entitled.

⟑ The very first moments I felt so much anger towards God. Brayden had died a few days before birth, so his body had already started to break down a little. I was so upset; he looked like he'd suffered and I couldn't understand how God could make his already tough struggle that much worse. I know that the emotions all came over me so fast and in such a rage that there was an immense mix of emotions, but after those first few seconds I found a sense of calm and was able to move past my anger. He was so beautiful. —*Camille*

⟑ They wrapped him up and brought him over to me and laid him on my chest. He was blue, so blue and purple. His breathing and his heart were so bad. I don't know what I pictured, but when I pictured him alive, I thought he would look more alive. We never saw his eyes. He never moved. —*Kathleen*

A Gift of Time

When they put Frankie on my chest immediately after pulling him out of me by C-section, I remember feeling stunned. Who was this little creature they had taken out of me? Was this the same little fellow who had been growing and kicking inside of me, whom I had been nourishing and sheltering for so many months? I remember looking at his body, taking in all of his features. I was relieved for the time to finally have arrived that I could see him. But I continued to feel almost numb. I think my husband felt the same way. —*Susan E.*

Visible Anomalies

Because the only preparation I had for seeing her was everything that was wrong with her, I was blown away by the fact that she looked like my baby, my little girl! No one had prepared me for the fact that I would be meeting my child for the first time and that it didn't matter if she had anomalies or not. I saw them, but they were not what I saw when I looked at her—I saw my daughter, and she was perfect and beautiful because she was ours. —*Alaina*

I had spent so much time during my pregnancy being afraid of what the birth and meeting my baby would be like. When I finally met him there was no fear, just sadness. —*Missy*

If you have been told that your baby has physical malformations, especially if the anomalies have been described to you insensitively or if you were unsure what to expect, you may have been afraid of what your baby would look like. Parents often find that their fears evaporate upon seeing their baby. Some even see perfection.

I had been scared of what our son was going to look like. When he was born, he was the most beautiful child I had ever seen. I had expected his skin to be rough, due to the lack of amniotic fluid, but it was like silk. Once he was born, we realized it would not have mattered anyway, he was our son and in our eyes he was perfect in every way, flawless! He was the way God had made him. —*Deanna*

I had planned to not even see her because I was so afraid. I had developed such a horrific picture in my head of what she would look

Welcoming Baby

like, but when I saw her face, peaceful and resting, it was almost like looking at my other children as they slept. Also, she had the most beautiful hands and feet. I just marveled over their daintiness and how perfect they were. —*Shayla*

⌐ We were afraid that she would look funny, that her head would look big. When we first saw her, we both said the same thing, that she was beautiful. She was perfect. It wasn't frightening in the least.
—*Bridget*

⌐ It was nice to see that her appearance wasn't so scary. She was the most beautiful baby I have ever seen. I can't imagine having another that didn't look like her. I know that the syndrome gave her most of her features, but I am able to look past those things and see her for who she was supposed to be. I will never forget how soft she was, so pure and innocent. —*Chelsea*

⌐ When I first saw Jonah, I thought he was absolutely beautiful. All the fears of his potential malformations were dismissed. His bilateral cleft lip was certainly noticeable, but he was the most perfect, most beautiful little guy I'd ever seen. I remember thinking that aside from his upper lip and nose, his body looked perfect, and I hoped that maybe his condition wasn't as bad as the doctors had all made it out to be. —*Heidi*

⌐ Certainly, the medical diagnoses were correct—her cleft was bad and her color didn't look too good, a symptom of the severity of her heart defects. She had the small head and close-set eyes that were typical of her condition, and one of her little ears wasn't quite formed properly. I actually never saw her ears. My 7-year-old told me about her ear—he thought it was so cute. We thought she was beautiful. She was perfect because she was ours and she had held on long enough to meet us. We discovered that when you love someone, you see them with more than your eyes. I hope she thought the same about us. —*Alessandra*

Some parents feel relief that their baby's appearance isn't so difficult to accept. Bracing yourself for that first look, you too may be pleasantly surprised by your baby's appearance or by your reaction.

⟿ At first, my OB said that Katherine Elizabeth was so beautiful. I thought she was lying, that she was trying to make me feel at peace, since we were not able to tell from the ultrasounds if Katherine Elizabeth would have any malformation of her head, face, hands, or feet. But when my OB lifted Katherine over the blue covering they had on me, I saw the most precious chubby beautiful little girl.

—*Lizabeth*

⟿ She seemed so small and innocent. She was able to breathe on her own and she was looking pretty good. I felt surprised and thought about how I sometimes had imagined a horrible-looking baby that I would not be able to love, and here she was and I loved her as much as my other children. —*Debbie*

⟿ I couldn't believe how happy I was. She was so tiny and so dear—her voice was sweet and gentle but loaded with meaning. Her cleft lip and palate looked worse than I expected—there was almost no upper lip there—but I couldn't believe how beautiful I thought she was. —*Alessandra*

You may be able to focus effortlessly on your baby's beauty even as you acknowledge obvious malformations. Or you may try to avoid your baby's malformations in order to focus on what's normal and precious. Either way, you are showing courage in the face of stark reality.

⟿ She looked very limp and pale. It was hard to listen to her try to breathe. I did see the abnormalities (squished nose and ears, large head) that I had been told of. Still, she was my baby girl and she was beautiful. —*Sherry*

⟿ I looked at her more closely. She was so tiny, especially her head. The cap I tried to knit as small as possible was still too large. I did not want to look under the cap. I tried to look at the rest of her body. I saw my daughter, a baby with a dreadful malformation, but my daughter first and foremost. —*Monika*

⟿ Her skin was dark with lots of vernix that hadn't been cleaned off. This was totally fine with me since that would have taken

Welcoming Baby

time. She was all swaddled up in a blanket with a hat on. She was breathing so shallowly but quietly. Her facial features were flat. She had the sweetest hands and feet. Later when I saw her with her hat off, her head was open on the top. It truly had to be a miracle that she was alive. The rest of her body was just like any other baby. —*Katharine*

The whole room was crying when Luke's head was delivered because they all had such hope, all but me. My crying was done and I wanted to meet my baby. The top of Luke's head was severely deformed. He had no skull from the eyebrows and ears up. What I saw, though, was his daddy's nose and my mouth and his daddy's toes and his little fingers, and I loved all of him and I didn't want to let go of him. —*Sue*

Especially if you feel well-prepared for your baby's appearance, you may find yourself focusing on other details such as vital signs, facial features, counting fingers and toes, or the way your baby feels to you.

I was glad for the preparation our last ultrasound had provided concerning his appearance. I was not shocked at all by him when I saw him for the first time. Instead, I was trying to figure out if he was alive or not. —*Karla*

He was so limp. His head was really big too, because of his condition. But I don't think that's the first thing I noticed. We opened his blanket up and we were looking at his fingers and his toes. When I think about him, I almost never think about the size of his head. I mean, yeah, his forehead was really big. But I think about his face. —*Jill N.*

Her little hands were in fists, as we expected. All along I would see them on ultrasound and I just wanted to kiss them. I loved them even though clenched fists were a sign of her condition. I loved them more than I can say because they were a part of her and my heart was and is full of love for her. —*Kristi R.*

If you aren't prepared for what your baby looks like, anomalies can be distressing to see. If you struggle with your baby's appearance, you may feel guilty for not accepting it more gracefully or lovingly.

 ⟶ I remember I asked my baby's father what the baby looked like; how big was his head? He said, "It's big." I asked him how big? He compared it to my son's basketball at home. When the doctors were able to measure his head, it was 53 centimeters [about 21 inches] around. I could not believe that the doctors were correct. I remember feeling embarrassed that this baby was growing inside of me. It was hard to look at him. I had not expected any of this, and I especially wasn't prepared for what he would look like. And now I have deep regret and remorse for the way I felt about my son. It wasn't his fault. *—Kimberly Anne*

If your baby's appearance or condition is troubling to you, you may benefit from taking your time to get to know your baby and the uniqueness of your baby's body to give yourself the chance to adjust to the reality. You can feel proud that you were able to nurture your baby during pregnancy in spite of the challenges he or she faced.

Sometimes the first sight reveals the severity of a baby's condition. Seeing with your own eyes can help you acknowledge and even accept the inevitability of it all.

 ⟶ After Gemma was handed to me and I saw how sick she really was, I told our baby girl, "It's OK, sweet Gemma, you can go to heaven now. Mommy loves you, baby girl." Not a single eye was dry.
—Courtney

 ⟶ I must confess that I was soothed to know that she would die soon. She certainly couldn't live; her condition was too hard.
—Monika

 ⟶ I thought I wouldn't be able to let him go. Seeing his anomaly, I felt pity for him. I wouldn't have wanted him to suffer here, and I realized then that sometimes death is the healing miracle a person prays for. *—Jo*

Whether your baby is born alive or still, with visible anomalies or not, you benefit from being able to spend the time you need to process your baby's condition and appearance.

Immediate Medical Intervention or Assessment after Birth

Depending on your baby's condition and your wishes, there may be immediate medical intervention after birth, and this will affect your opportunities to interact with your baby. When your baby receives intensive care, this can feel intense for you too.

⌐ I remember that she cried when she came out and we all started crying because it was some indication of hope for her. I just thought: *If she can cry, then she has some type of lung function.* There were a lot of people rushing around and I remember it being very eerily quiet after they had her on the table, which was really scary. I could hear the specialists talking but nothing made sense to me. —*Jessie*

⌐ Our sweet baby Josiah announced his arrival with a few cries. I cried with him. It was pure joy. His crying got weaker, and the NICU team was on hand to help stabilize him. He wasn't doing fantastic things so they brought him over and let me kiss him before they passed him through the window into the NICU. —*Behka*

⌐ My doctor put him on my belly while my husband cut the cord, and then he was rushed to be vented. I remember saying how much I wanted that baby! Now that he was there and I touched him, I wanted him to live so badly, more than I ever knew! —*Amber*

⌐ It took at least ten minutes to get her stable enough to be held, five minutes before we even heard a faint cry. So when I held her in my arms, it was a relief that she was breathing. She was very gray and her cleft lip was worse than I expected, but it was love overflowing. —*Gina*

When a baby is taken away while the mother is still in recovery, the mother can feel left behind. The father or other family members can accompany the baby and play an important role in making sure the mother gets to have some connection too.

⌐ The time right after Jordan's birth was really hard for me. He was in the NICU and my husband was with him. I was alone in the OR with the doctors for what seemed like forever, but was probably closer to forty-five minutes. Then I was transferred to a recovery room. My teenage son was videotaping Jordan in the NICU, his first bath, him being weighed and measured, his first diapering. He would run from the NICU to my recovery room to show me clips of Jordan's video so I could watch his progress. I was delighted for every update and just a bit sad that I was not able to be there myself. —*Jenny D.*

⌐ We had planned to have other doctors do a quick check to verify the diagnosis. So as soon as he came out, they took him to an exam room, and I followed him in there and snapped a few pictures while they did that. Then they wrapped him up and I took him back to the OR to show my wife. And then one of the neonatologists came over and whispered to us, "He doesn't have long." It didn't hit me much at that point, because I kind of assumed that already. So while they were stitching her back up, he was in my arms, and I held him down by my wife's face so she could see him. She had a hand free so she could move and touch him. It was pretty much me holding him that whole time. —*Greg*

Seeing Your Baby in the NICU

Your first sight of your baby may be in a neonatal intensive care unit. This sometimes is a necessary part of stabilizing and evaluating your baby. Particularly if you have chosen certain kinds of medical interventions, you may be able to easily see past the machines. Or perhaps the machines and other medical interventions get in the way, making your baby seem foreign at first. Shock is a normal reaction, but as your baby and the NICU setting become more familiar, you can warm up to your little one. If your baby was taken to the NICU against your wishes, your numbness or distress would be partly an expression of your grief about this.

⟿ She was hooked up to ECMO, which is a heart-lung bypass machine, and she had tubes and wires everywhere—but she still was one of the most beautiful sights I have ever seen. —*Elizabeth D. P.*

⟿ I was wheeled in to see her. She was dressed in only a diaper and countless wires were attached to her tiny body. She was a foreigner who had been taken over by scientists. It was a sterile environment and I had no emotion. —*Doreen*

⟿ At first I felt numb and no feelings or emotions. I went to the NICU to see her. She did well after her first surgery but it all felt unreal. After about the third day, I went to see her and they had her in a little cap and a blanket I had made for her. It seemed like all the ice and coldness around me melted away and I just felt a deep love and sadness for her. —*Debbie*

Fortunately, fewer health care practitioners insist on admitting dying babies to the NICU, unless the parents request a thorough evaluation. The days of intensive care at all costs and regardless of parents' wishes are coming to an end, yielding to an alternate path of allowing parents to honor their baby's natural life and death.

IF YOUR BABY LIVES AFTER BIRTH

Many parents worry about what their time together will be like if the baby lives for more than a brief moment after birth. But when the time comes, most parents discover it feels natural—and more magical than they dreamed possible.

⟿ It seemed like a dream. We almost forgot she was sick. We just savored every moment. We didn't have time to be scared. It was a blessing. —*Delsa*

⟿ It was almost like time was standing still. —*Heidi*

⟿ We continued to hold Lily and talk to her, basking in her existence. Even though I knew that she wouldn't be with us for very long, I couldn't help but be happy around her. She was doing the best that she could, and that was all that we could ask. She was the vision of sweetness and innocence. Indeed, she was pure, just as her name means. —*Katharine*

↝ It was the most happy time I ever had. We were so grateful that Anouk was alive. —*Monika*

↝ Seeing the nurses talking to and touching the baby made it seem OK for me to do that. I didn't realize that I should, that it would be good. One of the nurses picked up my baby and laid him over my right arm. And then she said with so much care, "Ohhh, he just opened his eye—he knows he's with his mom." —*Kimberly Anne*

Particularly if you've been able to adjust to your baby's diagnosis and feel prepared for your baby's condition, time after birth can be imbued with celebration rather than mourning. Your time parenting your newborn is a natural extension of the care you lavished on your baby during the pregnancy.

↝ The day he was born, that was the best day ever. I got to meet him. I got to hold him. Everybody came. Everybody in our family that we wanted there was there. By the end of the day, everybody was there, he was there. There were tears, certainly, because we knew what was going to happen. That was the hello day. It was very celebratory. —*Jill N.*

↝ Every minute I had with her was cherished. The night after she was born I could not sleep at all due to all the excitement and a bad head cold. I sat up most of the night holding Anya in my lap. She was so awake and active during this time. I remember spending quite a bit of time looking at her while she studied my face. —*Steve*

↝ I wasn't really sad after he was born—I was as excited as if he had been a healthy baby. I was excited every time he would breathe and make sounds, even though I knew every one was potentially his last. —*Greg*

↝ The time right after our son was born was very exciting. It was the same excitement I felt when our first son was born—we were proud parents, again! —*Deanna*

Welcoming Baby

↶ We wanted to throw her a birthday party in the delivery room. My husband and I had a special birthday cake made. We read *Goodnight Moon* to her while I was pregnant, so we had the cake decorated with a cow jumping over the moon. —*Delsa*

Because your baby's life will be short, every moment is cherished. You may feel filled with happiness and gratitude for all you get to experience with your baby. At the same time you may feel deep sadness, aware that your time is fleeting.

↶ I held her for a long time, a little difficult because of the C-section but the nurses tried their hardest to help with this. I was so sad that her life would end soon. I wanted to remember everything about her. I just stroked her head and cheeks, kissed her and told her how much I loved her over and over again. —*Sherry*

↶ The four hours of Maggie's life were so joyful for me. I felt grateful for every second we had her. She was extraordinarily present during her entire life—looking around, crying, smiling (sounds incredible—but it was true). —*Alessandra*

↶ This time was very precious. I was so happy to finally see her. Lily and I took a bath together. We invited the rest of our family in for a baptism, which our pastor came to perform. The rest of the day we made mementos of foot and handprints, which our 5-year-old son helped to create. We read to her. We invited a few other friends to come to meet her. We took lots of pictures in the early evening. Our time with her was just right and very serene. —*Katharine*

↶ The first twenty-four hours all I did was hold Grace and try and memorize her. I was expecting her to go any minute. It was surreal. When the next morning rose through the window, I couldn't believe I was getting another day. I thanked God for more time and soaked her all in. My family was with me and everyone held her. —*Chris*

↶ We just watched her so closely for the entire forty-five minutes. We saw her take little breaths. She couldn't do much else, but just watching the breathing was beautiful. It was truly amazing, the closest to a miracle that I'll probably ever experience. Ashley was wrapped in a blanket and I held her on my chest. I stroked her hair and touched her face the entire time. Her grandparents, the doctor, the nurse, and our minister surrounded the bed. I really believe Ashley could feel how much we all loved her. Earlier that morning the nurse didn't think Ashley would even make it to birth alive, so having those forty-five minutes with her was awesome. It was such a beautiful time, a memory we'll hold in our hearts for the rest of our lives. —*Shellie*

Fathers in particular can shine after the birth, because they, unlike the mothers, can be up and about immediately after birth.

My husband was so *proud!* He walked around holding his two baby girls. —*Allison*

My husband held Anya like a pro. He'd held so few babies in his life, and she just fit perfectly in the crook of his arm. —*Delsa*

My husband was a proud father. He said that it felt good to go back into the waiting room and tell our families the good news. —*Rebecca J.*

Our time with Baby Gianna was my finest hour—ever. —*John*

Difficulty Being with Your Baby

Not all parents find it so rewarding to spend time with their baby. For some, being with their baby feels too shocking or sorrowful to bear at first. Perhaps you had been in denial about your baby's condition or held out fervent hope that the doctors were wrong. Perhaps you had been distancing yourself in a futile attempt to experience as little grief as possible. Sometimes it's the father, who hasn't spent months feeling this growing life within, who is freshly grief-stricken by the reality. You may need time to adjust to what you are witnessing.

This time was incredibly difficult for my husband. He spent much of the time crying in the bathroom and could not bring himself to bond with the baby. —*Samantha*

During our visits to the NICU, I was overjoyed. I got my miracle I prayed for—I met him alive! My husband was devastated—he did not get the healthy baby he had prayed for. I spent our visits smiling and cooing over my miracle boy. My husband spent those moments sobbing at the sight of his much-loved son so very sick. Jordan was hooked to a ventilator, heart monitors, IVs, and a very tiny blood pressure cuff. I guess I didn't notice that stuff so much; I just saw my miracle staring up at me, squeezing my finger with so much love. My husband saw his tiny newborn, so very sick, supported in life by so many machines. We later read the NICU nurses' reports, which actually documented the differences in how we were coping. What they didn't know is that I had spent the previous twelve weeks sobbing and praying for the miracle of a moment to look into his eyes, while my husband had spent twelve weeks believing his son was going to be just fine. —*Jenny D.*

Feeding, Soothing, Sleeping

Perhaps the most precious moments are those that are the simplest: feeding, soothing, and admiring your baby as he or she sleeps.

As explained in Chapter 5, newborns typically aren't hungry for the first day or so after birth. In addition, for a dying baby, nourishment is unnecessary and could even be a burden. If a baby is not imminently dying, the mother can try bringing the baby to her breast or placing drops of milk in the baby's mouth. Even having your baby suck on your finger can be rewarding and memorable.

I cherished the times I got to breastfeed Anya. It was something only I could provide. It was our special time. I felt like I was giving her life. —*Delsa*

During our hospital stay, I tried breastfeeding but Sarina never really had the energy to suck. This was a big sign to me that she was truly sick. That and her tiny cry. She was very calm and peaceful, and her cry seemed so quiet. Not that of a normal newborn. We held her and rocked her and told her we loved her the whole time. We kept her wrapped up in cozy warm blankets and did all that was possible to keep her comfortable. She never seemed like she was in any pain, and the doctor continued to reassure us that she wasn't, that she would just get weaker and weaker until she would peacefully pass on. —*Christine*

⌐ At one point, we were concerned that the constant flow of oxygen from the mask was drying out his mouth, so we wet my finger with some water and moistened his lip and tongue. His tongue found my finger and sucked so strongly. I never would have imagined that this would have meant so much to me, but it did. Just feeling his tongue on my finger was a vicarious substitute for nursing him, I guess. I was also able to gently feel around in his mouth since the bilateral cleft was so foreign to us. For the remainder of his life, we kept a clean, moist finger in his mouth for him to suck. It was definitely one of our special bonding moments with him. —*Heidi*

Many families describe the sweetness of watching their baby sleep or cuddling in bed together as a family.

⌐ I would just lie there with my baby and my husband in the hospital bed and stare at my baby. I would wake my husband up from time to time because I was worried about Noah dying. I then would go back to staring at Noah and thinking that he was the most beautiful little boy that I've ever seen. I remember thinking that our son is a miracle. Here he is alive and in bed with me and we are covered in blankets and we are warm and we are OK for now. —*Jenny A.*

⌐ My husband, Sarina, and I settled into bed for our first night together. Sarina was sleeping peacefully between us, and we just stared at her. We told her how perfect and beautiful she was, and that we loved her very much. We touched her and held her perfect little hands. We hardly slept that night because we didn't want to be asleep when she died. —*Christine*

⌐ He was most at ease when he was resting on my belly. It was like he knew that was home for the last nine months. The first day, he really only relaxed when he was with me; however, by the second day, he was very relaxed when he was with his daddy as well. —*Heidi*

Welcoming Baby

Spiritual Rituals

For many families, spiritual ritual is deeply important and meaningful. (For more information, see the discussion in Chapter 6.) Whatever your religion, tradition, or beliefs, ritual can confer acknowledgment of your baby's life and validation of your role as parents.

⟿ While our priest and dear friend was reading the Rite of Baptism, his voice began to crack with emotion, and I could feel a lump forming in my throat. —*John*

⟿ The baptism was wonderful. All stood in a circle around the room. My husband held Nora and I held Anika. I don't remember much except the feeling of being serious, the joy and happiness at the same time. It felt right for them to go through this ritual together. My twin girls. —*Kristi F.*

⟿ The day after Sarina was born, we had her baptized. We did this more for my husband's parents than for ourselves, since we are not very religious. However, it is something I am so grateful we did. It was something special and meaningful in Sarina's short life that we have to hold onto. —*Christine*

Photographs

⟿ Everyone took pictures, rolls of pictures. I remembered looking at some of the photos online and saying, "How can these people be smiling?" But there I was, holding my daughter and smiling. I had Emily, for however briefly. Why wouldn't I smile? —*Jane T.*

⟿ We took *lots* of pictures. I felt like she was having some kind of modeling shoot. —*Katharine*

As described in Chapter 6, taking photographs of your baby—whether the baby is alive or not—is not only perfectly acceptable but tremendously important for many families. This is your time to capture images of your baby and everyone expressing their love and devotion.

Time with Siblings

⌒ I worried a great deal about our sons, ages 6 and 2. I didn't want for them to be traumatized by this experience. After reading a great deal and talking with other families who had gone through infant loss, we decided to have them see Gianna and we are so glad we did. We have video of my 2-year-old lovingly caressing his baby sister's beautiful, perfect toes while singing "Tickle, tickle, tickle"; snapshots of our 6-year-old kissing his baby sister's sweet face and head full of dark hair. The moments we shared with Baby Gianna, despite the heartache, were the best thirty minutes our family has ever experienced. *—Jennifer*

As discussed in Chapters 3 and 4, much can be done to prepare siblings for meeting their baby brother or sister. Fears about including older children typically dissolve once the time finally arrives. Parents are often relieved and even awed to witness how natural, loving, and matter-of-fact older children can be.

⌒ I was overwhelmed at seeing the delight her brothers—7 and 5 at the time—took in meeting her, talking to her, holding her, loving her. The boys were at the hospital within a half hour of her birth and adored her. It was incredible to see the three of them together. There was one point when Harry was holding her and Charlie was next to him, with one hand on Maggie and the other on Harry—the three of them formed a perfect triangle, each of them sharing and receiving a lifetime of love. It was absolutely beautiful. My three perfect children all together. The pictures of that extraordinary scene are my most prized possessions. *—Alessandra*

⌒ When my older daughter held her little sister and sang to her, it felt like the whole world stopped for a few minutes. I cannot describe how wonderful it was. I wish everyone could have been there to experience it. I felt so lucky to have the two of them as my daughters. *—Holly*

⌒ I have a vivid memory of my two older children meeting Habib for the first time. My 4-year-old daughter was holding him

Welcoming Baby

in her arms and staring at him. My 2-year-old son was standing next to them and looking at the baby, and then he carefully lifted his index finger and gently touched his cleft lip. I also remember Habib's innocent, calm face, which seemed like it had completely surrendered. —*Azima*

⌐ Our older girls saw only a sister who needed to be loved and touched. It was sweet how they made sure her proboscis was somewhat straight on her face as we took photos and bathed her. When my nephews came to visit the next morning, the 5-year-old held her, then turned to his 2-year-old brother and said, "She's just like us except her nose is up higher." —*Brenda*

Children generally love to be involved and to have something to do. Depending on their ages, you can enlist them in helping you with the baby, just like any proud big brother or sister. This is their chance to make memories too.

⌐ Our older son spent time showing Lily our book that we had been working on with messages, art, and pressed flowers. He taught her all of the flower names that he remembered and that his favorites are zinnias. We read her a couple of books, and he shared his baby toys with her. Before our wonderful nurse left for the day, she helped us do Lily's "arts and crafts" projects. Our older son enjoyed this part a lot. We got a shell filled with plaster of Paris and then imprinted with her toes. We made a plaster of Paris kit of handprints and footprints, and he helped. —*Katharine*

⌐ When one of the nurses was giving Aubrielle her bath, she noticed that our older daughter was very interested. So the nurse grabbed a chair for her to stand on, then helped our older daughter give Aubrielle her bath. I loved watching. It was beautiful and special. —*Holly*

Time with Family and Friends

Inviting family and friends to meet your baby widens the circle of support around you and your baby. Photographs depicting them tenderly holding your baby can be especially affirming.

A Gift of Time

⌐ A favorite memory is when my parents came to meet Thomas while we were in the recovery room. We have this wonderful picture of it; I am holding Thomas and they are next to my bed looking at him and smiling. My dad is even holding onto his hand. If you didn't know the real story you would just think that they are just like every other set of "normal" grandparents admiring their new grandchild. —*Kathleen*

⌐ We had planned to have our older son there when the baby was born. The plan was that no one else would be there, just us. Once we had our baby, our feelings changed and we were overcome with the excitement of our second beautiful child. It didn't matter what the diagnosis was; he was our son and we were proud and blessed to have him. We immediately called everyone in the family and invited them to come. —*Deanna*

⌐ Friends and family started coming. Everyone held him and we took many, many pictures. It was a special, reverent time. —*Tracy*

⌐ Luke's birth was actually joyful, and when our other kids came it was like a party room! My mom had had a very difficult time during my pregnancy, so seeing her holding her grandson was wonderful. She really hadn't wanted to hold him, but she needed to and said it was one of the best things she did. —*Sue*

Additional Medical Decisions for Your Baby after Birth

If your baby is not imminently dying, you may need to make additional decisions about medical care after birth. The desire to protect the baby from pain is paramount for many parents. You may be able to protect your baby from some painful procedures entirely.

⌐ The neonatalogist wanted to draw some blood to run tests and confirm the diagnosis after our son was born. I refused to allow my son to be stuck with a needle for that. I made them use a cord blood sample, which ended up costing my husband and I quite a bit extra. I didn't care. —*Kathleen*

⌐ As we had been all during the pregnancy, we were concerned about any pain he may be experiencing. One of our nurses responded to our concerns so beautifully, saying that he would have been in a lot more pain several months ago if we had made a different decision—and he would not have known our touch and the extent of our love for him. Hearing that from the nurse helped console us. —*Heidi*

Sometimes a baby is born with a condition more—or less—severe than anticipated, and parents may change their minds about medical intervention. If your baby needs to be evaluated or if you put off decision-making until after birth, you may be asked to make some decisions right away. Or you may be asked simply to confirm the wishes already spelled out in your birth plan. Communicating your wishes regarding resuscitation, feeding tubes, or other life-prolonging treatments can confront you with the stark reality that your baby is very ill.

I didn't even really think about the fact that after she was born, medical decisions might even be harder. I thought the hard decisions were already made, but I think it was harder after. It was harder for my husband, for sure. Because then it's not just someone else's baby you're talking about, or someone on a Web page. It's your own baby, right there in front of you. —*Bridget*

The neonatologist came to me with a sheet of paper for me to sign. I remember him reading it to me, but I didn't want to listen. It was the DNR—do not resuscitate. As I held onto the pen, looking down and seeing my husband's signature already on it, I knew this was for real. Regardless of our son looking and sounding so healthy, he was terminally ill. This was not a dream. My son, my baby was going to die. —*Amy*

By the time their baby is born, parents vary in how much they've been able to come to terms with decisions about medical intervention. You may have done all your medical research and soul-searching during the pregnancy and feel at peace with your desire to surround your baby with only love and comfort. But if you decided to wait and see, saving decision-making until after your baby's birth, you may find yourself struggling with an urge to intervene. Or if you'd hoped and prayed for a miracle during your pregnancy, you may feel distraught as you are confronted with the reality. Even if previous decisions were confirmed by your baby's condition after birth, you still may feel compelled to take action. This normal and common impulse is a reflection of your natural parenting instinct to fight for your child's life. If it was possible for your baby to live, not just survive but also thrive, of course you would order up the interventions that could make that happen. But in the absence of any realistic or humane options, allowing your baby to live out his or her natural life is a true measure of your parental devotion. There *are* fates worse than death. As many parents observe, resisting this urge to intervene and instead enveloping their baby in comfort may be the most unselfish act they ever carry out.

⌒ We held our breath. But Nora wasn't going to die right away. It took a while to get used to that. But the next day after she was born, the doctor heard the heart murmur. I was sad. I had held out hope that they were wrong, that she didn't really have hypoplastic left heart syndrome. We decided that it was pointless to drive for another consultation with experts. We would just use up valuable time. It was hard to completely let go, but it was what we wanted for Nora. We wanted her to be loved and held and cuddled, not inspected and poked and analyzed. —*Kristi F.*

Palliative Care

Now that your baby is born, more conventional hospice and palliative care treatments can be pulled into action. (For more information, see the discussion in Chapters 2 and 5.) If it appears that your baby will live for more than a few hours and if you haven't already made contact, ask if your hospital has a pediatric palliative care team or call a hospice and ask someone to visit you and your baby in the hospital.

TAKING BABY HOME

Some babies can be discharged from the hospital and go home. Perhaps this is something you've dreamed of doing; perhaps this is unexpected and even frightening. If you hadn't planned to bring your baby home, leaving the security of the hospital may feel like you are casting aside your safety net. But in many cases, when the mother is able to go home, the baby is able to go home too. Sometimes this decision can be made within a day or two after birth.

⁓ After a day and a half in the hospital, we made the decision to take Sarina home. It was a big decision, but it felt right. Before her birth, I was certain that I wanted the whole experience to take place in the hospital, where there were nurses and doctors to help us out no matter what. However, after she was born, it just felt right to take her home, to show her where "home" was, to make memories at home as well. She was part of our family, and would continue to be even when she died, so taking her home made it more real, it gave us more to hold onto, more to remember. —*Christine*

⁓ After many conversations with caregivers, we decided to bring him home, and if he was around long enough to be strong enough for a surgery, we would bring him back. Josiah was not given a body that would last a normal lifetime. His time would be short, and we wanted it to be sweet. We didn't want to keep him here longer than his body could last, causing unnecessary suffering, but we also didn't want to cut his life short by not doing something we could have. It was a fine line, and we were going to let Josiah decide. We were bringing him home, giving him the freedom to live as long as he could—and also giving him the freedom to go when his body couldn't do it anymore. —*Behka*

⁓ With quite a bit of trepidation we brought Lucy home about forty-four hours after delivery. She was failing, and I was afraid that she would die in the car seat on the way home. At the same time we didn't really want to take the pediatrician up on her offer just to stay in the hospital until she died. We had no idea when that would be. —*Jane G.*

If your baby is in the hospital for days or weeks, you may settle into a routine and become attached to the staff caring for your baby. Going home can be an intimidating proposition. How can your baby need round-the-clock medical care one day and go home under your care the next? It's important to know that you can acquire the necessary caregiving skills while in the hospital. Then you'll have those skills along with the many comforts and advantages of being at home. You can also enlist the help of home health care or hospice.

I never dreamed or planned of anything beyond Grace's birth. I never bought any baby things. With the change in Grace's condition, I was totally unprepared. After day 5, I had to leave the hospital without my daughter. She stayed in the special care nursery. I would go up each day and spend eight to ten hours with Grace. The nursing staff was so kind to us. They let me know that if she was having trouble at night, someone would hold her. They comforted me in letting me know that Grace would not die alone if I couldn't be there. We became very comfortable in the nursery. I learned how to care for Grace and become her nurse. I learned how to insert a feeding tube, how to read and monitor the apnea machine, and how to be a mom to a little girl with special needs. After about two weeks, hospice started to talk to us again about taking Grace home. I was very scared because we had become so comfortable in the nursery. I knew we had to take her home, but I was terrified about having Grace die at home especially with my older girls at home. A hospice worker counseled us and explained that we had included the girls in the whole story and to leave them out of this part would be hard on them. They had been away from me for about a month, and it was time for us to be a family again. She and her gentle way, along with the nurses, calmed me down and a week later we did bring Grace home with hospice support. Grace came home on her one-month birthday. It was bittersweet to leave the nursery because we had become so close to the staff. —*Chris*

Once you've decided to take the leap, it's time to go home. It's a satisfying parental milestone, even though it can be tinged with mixed emotions. You may be nervous, but your nurturing instincts can soon take over, building your confidence. You may adjust more easily than you think is possible.

As the aide pushed me into the elevator, I was holding my two precious babies, dressed in their pink and blue, and the other occupants started oohing and aahing over my twins. In some ways that was special—it was the only time that anybody really was excited for my twins in a "normal" way, but it was so sad, because only I knew that I was bringing one of my twins home to die.

—*Jane G.*

I remember taking both girls out to the car. My husband and I were nervous to be alone with them, without the support of the hospital and with the unknown of death. Once we got home, though, it felt so right. —*Kristi F.*

It was so natural for us to bring her home. We just put her in the back seat—didn't even think twice about it, even with all her health problems. We just loved her. It just kicked in and it just became natural. —*Bianca*

With your first kid, bringing the baby home is a terror because you don't know what you're into as a new parent. You've got this fragile thing you're responsible for. With the second kid, there's still some of that, but you're trying to figure out how you're going to juggle the second kid with the first kid. With Adriana, our third child, we had five and a half months to think things over. We knew what the score was. There was a lot of pressure taken off. She wasn't going to live very long, and there wasn't a damn thing we could do about it. So we were just going to take good care of her during the time we had her. And that was that. —*David D.*

Practical Considerations

We didn't know what to expect, so I never really thought about what would happen if she did come home. What do I do? I didn't read any of the baby books and those things. That was a bit of a panic moment; what do I do now? But we kind of let her do what she was going to do. —*Bridget*

Since we did not expect him to live long enough to come home, we were not ready. While I was in the hospital, I called a friend to

A Gift of Time

buy a few essential items and bring them to the hospital so I could take the baby home. The Perinatal Comfort Care program gave us a car seat. The hospital gave us some diapers, formula, feeding tubes, and syringes to take home so we could feed him. At the hospital we signed a DNR (do not resuscitate) sheet, in case we called the paramedics at home. I was definitely not ready for that. —*Azima*

If your baby is able to come home with you, you'll have practical considerations you may not have planned for: feeding, clothing, diapering, bathing. You'll likely want to spend your time with your baby rather than doing emergency shopping, so this is a perfect time to enlist family, friends, neighbors, even co-workers in helping you stock your nursery. They may be delighted to spring into action for you.

My wife's parents stayed with us the first week, and we sent them to Target every day. We had nothing, because we didn't want to come home to a baby room and have no baby. —*James*

We were so careful about not buying too much: Let's just buy one package of diapers. OK, one more package of diapers. —*Jill K.*

Normal adjustments to newborn feeding may be complicated by physical conditions in your baby such as a cleft palate or lack of a strong sucking ability. Your caregivers or organizations devoted to your baby's condition should be able to offer practical suggestions.[3]

The nights were the hardest—neither my husband or I wanted to fall asleep; one of us was always awake. Sarina seemed more restless at night, and we worried that she was hungry and in pain. The nurse gave us glucose water to keep her hydrated; Sarina didn't seem to want to drink from the breast or from the bottle. —*Christine*

I couldn't breastfeed her because she didn't have the suck reflex; she wasn't strong enough for that. I pumped and fed her through the feeding tube every three hours. —*Bianca*

Hospice in Your Home

Hospice support can significantly lessen your anxiety and raise your feelings of confidence in caring for your baby. Ideally, pediatric hospice care is in your area. But even hospice programs more accustomed to caring for elderly patients may be able to tailor their resources for you.

The hospice team was key in giving us the support we needed to continue. There were two nurses, a social worker, a pastoral care worker, a nutritionist, and a pediatric intensivist. The nurses would stop by every morning to check Grace. Basically, we were doing the care ourselves. Things were getting back to "normal." It was so good to be home. I never dreamed I would get the time I was getting. —*Chris*

Our hospice nurse visited us two to three times per week. We were provided with all of the medications to take care of Noah. She brought gauze and bandages to ensure that Noah's encephalocele was covered to prevent infection. The hospice nurses all supported us with the utmost professional care to ensure that Noah was not in pain or suffering and that all of our needs and concerns as parents were met. —*Jenny A.*

Sarina lived another day and a half at home. I was more comfortable at home, in our own bed, and a nurse came to visit us often to make sure everything was OK. —*Christine*

Time Together at Home

Whether your baby's time at home is relatively brief—a day or two—or stretches into weeks or even months, this is your time to savor. There are many precious, intimate moments to be had.

Nora had her eyes open a lot. She was taking everything in. She was relaxed and easily soothed. We all slept together, and it was heaven for me to have our older son and my husband and the newborn twins all next to me, quiet, relaxed with nothing to think about except to just be and soak it all in. My husband and I would take turns holding Nora as she was awake a lot at night. I didn't really sleep since I didn't want to miss anything with her. —*Kristi F.*

⌐ My most cherished memories are at night. I would sleep with her on my stomach and spend the whole night just holding her.
—Debbie

⌐ My most precious memories of Grace have to do with being her mom, doing the things for her that I did for my other two. Unwrapping her, bathing her, changing her, putting lotion on her, and holding on tight. She was a little baby who was loved. I also look back and smile at the things we did that were "normal" like going for a walk around the block. The nights were my quiet time with Grace alone. I would sleep on the couch with Grace on my chest and feel her warmth, her breath and her heartbeat—and thank God for another day. —*Chris*

⌐ After my wife gave him his baths, I would pick up my little Noah Sam and hold him in both of my hands because he was such a cute and tiny little baby. I would cradle him close to me and I would kiss him over and over again and I never, ever wanted to put him down. He was my sweet and innocent little boy. I loved to hold my son. That was my favorite time of the day. Because of his condition, we were never sure if movement would hurt Noah. Eventually we learned that we could gently pick him up and lay him against our chests. Noah loved the warmth and closeness from being held close to us. He even slept the best when he was lying on one of us. I would lie in bed for hours and burp him after I fed him his bottle and then I would let him sleep all nuzzled close on my chest. Those times with Noah, I will never forget. They are forever a part of me. —*Todd*

As you get to know your baby, you may be able to discern subtle aspects of your baby's personality or your baby's responses. You may even have enough time to celebrate some milestones and holidays and include your baby in family fun. When you have more than a few days at home with your baby, instead of only focusing on impending death, you get to focus on life.

◞ We did one-month birthdays. We did week birthdays. We did day birthdays. —*James*

◞ We thought, *Wow, we made it to Thanksgiving. Wow, we made it to Christmas.* Each day was a milestone. —*Bianca*

◞ Day 21: Life is a party! So far, Josiah had eaten out at Olive Garden with mom and dad, attended his siblings' baseball games, had a movie night with the family, and received many hugs and kisses from his family. To make as many memories as possible for our children, we had them each choose a fun family activity they would like to do, so basically we were on "party schedule" for the next while. It may sound heartless, that we had a dying baby and we were out setting the world on fire. But we wanted Josiah to experience as much of life as possible, and again, doing things is empowering. Just sitting around waiting while death is at the door is an exhausting experience; we tried it that way with our other baby who died. —*Behka*

Despite the savoring and celebrating, there are challenging times. You're deeply concerned about your baby, and you know the end is coming. At the same time, you can be grateful for the opportunity to experience it at all.

◞ Even as she was going downhill, we knew we'd beaten a lot of odds. —*David D.*

Siblings at Home

◞ Once we brought Rose home, my other children were so wonderful. They wanted to hold her and help with her tube feeding. Rose didn't have thumbs and they were curious about that, but it was pretty matter-of-fact: They'd tell people she didn't have thumbs. We tried to keep our normal schedule as much as we could. We brought Rose to the park and to gymnastics. I do remember feeling torn between having enough time with my other children and enough time with Rose. That's why it was so comforting to sleep with her all night. —*Debbie*

It was confusing for our other children because we said we probably won't be bringing home a baby from the hospital, and then we did. And then they didn't understand, because she looked normal. —*Bianca*

If you have other children at home, you'll have even more factors to juggle. There's the daily routine of making sure everyone gets fed, dressed, bathed, and attended to, which as anyone with young children knows is a full-time job in itself. Family and friends may be eager to help you with cooking and household tasks, and they also may be delighted to take your other children for an outing or simply keep an eye on them in your home so you can tend to the baby.

Even more important is helping siblings manage emotionally. They may need to be reminded that it's OK to cry—and it's OK to laugh and play. You can remind them that it's OK for mom and dad to cry too; everyone is sad that the baby won't be able to stay long, but you'll all get through it together. They can feel like a special big brother or big sister by helping fetch diapers or singing to the baby. Even if they aren't old enough to remember these experiences later, someday you can use photographs and storytelling to show how important they were in the life of their baby sibling. If you are fortunate to have a child life specialist available through your hospital or hospice, their counsel and support can be invaluable (see also Chapter 3).

Family and Friends at Home

Time at home also allows you the opportunity to invite family and friends to participate further in the life of your baby. One of many benefits is that your baby becomes tangibly real to others, more than if they were unable to meet your baby in person or only saw photographs.

I enjoyed sharing her with my family once we got her home. I sat and watched as everyone took turns holding her and telling her stories. —*Steve*

⌐ Because we got so much time, we opened our home and hearts to many, many people as we shared our daughter, Grace. Sometimes I think I was selfish because I wanted many people to hold her. My rationale was that by holding her, Grace became real to them—and that all of these people would remember her with me when she was gone. She was really here and she mattered. Grandparents, cousins, friends from work, neighbors, and friends of the family all came into our home and held her. The simple act of holding this precious, fragile child was a witness to her life. I took a picture of each and every person who held Grace. Those pictures are precious to me now. —*Chris*

Depending on how stable your baby is, you may want to share him or her with a wider audience such as your neighbors, co-workers, or religious community. Doing so can have the powerful effect of building a broader social network that you can lean on for support.

Uncertainty

⌐ It was easy in terms of taking care of him physically, but emotionally, it was extremely difficult. Every moment, I would wonder if this was it. Every day, I would wonder if he would live another day. In essence, I was waiting for the angel of death to arrive and take my baby's soul away. —*Azima*

⌐ I remember thinking, *OK, we've had another breakfast with him, will we have another lunch too? —Melanie*

⌐ After about the fourth day, she was still alive—a miracle. All I knew is that the doctor told us that we could stop counting minutes and hours—instead we would be counting days, weeks, and maybe months. I didn't know if I was happy or scared to death. —*Chris*

Anticipating the death of a loved one is always difficult, whether the ailing person is a newborn or is very elderly. Predicting how much time a person has left to live is a notoriously fallible endeavor. You may have been given a ballpark estimate, but in many cases it's little more than a guess. Living with this uncertainty can pose its own challenges.

⌐ Everybody talks about living in the moment. But it's impossible to do on a day-in, day-out basis forever. You can't exist in that moment for an extended period of time, because you have to pay bills. For us, we just gave up on the thought of time. —*James*

⌐ We didn't know what to expect, so we didn't plan for anything in particular. We were told that Ramona would not have a long life, but they couldn't say just how long it would be. So I had to live every day as if she could be gone the next day. I tried to spend as much quality time with her as I could and wanted to make her as happy as I could. After a while, I just tried to live like a normal person. —*Rebecca J.*

If your baby continues to live longer than expected, this will require another major adjustment and reorientation for you.

⌐ It was very difficult to shift gears so completely and adjust to Paul living. We were stunned. We were definitely not expecting it and not prepared for it. We sat in the cardiologist's office not really knowing what to say. What can you say? "Wow, that's great" just doesn't fit. So here we are today, four years later, and still our life with Paul is a continual adjustment. I think we do very well most of the time, but I do often think about the fact that Paul is dying. Having said that, we are also deeply grateful for the time we've had, and we know what most families have been through with the same diagnosis. Being told we could expect to have him for ten years was like winning the lottery. We love him and we'll continue to give him all the tender care we can until our good Lord wants him home. —*Melanie*

Negative Reactions from Others

One gift of having your baby live long enough to go home with you is that you might have the pleasure of taking your baby with you on errands or just a visit to the doctor. Simple, everyday life takes on added sweetness with your baby in tow.

Unfortunately, it's possible you might run into intolerant people who refuse to recognize the intrinsic value of your baby.

⌐ A woman said to me, "Oh, how old is your baby? What's wrong with her?" I said she has Trisomy 18. She said, "What's she going to be like when she grows up?" I said, well, she's not. She's going to die. She said, "Did you know before she was born?" I said yes, and she said, "Oh, that's too bad. You must have found out when it was too late to have an abortion." I just stood there and thought, *I can't believe you just said that to me. How can you look at my daughter and say I should have had an abortion?* I just said, "We chose to have her for as long as we can." I wanted to say something nasty, but I couldn't think of anything fast enough. —*Bianca*

Comments like this are a reflection of prejudice and ignorance, not in any way a valid reflection on your baby or on you as a parent. Your love for your baby may or may not persuade an uninformed bystander to reconsider his or her biases, but that's ultimately beside the point. The point is that your love for your baby makes all the difference in the world for the two of you.

Medical Decisions at Home

Jill K.: Alaina got a feeding tube when she was 4 months old. Prior to that, her feedings would last three hours. I don't think at the time we realized how different that was. We just thought, well, everyone deals with getting up at night, we just have to buck up and deal with it too. Finally they said she was using more calories eating than she was taking in. They asked if we wanted to think about a feeding tube.

James: That was the only intervention we did with her. One thing we struggled with was, it's a slippery slope. How much further do we go here? How about if she has trouble breathing? Where do we stop? It was a hard step for us, but I think was justified, because after she got the feeding tube, she really grew, and she was happier.

If your baby continues to live longer than expected, more medical decisions may need to be made. You may want to consider interventions that improve quality of life—for your baby *and* you. For example, feeding tubes, supplemental oxygen, and seizure medications can be part of palliative care, not aggressive attempts to extend life, and they won't interfere with your baby living a natural life. Or perhaps an antibiotic might be needed at some point to eliminate a simple infection and keep your baby more comfortable. After making it this far, it's likely that you have a team of caregivers whom you trust—and who have fallen head-over-heels in love with your baby. They can be your sounding board and can offer you sage advice. Just like you've done since the day of your diagnosis, you can continue to let your baby lead you.

Holding Back and Coming to Terms

When Alaina was lasting longer than two weeks, one thing I was struggling with a lot, and I spoke to the perinatal hospice chaplain about it, was that I wanted her to die. Because I was ready to suffer the loss and grief, and the waiting was getting excruciating. The best thing he did for me was to tell me I'm not insane. I'm not crazy for these thoughts. Everyone going through something like this has those thoughts. —*James*

No matter how long your baby lives, it's a normal to try to keep some distance in an attempt to protect yourself emotionally. Or the uncertainty of when your baby will die can wear on you and the stress can lead to trouble with depression or anxiety. It's even possible that well-meaning family and friends or caregivers may suggest it will be easier for you if you don't get too attached to your baby. This is reminiscent of advice you may have received to terminate your pregnancy and to forget about it and move on. Not only does it have overtones of that outdated advice, it doesn't work. You already are attached, whether you're acknowledging it or not. The question is what to do about it.

I wasn't opening myself up to Alaina. I wasn't allowing her to get inside, because I thought it would be so much harder. And it was. But it was so worth it. —*James*

eight

⁓

Saying Goodbye

Holding On and Letting Go

⁓ At the end, Nora was in my arms. Her twin sister lay between my husband and me, and her big brother was on the other side of my husband, sleeping. Nora's eyes were open, waiting for the light and for the day to come. The sun was making it bright outside, but there wasn't any sun because it was very foggy. My husband said that the spirits are closer when it is foggy. Her color was pale, but she wasn't blotchy like she was before. Her breaths were small and close together. My husband and I each had one of her hands in our fingers. We lay there and then I looked and her mouth was closed. She had been breathing through her mouth. I asked my husband if she was gone and we felt her chest and she was. It was so peaceful that I don't know the moment she died, but it also felt like a time longer than a moment. I cried and held her and cried. My heart broke. All that we had dreaded, it was over. We wanted it to be over, but we didn't want it ever to be over. —*Kristi F.*

For the vast majority of families whose baby has a terminal prenatal diagnosis, the diagnosis does turn out to be correct and the baby's life does come to an end. It is normal to have fear and anxiety about your baby's death, especially if you have never witnessed someone dying or seen someone who is dead. Reading other parents' descriptions of their baby's death and their experiences of saying goodbye may help ease some of your apprehension about your baby's last moments. Other parents' stories also may give you ideas for making the most of the time you can spend with your baby's body, as well as ideas for commemorating your baby's life with a funeral or memorial service.

⁓ It is like walking in another dimension. —*Dana*

If your baby is born alive, you may have the honor and the sorrow of witnessing your baby's death. Emotionally, parenting a dying baby entails simultaneously holding on and letting go. It is a bittersweet time.

If your baby lives for more than a few hours, you may need some respite and time to take care of your own physical and mental health. It is the nature of anticipatory grieving to occasionally disengage. You need to be able to step back, process, and refuel, to be ready to reengage with your baby and the situation at hand. This dance of holding on and letting go is a way to navigate this time and cope with the upcoming final separation.

As the end draws near, you may get to a point where you know it's time to tell your baby that it's OK to go. And your love remains.

THE DYING PROCESS

The human body gives signals when it is beginning the normal, natural process of shutting down. Here are some of the physical changes as a body prepares to stop:

- *Coolness.* Hands and arms, feet, and then legs may become increasingly cool to the touch, and skin color may change. This is normal and means that blood circulation is being decreased to extremities and reserved for the most vital organs.
- *Sleepiness.* Metabolic changes mean that the baby may spend an increasing amount of time sleeping.
- *Incontinence.* Of course, even a healthy baby needs a diaper, but muscle relaxation may cause urination or a bowel movement close to the time of death.
- *Changes in breathing.* Breathing may become shallow or irregular, sometimes with pauses in breathing of five to thirty seconds or even up to a minute, followed by big breaths.
- *Lack of hunger or thirst.* This would be noticeable if your baby lives long enough to settle into a feeding pattern. As death

Saying Goodbye

nears, the body naturally begins to conserve energy and needs little or no food or drink.[1]

While your baby is dying, you may feel attuned to every nuance. It can help to remind yourself that your baby's body is following the natural flow of the dying process.

EXPERIENCES WITH BABIES AS THEY ARE DYING

For some babies, the time between birth and death is as fleeting as a breath.

⌐ Frankie lived for one minute, if that. He took one big breath when they pulled him out of me, they placed him on my chest, his mouth moved a little, and then he died. He was a mystery, I remember feeling. There wasn't nearly enough time with him—of course. —*Susan E.*

⌐ They took Eli to the warming table, and his heart rate was only thirty beats a minute. The nurse wrapped him up and asked my husband to take him back to me. We just held him. He never took a breath, he never cried. We held him, we talked to him, we sang to him. We told him we loved him. After we could tell he wasn't going to stick around, we told him it was OK to go. It was peaceful to watch him go. There was no sense that he struggled. There was no sense that he was in pain. —*Jessica*

Some have a few more minutes or hours.

⌐ The doctor really wanted to keep the room very quiet. There were no monitors or anything like that, no life-sustaining efforts. She wrapped him up and gave him to us and she left the room, and we held him for probably twenty to thirty minutes. It was hard to know exactly when he died because his breathing was really shallow and his heartbeat was really slow. I had feared that Michael would resist death and that we would watch him struggle for life. But it was so peaceful—he had no fear of death. It was all so much more peaceful than I ever could have imagined it would be, and not the least bit frightening, as I had feared it would be. —*Missy*

⟿ His heart rate was faint, and his breaths came very seldom and were labored. My husband kept thinking that with each breath he was coming around and kept trying to encourage him, but I think I just knew we were losing him. The nurse tried, albeit compassionately, to explain that the breaths we were hearing were his last—that this is what breathing often sounds like when people are passing away. All I could do was cry and moan softly. I didn't even sound like myself. I had never known pain like that. —*Christie*

⟿ Emily remained with us for two precious hours. During that time, she had an attitude of paying careful attention to all of us. She opened only one eye, but she did seem to have some hearing because she reacted to my voice and the things I said. I told her that if she had to go, it was all right—she could go. A little after 1:00 in the morning, just as the videotape ran out, she left us. —*Jane T.*

⟿ Her passing was very peaceful and gradual, as the neonatologist had told us to expect. Despite our sadness, our short time with Gianna—about thirty minutes—was filled with love and joy. It was much less traumatic than I had expected. Everything was so beautiful. It was full of love and tenderness. —*Jennifer*

Hearing is believed to be the last sense to fade before death. You may wish to talk or sing to your baby.

⟿ I remember saying over and over, "Isaac, it's your mommy. I love you so much, and I am so, so proud of you." I remember thinking, *If I could have only a few seconds to talk to Isaac, what would I want him to hear and to know?* And that was it—that I love him, and I am so proud of him. —*Stacy*

⟿ Jonah stopped breathing and his fingers and toes began to turn purple. My husband was holding him. I dropped to the floor and grabbed his little hands. We both began to cry and begged him to take another breath. After what seemed like forever, he did take a big breath, to our relief. However, we knew this was probably

Saying Goodbye

the beginning of the end. He continued to experience apnea like this sporadically for almost six more hours. Each time we would beg him to take another breath, don't leave us now! Yet, sometime around midnight, my husband and I experienced a sense of peace and we knew we could not keep begging for more time from him. My husband continued to hold him and I had Jonah's hands in mine. We told him it was OK, that he could go now. It was the hardest thing I've ever done, but we knew it was time. We talked about heaven, and I remember Jonah looked right at me as if to say, "Keep talking! This sounds great!" We continued to sing and talk to him about how thankful we were for the time we got to have with him. I kept squeezing his little hands three times for "I love you." The apnea became much more frequent and the length between taking a breath more distant. And then, he just quit taking in breaths at all and his chest quit rising. He was gone. —*Heidi*

⌐ My husband and I sat, locked our arms together, and at that moment, Kevin took his last breath. He looked so peaceful and comfortable. He looked like he was sleeping. My husband held him for a little while, and as he did, he wiped a tear from his eye and placed it onto Kevin's cheek and said, "Take my tears with you." —*Amy*

⌐ My husband and I took turns all day lying next to him on the bed, and I read scripture to him and sang to him. I would brush my cheek against his so he could smell me, feel my cheek, and know that I was near always. My husband told him stories about his mommy and daddy and our love and about how much we loved him. He sang to him and kissed him and talked to him so softly about every topic under the sun. One thing that my husband and I did was constantly reassure Noah that we were going to be OK and to not worry about us. We told him about how beautiful and peaceful heaven was going to be, and we told him that he would no longer be sick. We told him that when he was ready, to let go and go. I told him that I would miss him desperately but that I did not want him to suffer. Noah passed away in my arms as I held him. His last breath came out of his little body like he was so tired that he just could not work anymore. I wept like I have never wept before. —*Jenny A.*

A Gift of Time

Jessica: We told him about all the people who were at the hospital to meet him, everybody who loved him. And we told him it was OK to go home.

Brad: We told him we were proud of him for fighting.

Jessica: We sang "Great is Thy Faithfulness." And when I was crying too hard to get through it, the nurse picked it up and she finished it for me. Like the tears I cry now, they weren't bitter tears, they were tears of acknowledgment and pride and sorrow that we wouldn't get to see him walk, wouldn't get to hear him talk, kind of a final acknowledgment of those things. I think we sort of felt him go. It was peaceful. It wasn't traumatic, it wasn't scary. It was just us loving our son. We weren't heroes. We were just parents.

You might not even be aware of the moment of death.

It surprised me that there was no moment when she was really gone. She just sort of faded, and I could not tell that she was really gone except that she did not breathe any more. —*Laura W.*

She slipped away so peacefully. We didn't actually know when she died. It was not traumatic at all. I expected that it would be more difficult for all of us. —*Katharine*

Maggie began having apnea spells shortly after her birth. The last time, we were pretty sure she was ready to leave. We told the boys that we thought she was getting ready to die and asked them if they wanted to be with us. They didn't (at that point, they were crying) and my parents took them into the hall. She was tucked safely in my arms. My husband had his hand on her. I don't really remember if I was crying—I think my husband was. She took a few breaths, closed her eyes, and left. It was so peaceful, we wondered if she was really gone. It wasn't dramatic or loud as we worried it might be. And most importantly, she didn't seem in any pain at all. That was such an extraordinary relief. We waited a few minutes to be sure and then my husband called the doctor, who confirmed her heart had stopped beating. —*Alessandra*

Saying Goodbye

He just kept getting weaker and weaker. The nurse would come check his heartbeat to see if he was still alive. The last time, she checked then shook her head and said he's passed. My sister and I held each other and sobbed. My husband later told me that he thinks Daniel passed in his arms. I said I'm so happy that he was in someone's arms, no matter who that person was, who loved him. Daniel did not suffer and it was peaceful. —*Tracy*

She just died peacefully; she was just still and quiet and slipped away without us noticing the exact moment. She was passed around from person to person and I am not certain that I was holding her when she died. I wish I knew that I was the one holding her when she died. —*Sherry*

If family and friends are sharing these sacred moments near your baby's death, it can be a profound experience for all of you.

My husband looked at me and asked, "Is he gone?" All I could do was give one nod. Oh, the tears flooded, and, yet, Noah finally looked so peaceful. I touched his chin and kind of closed his mouth. I held him to my cheek, not wanting to ever forget the feel of his soft warm skin against my cheek. I inhaled deeply to remember that sweet new baby smell. I wanted to hold him tight and put him over my shoulder to rub his back. My mom leaned over my shoulder looking at her grandson and whispered, "Who would have wanted to miss out on this day!" —*Kristin*

After I took my time with Jordan, I passed him to his big brother Christopher. This was the only time Christopher was able to hold Jordan, and you could see such an amazing love between them. Here was this 16-year-old boy, 6 feet, 3 inches, tall, kissing his 13-inch brother goodbye. I can't begin to describe the love and sadness in the air. Benjamin was next to hold his little brother. He repeated the phrase I had heard from him so many times in the past two days, "He is so tiny." Next, Zachary held Jordan and didn't want to have to let go. The only thing harder than kissing your son goodbye, knowing he was dying, is watching your children kiss their younger sibling goodbye. No parent should ever have to see such a heartbreaking moment. Still, I think it was one of the most beautiful moments my sons and I will ever experience. —*Jenny D.*

⌐ It was so different from what I anticipated. I thought she would only live a few short minutes. I hadn't thought our families would even have time to see her alive. She lived for about forty-five minutes. We all watched her breathe, we cried, and we stroked her thick, dark hair. She died at the end of her baptism—she just stopped taking breaths. It was so peaceful, like she was going to sleep. Even though it was such a sad moment, everyone who was around the bed felt like it was the most profound experience of our lives. We're so glad we were there to surround her with love and let her go so quietly. —*Shellie*

Death at Home

For families who can take their baby home, death may happen there. The intensity, sadness, mystery, and nervous anticipation may be no different between home or hospital, and you may find it reassuring to be surrounded by the familiar comforts of home. It can help to have the support and counsel of health care providers and close family and friends during this time.

⌐ It wasn't terrifying. I think I knew that it was going to be soon. She had lost more weight and, in talking with the hospice nurse, I knew it wouldn't be long. I just had a sense. So we were getting ready for bed and I said to my husband, let's go into the nursery. We went in and held her and read her stories and talked with her and played her music. We stayed there for a few hours. I had been praying with her and telling her all along that when it was time for her to go that it would be OK. I don't think my husband had really been to that point yet; I think he was still really struggling. But that evening he was more accepting, and he had told her the same thing. I think she knew then that she could go peacefully. We went to bed around 11:30, and I fell asleep. My husband was just holding her in bed. I think he fell asleep but then he woke up because he said her breathing changed. He picked her up and she took one big breath and kind of sighed and that was it. —*Bridget*

Saying Goodbye
———
253

I called my husband at work because she was not breathing right. I said, "I think this is it." He came home and he held her. The kids were downstairs playing quietly and not wanting anything. It was almost like they knew. —*Bianca*

My baby started to have episodes of apnea, which got longer and closer to each other. He would turn completely blue. That sight sent shivers down my spine. It started in the morning of the last day of his life. Then he started breathing again only to have another episode in early afternoon. This episode scared everyone so much that my father-in-law called the paramedics. The paramedics affirmed to me that the baby's dying process had started. The Perinatal Comfort Care counselor came and spent some time with us. This apnea continued throughout the evening and into the night. Around 3:00 a.m. he had an episode which lasted for about five minutes. I remember thinking to myself, *How can a person not breathe for so long, and wouldn't that person's brain be dead by now?* He started breathing again, taking shallow, slow breaths. And then he had his last apnea around 3:20 a.m. I was staring at him and waiting for his blue skin to turn to normal. At 3:27 a.m. his skin color changed from blue to pale and I did not see him take any more breaths. I looked at my husband and said, that's it, he's gone. —*Azima*

We knew her death was coming. On the fourth night with her, we were kind of expecting it. It was hard staying awake at night, though. That night I was feeling pain, my milk was coming in, and I had a terrible headache; the past couple of days had taken a toll on me. Sarina was in our bed between the two of us. We snuggled close to her. I remember trying to stay awake. Then suddenly at around 2:00 a.m., Sarina let out a cry—a cry that was quite loud and seemed urgent. Both of us woke instantly. It was then that we knew the time had come. My husband picked Sarina up while she breathed in and out a few more times, and then it was over. I don't like to remember this moment; it hurts way too much. I prefer to remember the day she was born. However, I like to think that Sarina cried to wake us up, so we would be with her when she died. —*Christine*

We asked my older girls what they wanted us to do if Grace died at home during school hours. They told us to come and get them. Grace had a difficult night before she died, with several apnea episodes. Surprisingly, I was very calm that night and didn't wake my husband. She kept reviving herself. We had gotten used to all the apnea episodes; this was part of her condition. The next morning, my husband and I looked at Grace and thought she looked bad— very pale and limp. We gave her a bath; she loved her bath and usually would perk up. My parents came over, and my mother blessed Grace. At about 10:00 a.m.—exactly two months from her birth— my dad mentioned to me that he thought she had gone. I told him no, she was still warm. I couldn't believe it. It was peaceful, calm, and very gentle. We got the girls from school and my family all came over along with the hospice nurse. I finally had the end of the story. It was nothing that I could have planned. It was just right and it was not scary—it was beautiful. We were together in her death as we were for her birth. —*Chris*

Steve: We woke up to Anya crying unusually. At first I thought it was funny, because she sounded like a little bird, but then it occurred to me that she was having problems. I took her and rocked her in a rocking chair and was able to calm her down a little bit. After Anya was given morphine and oxygen, we took her into our family room and listened to some peaceful music while we waited for the sun to rise. Our parents and my wife's aunt and sister were present, and my wife held Anya in her arms until she passed away. She was holding my finger and we told her it was OK to go and that we would miss her. The sun was just coming up. Our hospice nurse arrived and declared that Anya had died, and we all wept for some time.

Delsa: I still get a pang in my chest when I think about the last few hours. I remember Anya crying differently. She'd been breastfeeding with no problems the day before. This time, I couldn't get her to feed. I think I was in denial. I remember my husband saying, "Let's call hospice." I didn't think we needed to resort to that, but I called. The hospice nurse advised I give her morphine and oxygen. I asked if I could give her Benadryl instead. To me, morphine meant she was dying. I wasn't ready. We were so sad, but I remember thinking, *I can't cry. She's still alive. I can cry when she's gone.*

After she died both of us held her and told her we loved her. We changed her diaper for the last time and put her cute pink pajamas on and wrapped her in a special blanket. Right after she died, my husband lit a candle, and we left that candle lit until they took her away the next day. We put her back in bed with us. We cried ourselves to sleep holding our precious daughter. The next morning, my husband's parents called the nurse who was in charge, and she brought over the doctor who confirmed Sarina's death. The candle is blown out, not to leave us in the dark, but because the morning has come. Sarina's life may be physically gone, but she is part of the world in a new way, in our hearts and in our memories. —*Christine*

Death in Unexpected Circumstances

There is no blueprint for how your baby's death might unfold. It might happen in completely different circumstances than you'd imagined. Here's how it was for Alaina's parents:

Jill K.: I was calm-worried. I thought something might be really wrong.

James: So we decided to go to the doctor's office for a checkup. When I took her outside to get in the car, I realized, holy crap, we've got to go. She's pale. That's not the right color.

Jill K.: We found out that Alaina was in heart failure. The doctor said that if we gave her diuretics she might have some more good days. It wasn't about making her life longer but about making her feel better. We had to decide whether to go to the hospital. We considered it, and where we came down was if it was an infection that could be fought with medication, we could have considered treating it. But it was the heart.

James: We left the doctor's office and walked to the elevator. I was looking at Alaina and she was looking distant. She was looking at the light. She wasn't looking at me anymore. I said, "Jill, look, she's looking at the light. I think she's going to go.

A Gift of Time

Let's say goodbye." I just whispered in Alaina's ear: "I love you and if you want to go right now, it's OK. Don't feel like you to have to wait for us." We put her in her car seat and got in the elevator. Jill checked on her to make sure she was still breathing. And she wasn't. She died in the elevator. And it was the only time she could die. They say that people don't like to be watched to die. The only time she wasn't going to be completely watched was that moment in the elevator.

Jill K.: If we hadn't read stories like that, I think it would be hard. I would think, *I can't believe I wasn't holding her when she died.*

James: We could feel her spirit in that room, in the lobby. It was so tranquil and so calm. I didn't even cry at all. My baby was dead in my arms, and I wasn't sad or terrified. I was so peaceful. It was just like, OK.

Jill K.: Both of us felt she was right there, right over my shoulder, saying, "I'm here. You're fine."

Discontinuing Medical Interventions

For families who initially choose medical intervention, when tests or aggressive measures don't yield the hoped-for results, it becomes time to make decisions about letting go.

We wanted all measures taken at birth to keep her alive and to get her breathing. On two separate nights Amaya coded three times. On the second night, the third time she coded it took chest compressions to get her back. She only weighed four and a half pounds and was so tiny. The next night we decided to not take further measures than oxygen, stimulation, and bagging should she code again. That was the hardest decision of our lives. —*Gina*

We had planned that we were going to aggressively treat our daughter and that whatever machine she need to be placed on to help her survive, we wanted them to place her on it. At the same time we had also said that at any given moment my husband or I could change any decision we had mentioned on the birth plan, and that is what happened. At the end when my husband saw that Katherine Elizabeth's heart rate was dropping and how her little body was shaking with the ventilator machine, he could not bring himself to have them place her on any other machines, especially the ECMO machine. So with the biggest pain in his heart he told them to unhook her and let her rest and fall asleep, and in less than five minutes she passed away. *—Lizabeth*

∽ When we got into the NICU, it pretty much hit us that this was it. I knew he was going to die when the doctor asked me if I wanted to hold my baby. When I was finally able to hold my son, it felt amazing. I wanted to hold him so badly for so long that when I finally did, I actually felt so much joy. Even knowing that he was about to die, it still felt so amazing finally holding him! His vent tube prevented us from moving him too much, but he was there, in my arms. Not long after that, we decided that we wanted his vent out. He was pretty much gone by then anyway, and we wanted to see his whole face. I handed my baby over to his daddy. I was the one who got to bring him into this world; I wanted his daddy to be the one who held him as he left. *—Amber*

∽ After a few days, we were told that she would need a tracheotomy and a breathing tube, which she probably wouldn't be able to get off of. We decided against the invasive medical intervention and took her off the life support. They said that she would pass within an hour or two, but she lasted two and a half days more. My husband and I were sitting with her on her hospital bed and holding her hands. We talked to her, telling her that we loved her and that it was OK to finally let go of her life. She had fought and held on for so long! She slowly wound down, and five minutes before she stopped, she made a noise as if she was telling us something. And then we watched her stop living. There was no pain or funny breathing, no seizures. It was very peaceful. Even though we were sad, we knew that our prayers were answered—for her to be comfortable, without pain, uneventful, peaceful. *—Rebecca J.*

∽ My husband faced me on my hospital bed and we joined together, the three of us in an eternal embrace, as the doctor removed Jordan's ventilator and turned off all of the machines attached to him. As the beeps and buzzing of the machines went silent, we heard a spontaneous song rise up as our friends began singing, "We

A Gift of Time

Are Standing on Holy Ground." My husband undressed his son so we could spend our final moments with him without anything blocking our view of our son. We both placed our hands on his chest so we could feel his final breaths and the final beats of his heart. My husband's tears were flowing down and falling on Jordan's tiny arms. —*Jenny D.*

Discontinuing or declining further medical intervention can be agonizing. It may feel as though you are making the final call between your baby's life and death. Others who don't understand your baby's condition—perhaps not having seen the baby, not witnessing what the interventions have been like, or not being fully informed about the burdens versus the benefits of the treatment—may question your decision. They might be assuming that modern medicine can fix everything. They might wonder why you went this far with your pregnancy only to "give up" on reaching for a miracle and "let your baby die." Deep down, you might share twinges of those feelings too.

It's important to remember that ultimately it is the terminal condition, not your decisions, that brings your baby's life to an end. You are not taking direct action such as administering a lethal dose of medication or withholding nutrition and hydration with the intent of causing death. You are accepting the reality that medical science is no match for your baby's problems, focusing on palliative treatments that alleviate pain, and realizing that sometimes the purest act of love is letting go.

If Your Baby Struggles

He was unable to breathe. I felt like I failed him. What kind of a mother cannot help her child? All I could do was hold him and tell him how much I loved him. I told him that it was OK to go and that we would be together again someday. —*Brooke*

Vayden's immature lungs were the main cause of death; it was hard for me to hear his struggling cry and gasps for air. I will never forget that painful sound. I wondered if he was in pain as he struggled. It was heartbreaking. —*Stephanie*

Saying Goodbye

⁓ I remember it was shortly before he died that his fight for life became very painful for me to see. I don't remember if I actually said it out loud, but I was thinking it in my mind: *Thank you, thank you for trying so hard for me. It's OK, it's OK, you can go—no more struggling, Noah. I love you!* —Kristin

⁓ Gabriel started struggling during his feedings, so we had to resort to tube feedings. This was stressing me out. I was feeling like he might be trying to slip away and I was beginning to get sorely attached. I didn't want to let go. By nightfall, his color was not good. His temperature was lower and we wrapped him in a third blanket. As the night went on, Gabriel started with small little seizures of turning purple. I didn't understand. I thought maybe he was choking or not getting enough air, so I would raise his little head and soon it would pass, and he would be OK. About midnight, we settled down and decided to get some sleep. I was a wreck. I had cried all afternoon until my eyes were swollen. I nestled Gabriel beside me in the bed and drifted off to sleep. Then about 1 a.m., he woke having a seizure. The nurse said it was just a matter of time now. Frantic, I got out of bed and began rocking him. Praying, crying, and asking God for his mercy in between every seizure, until he seemed to have the most terrible seizure of all. Then he laid there still in my arms. —Sonya

If your baby appears to have difficulty breathing, it can help to remember that irregular breathing is a normal part of the body shutting down. It does not necessarily mean that your baby is suffering. Witnessing this is often more distressing for the parents than for the baby. If you are concerned about the sounds or if you perceive that your baby is struggling, medications can help your baby appear to be more comfortable.

As you watch all this unfold, you may feel anguished and consumed with worry that your baby may have suffered. A primal parental instinct is to protect your child. You may feel a sense of failure. You also may feel deeply cheated: How could it have ended this way, when you worked so hard to continue the pregnancy and hoped desperately for a peaceful end?

But you can also look at it another way. Sometimes life is very hard; sometimes parenting is very hard. Even parents of healthy children cannot protect them from all of life's storms. Perhaps parenting in its purest and noblest form is simply being there during those hard times, showering your child with all of your love and comfort. You parented your baby in unique ways that *this* baby needed. If your baby struggled, who better to embrace your baby and whisper words of love and encouragement than you?

It may also help to remember what your alternatives really were. Isn't it better for your baby to leave this life in your warm embrace, rather than being attached to cold machines? Isn't it better for your baby to be lovingly cradled by you during this final struggle, rather than being aborted by a stranger, never to feel your tender touch?

You have not failed as a parent; you have risen to an awful, painful test and conquered it, parenting your baby in an extraordinary way.[2]

Spiritual Aspects and Experiences

Many families say that being present with their baby during the dying process and at the moment of death is a profound spiritual experience.

We removed Remi's breathing support. The neonatologist gave her a lot of morphine and another medicine to ensure that she wouldn't be aware at all. Remi was so peaceful and beautiful. My husband and I held her, turned the lights down low, played lullabies for her, and danced with her. About six hours later, at 12:30 a.m., Remi passed away on her daddy's chest. I can't even explain the feeling in words. It truly was a connection with her and God that we have never felt in our lives. This act, helping her leave the world in a loving and peaceful way, was more spiritual and amazing than childbirth. It was a connection with her spirit that I can't explain. —*Jessie*

After the nurse turned off the machines, she took Thomas to the room where I was waiting in a rocking chair and laid him gently in my arms. I began rocking him and singing. I was filled with an indescribable peace and joy, as it occurred to me that I had been given a great privilege. I had been chosen to sing to this beautiful baby as he went straight from my arms to heaven. I had my answer to the question, "Where is your God now?" He was right there, and he had been there all along. I could feel his presence that day, so close, as if I could touch him. —*Kelly G.*

⌛ Anouk's death was the most peaceful moment of my life. Early in the morning, I was lying in bed and had Anouk beside me. She had been very quiet almost the whole night, but suddenly she woke me up with little cries. I sat up and took her in my arms. My husband sat beside us. We noticed that her breathing was very bad; the intervals were very long. We realized that she was dying. She was very peaceful at that time and had stopped crying as soon as I took her in my arms. So we prayed together and told our heavenly father that we were ready to let her go. After that prayer, she took one more breath and died. A few moments later, I saw an image of God at the top of the other side of the room. I didn't see a face, but in my heart I knew who it was. Then I saw Anouk's spirit leaving her body and join God's lap. I saw her there, on God's lap, with his arm around her and I knew that she was at her place. I didn't have to worry; she was safe. We were alone in the room and my husband didn't see anything. I didn't share that vision with him right away, as I felt that it was a gift of God for me. During all those months between diagnosis and birth, my comfort came from the hope that Anouk's life would not end with the death of her body, but that she would have eternal life. And at that moment God gave me that vision to let me know that she was indeed with him now. —*Monika*

⌛ It was far sweeter than I could have ever imagined it to be. Zachary's eyes were fixed on my face and then he looked at my husband. Then he looked over our shoulders and fixed his eyes on someone we could not see, but we knew He was there. Then that precious 3-day-old baby lifted up his arms, took his last breath, and entered eternity. —*April*

⌛ Her eyes had lost their fight, and as the night wore on her breathing became louder and louder. We just sat and rocked her. We were both very tired so we brought Louise's bed into our bedroom. At about 2 a.m. I was awakened by voices saying, "Shh, shh, she's waking." When I opened my eyes, I saw only darkness and heard only silence. I realized I didn't hear Louise breathing anymore, and I woke my husband. He went to her bed and he started to cry. He brought her back to our bed and she was so peaceful. We laid there for what seemed like hours and then we woke our parents. We sat just holding her and crying together. —*Tracey*

I had packed Josiah in the stroller and took him for a walk around the block. We returned to a quiet house; my other kids were out playing. I was changing his oxygen supply from the portable tank to the in-house machine when I felt a sudden urgency to pick him up, not because he was suffering, but because I felt a spiritual excitement happening. It is hard to describe, but I felt a spiritual rejoicing from beyond our world. I felt the veil to the next life being opened and someone else join us. I felt Josiah's spirit leave his body and a joyful recognition of whomever was with us. Together, they went toward that spiritual rejoicing, that parting in the veil. Then Josiah was gone. I didn't have to check for a heartbeat because I felt him leave. And then complete peace. And joy. The same joy I felt the day his cry announced his arrival into this world, I felt as I witnessed his departure. Amazing. To understand the parting of the veil, imagine you are walking by an arena on the day of a big game. For a brief moment the door opens, and you can hear the roar of the crowd. You can feel their excitement and unity. You can feel their anticipation. You have no idea how many people are in the arena, but it is a mass. You have no idea what they are watching or what great thing just happened, but you know there is something exciting going on. All these things you can feel and know even without going inside. This is how it felt. It was the spiritual roar of the spiritual crowd. There were many. They were gathered together in an actual place doing something. There was excitement and anticipation. It was Josiah's destination when he left. Life after death is not just a good idea that we tell ourselves for comfort after a loved one dies. It is real. I felt Josiah leave his body, recognize whoever was with us, and go to that spiritual rejoicing. It was a beautiful experience. —*Behka*

Saying Goodbye

You have another gift of time with your baby after he or she has died. You can use this time to care for your baby's body, take photographs, and make as any memories as you wish to help sustain you later.

⁀ I was determined to remember everything about him and make concrete memories, impressions on my mind and soul that I could carry with me the rest of my life. That was such a compressed window of time to make a lifetime of memories, but that feat proved to be one of the miracles of a mother's heart, because in the time I had with him, I stored up treasures, secret memories of just the two of us that I would not trade for anything. —*Annette G.*

If no one has encouraged you or assisted you in taking advantage of this time after death, you may at first feel apprehensive or feel that you need permission to do so. But your parental instincts may draw you to your baby anyway.

⁀ I was left in my room with my dead baby. For the longest moment I just sat there looking at his bassinet. After a moment I asked myself, *What are you doing? That's your son, go get him!* I went and picked him up, cradled him to me, and just sobbed. I remember saying, "Oh, my sweet Noah!" My heart wanted him back so badly. I finally got to hold him as a mother should—close to my heart. —*Amber*

Physical Care for Your Baby's Body

Even after your baby has died, caring for your baby's body is entirely normal and natural. Once again, you are parenting your baby in profound ways that you wouldn't have expected or wanted but in ways that are uniquely tailored for this baby. Even if you've never changed a diaper or given a baby a bath before, even if you feel awkward and unsure, who could be better to care for your baby than you?

Many parents describe bathing their baby as meaningful. It is a sacred ritual in some cultures and religions to wash the body in preparation for its final resting place. Tradition or not, bathing your baby is a parenting task that gives you the opportunity to care for your baby's body.

⌐ It was precious and sacred. We had a bowl of water sitting on the table near the bed and they gave Nathaniel to me. As the morning sun streamed in the window, my husband and I bathed him with baby bath soap (I brought some with me to the hospital because I wanted to remember the smell). After we bathed him, I dressed him. I put on a little diaper, undershirt, and a soft cotton outfit. I sang to him, rocked him, and held and held and held him. It was more beautiful than anything I could ever have imagined. —*Annette G.*

⌐ One of my most cherished memories is that of my husband very tenderly giving Thomas his first and last bath after he died. I was stuck in bed due to my C-section. It was actually a good thing that I was. I think it gave my husband some good "quality" time to bond with his son. I had carried him for 36 weeks and was able to feel like I had nurtured him during that time. I think it's different for fathers. Our nurse that night helped my husband since I couldn't. I will never forget her quietly standing there, with tears streaming down her face, helping out. —*Kathleen*

⌐ When my husband and I gave Frankie a bath, it was hard for me to reach and I still felt quite drugged, but I did the best I could—my husband did most of it—and I loved it. Then we dressed him in the clothes we had picked out together and in the bunting that my mother had sewn for him. He had a lot of dark hair, just like my husband did as a newborn. So the nurse gave me a comb and for the next two days I combed his hair over and over again. (I slept with his comb for a week after I came home from the hospital.)
—*Susan E.*

In addition to collecting keepsakes such as handprints and footprints or a lock of hair, there are many other meaningful things you can do during this time.

I wanted to give her a birthday party, which we did a few minutes after she had passed away. It was so special for me, to have a party for her. My sisters got balloons and cupcakes, and we sang happy birthday. I wanted to enjoy my time with her and celebrate her life. I did not want it to be a depressing time, but a happy one. —*Holly*

It was so beautiful, even after she passed away. Later that night I had my first and only dance with Gianna, and I reminded her that her father was a handsome man. —*John*

Your Baby's Appearance after Death

You could tell when he was alive—he was warm, he still had color. It's amazing how much he changed within even a half hour of being gone; he changed so much. He was still him, but he wasn't quite the same him. —*Jessica*

It can help to know that your baby's appearance will change after death. Skin color will become pale, fingernails and toenails will turn pale or blue, lips will turn dark red, and skin eventually will appear mottled where blood settles. If the baby was unable to breathe well or was stillborn, the baby would not have had a vigorous coloring to begin with. The baby's body will at first be very limp, with muscles gradually stiffening over the next few hours as rigor mortis sets in. The body temperature will begin to fall and the body will begin to feel cool to the touch.

He changed before my eyes. I was not afraid. I was relieved that he had gone and that I did not have to worry about him anymore.

—*Jo*

I had never seen someone after they'd died, so I was quite scared about what my reactions would be, but she looked so at peace—no more pain, and she was beautiful. I think I thought that people who died had a tortured look on their faces or something. —*Tracey*

Lucy's appearance changed much faster than I expected. I had planned to make footprints and handprints and take pictures of her after she passed, so that I would not disturb her during her life by dressing her in fancy clothes. The rigor mortis set in very quickly, and she lost her beautiful smile, and I was unable to make handprints. —*Jane G.*

⌐ I wasn't at all prepared for what would happen to our little girl's body after she died. So many people encouraged keeping her for as long as we could, yet never explained what it would be like. All I can do is relay our experience. For us, after Gemma died she was no longer there. We were left with a very sick little body, which was hard to look at. I don't regret studying her little body or keeping her there for five hours after she died. I just wish I would have known what was going to happen to her. She quickly became hard, cold, stiff, and very purple. Her body was lifeless and she was *not* the cuddly little newborn I was hoping for. For some reason I was expecting her to become like a doll; instead she just seemed very dead. —*Courtney*

⌐ He was a gray color by the time he was cleaned and brought to us again. I remember I was so afraid to touch him. I was afraid to touch my own son. Not because I didn't want to but because he was so fragile I didn't want to hurt him. I know that doesn't make sense because he was already gone, but still I didn't want to hurt him. —*Rachel*

Especially if you are prepared, seeing these physical changes is not frightening. It can even help you accept the fact that your baby is no longer living and is no longer present in that earthly shell.

Keeping Your Baby with You

Don't be afraid to look at your baby's body—really look. This is your last chance to imprint these memories in your mind. See those little limbs that have been nudging you for months. Admire the precious features of your baby's body. It's OK to unwrap your baby; you can ask for warm blankets to help retain body heat as soon as you are done. It's OK to examine the parts of your baby that didn't form perfectly—or to focus on the things that did.

Saying Goodbye

〜 Once I got her in my arms, I shocked myself. I was calm, I stopped crying, and I remember smiling at her. She didn't seem to be dead to me. No, she didn't move or cry, but she was my baby and she was so perfect. I kept trying to remove the blankets that were wrapped around her to see how her little body looked. She had the longest arms and legs just like her mommy. Her body was blue, but I didn't really notice it. —*Annette H.*

〜 I really wanted to unwrap him and lay him on me, but I was afraid because I knew there would be issues with cold. One of his hands was hypoplastic; it was basically underdeveloped. We knew that from the ultrasounds. I'm not sure if the nurses knew if we knew, but when they wrapped him up, they tucked that arm in and kept his good arm out. So the very first thing I did was look at his underdeveloped hand. I wanted to see his little hand. It was very cute; it looked like he had a little mitten on. It was one of my favorite parts of him. —*Kathleen*

〜 It wasn't until after Emily was dead that I really inspected her. She had all the right numbers of fingers and toes. She had huge feet, just like her brother, and perfect piano-player hands with long fingers and pretty fingernails. Her eyes were brilliant cobalt blue, and her hair was dark brown. I finally had the courage to remove her cap and look at the damage to her head. Her face stopped right above the eyes: she had no eyebrows at all. In back, though, she had incredibly good skull formation for an anencephalic baby. There was an open part at the top, about as big as the circle of my thumb and forefinger. Her brain was exposed, covered only by a thin membrane. I could tell her brain had hemispheres—the doctors had been wrong when they said only her brain stem would form. She'd had a sucking reflex. She'd had hearing. She might have understood who we were. —*Jane T.*

〜 For the first time we saw our daughter at peace with no intrusive medical devices. We were able to swaddle her and walk around with her in our arms free from breathing tubes, catheters, and IVs. I wanted to skip up and down the halls of the hospital; I wanted everyone to see what a blessing she was! —*Jessie*

A Gift of Time

There's no hurry to give up your baby. Even if your desires make the medical staff uneasy or if anyone tries to convince you to let go, you can keep your baby's body with you for many hours, even overnight and longer.

⌐ When we went to bed the night of his birth, I held him and had him in the bed with me, and that felt like sheer heaven. I kept waking up, and when I did I would realize that he was there and I was so happy, even if he wasn't alive. I don't know if I've ever in my life felt so fulfilled. —*Susan E.*

⌐ We ended up keeping him with us that night. I didn't think I would want him in there after he had died. It seemed weird to me. But when it happens, it's totally natural. It seemed like absolutely the right thing to do. Of course we wanted him with us. I slept with him that night. —*Kathleen*

⌐ My husband lay in the bed with me and we held Caelyn between us. For a moment we were a family. I wanted to stay in that bed with my family forever. —*Chelsea*

⌐ My husband and I spent an hour with Hope Elizabeth all to ourselves. We held her and took pictures, we prayed over her, and we loved on her. We really couldn't quite get enough of her. Our nurse came to the door every twenty to twenty-five minutes, wanting to know if we were finished with her—to which we kept responding no! After our hour, we invited our families to come in and meet her. After everyone had gone home, we allowed our nurse to take her. Looking back, I wish I had kept her with me for the rest of my stay in the hospital, but because our nurse kept asking if we were finished, we thought we had to give her up. —*Alaina*

⌐ I held him most of the time throughout the next day, and the next evening the nurse put a birthing bed right next to my bed for my husband to sleep in so we could sleep together. How wonderful of that nurse! And then my husband put a silly British movie in our laptop to watch, we put Frankie right between us, and the nurse made us a little microwave popcorn to go with our movie. I was in heaven then, too, loving that our little family was together. I will

Saying Goodbye

cherish that time forever and also will be forever grateful for that nurse who created such a nice setting for us. —*Susan E.*

⁓ I had requested that he stay with me the night. I held him and rocked, sang lullabies he would never hear, sobbed, and said my goodbyes. When I was ready, I laid him down and slept the best sleep I had had in a long time. —*Sue*

If you or your caregivers are concerned about possible infection, the risks of handling a baby's body after death are insignificant, according to the Pregnancy Loss and Infant Death Alliance, while the benefits of spending time with your baby are many.[3]

Time after Death with Family and Friends

Keeping your baby's body with you provides time for your baby's siblings, other relatives, and friends to meet and honor your baby.

⁓ When our two older boys arrived they were naively curious, and it was comforting to see their interest in seeing their brother and to see them try to understand that he died. I'll never forget my 2-year-old son walking into my room saying, "Baby Noah all done dying!" At that moment I was sad and happy at the same time. Grief is strange! We got out the camera and took pictures of each of the boys with their youngest brother. They each held Noah and gave him hugs and kisses. I'm thankful it was so intrinsic, not inhibited by thoughts of Noah's body being creepy or gross. —*Kristin*

⁓ When Rose died, they all cried. Our 6-year-old daughter was upset that Rose would be in heaven before her, our 5-year-old son was upset because Rose never got to see our farm we were planning, and our 1-year-old daughter cried because everyone else was crying. —*Debbie*

⁓ The nurse came in to let us know that my whole family was here to visit. They all began to cry when they saw Mariah in my arms. I felt so much peace and talked to them without a single tear. I unwrapped her for them to see her little body. I first asked my mom if she wanted to hold her and she did. They all took a turn and wanted a chance to hold her. While wiping many tears, they all stood around my bed as we held hands and prayed as a family. I was so glad to have each of them there with me. —*Greta*

⌐ One good thing that we learned from our past experience when our baby daughter Lillie died is that family needed to be there. This time, we had called our parents to tell them that William had died and we were having a C-section that day, and they were all there in our room when we returned from surgery. They all got to hold him. No one from our family, other than my husband and I, had held Lillie. —*Pam F.*

In a few cases, depending on the baby's condition and taking into account their other children's ages and abilities, parents decide against having siblings see the baby's body.

⌐ Going into delivery I had my heart set on having our older daughter see and hold her little sister. Once we saw our baby, we didn't know if it was a good idea. We talked with the chaplain for a while, asking for her opinion. She had us think it through both ways and asked what would be our greatest regret. My husband and I agreed that we didn't want Mariah's condition to scare our older daughter. She might not forget the baby's red, peeling skin very easily. As much as I wanted her to meet her sister and say goodbye, it wasn't worth the chance of scaring her. —*Greta*

Even if you do decide that your baby's condition might be too over-whelming or upsetting for your other children, you can share some time together without the baby's body present, and your matter-of-fact explanations can be reassuring.

Photography after Your Baby Has Died

Photographs taken after your baby dies are important, particularly if your baby's life ended very soon after birth. (See Chapter 6 for practical tips on photographing your baby.) Because you can keep your baby with you for many hours after death, you have time to take more photographs of your baby's features and the details that are important to you. If your baby was in the NICU, now is your chance to take photographs of your baby free of the machines, tape, tubes, and wires. You can also use this time to capture important relationships between your baby and others. While some photographs will show expressions of grief, others can show the various expressions of tenderness and wonder, capturing the full range of your baby's impact.

⸺ If somebody had told me about bereavement photography before this experience, I would have thought those parents were crazy. That is sick, that is wrong, that is just not normal. But having gone through it, it is the most normal thing in the world. It's OK. —*Kathleen*

⸺ A photographer silently waited with her camera, and when we were alone she took what I now consider some of the most beautiful memories I could ever have of that brief time I had with David. She captured something beautiful from something that was heartbreakingly awful. —*Rachel*

⸺ We kept Grace with us for a few hours after she died. We bathed and dressed her in her baptism outfit. We took pictures and made our last memories. Those pictures are still hard for me to look at. There is such pain in our faces. —*Chris*

⸺ We took pictures from every angle and with every person who was there. You can never take too many pictures. The important thing to remember is that you can always put them away if they are too difficult to look at, but if you did not take them you have nothing. —*Donna*

⸺ Because we knew that Michael likely would not be born alive, we did not bring a camcorder or camera to the hospital with us. I could not conceive of documenting what I thought was going to be happen. But then of course when we got there and it all happened, it was so peaceful, and I was filled with regret that we hadn't brought a camcorder or a camera. One of the greatest kindnesses I have received in my life is a set of photos of Michael that a nurse took for us that night. That nurse, without saying anything to us about it, seemed to be able to recognize that we weren't in a place where we were going to be able to take pictures but that we should. —*Missy*

Hospital Care

⟿ The hospital staff had clearly been trained. I was put on another floor and a discreet sign was put on my door to let everyone know that we had suffered a loss. —*Jamie*

⟿ The postpartum care I received was wonderful. The nurses and my doctor were great. Aside from the physical care I received, we also received extensive emotional and spiritual support from the nurses, hospital chaplain, and people from our church as well. I feel like the hospital staff empathized with us every step of the way. —*Heidi*

Any mother who's just given birth needs some postpartum physical care and monitoring. Some hospitals offer the choice of staying in the maternity area or being transferred to another unit. Issues to consider include whether you want to be surrounded by other parents with living babies and whether you will have a private room. Another important factor is that nurses in a maternity unit are experts in postpartum care and may be exceptionally good at caring for parents who have experienced the death of a baby, while those working in other units may be unfamiliar or even uncomfortable with patients like you. If the maternity unit nurses do seem uncomfortable, remaining in the maternity area still can help affirm that even if your baby is no longer living, you are still a new mother and father.

⟿ My nurses were so wonderful. I knew that I had the option to go to another floor, but the postpartum nurses were so great and understanding that I decided to stay there. I did not have to share a room with another mom, and my husband stayed with me. One night I woke up crying because I missed Aubrielle, and my husband was able to be there to comfort me. The next day, when I was allowed to walk around and take a shower, I took a walk around the floor with my sister. We stopped and looked at all the new babies in the nursery. I realized at that point, looking at all the precious babies, that I could do this again. It was not hard for me to see all the babies. It helped give me hope. I was glad I stayed on the birth floor. Despite losing my daughter, I could still be happy for those who had their babies with them. —*Holly*

After I was moved to the postpartum side of the ward, the nurses did not seem to know what to do with me. Mostly they avoided coming into the room. However, they did honor my request to keep Nathaniel with me as long as I wanted. —*Annette G.*

In addition to your physical postpartum care, emotional support can be just as important.

The hospital was so caring and sympathetic. Everyone on staff treated us with so much respect and kindness. In fact, they called us every day for a week after coming home. —*Allison*

After Thomas died, my nurse asked how I was feeling. I told her I felt relieved. That seemed like the absolute wrong emotion to be feeling. She explained that it was completely normal for me to feel that way. She likened it to how people feel after a loved one dies from an extended illness like cancer. I think she was right. For so long I had been living with the fear and anxiety of not knowing what was going to happen. I was under a tremendous amount of stress. And while I did not wish my son to be dead or his life to be brief, it was a bit of a relief, at least initially, to know that all the wondering was over. —*Kathleen*

The nurse told me that she had lost a baby too. Now I could understand why she had been so understanding. I remember when she had to leave, and she knew I would not be there when she came back on shift. She told me that I didn't know how strong I was and that I was going to be OK, and then she left. —*Rachel*

When your caregivers affirm the preciousness of your baby, it can be powerful for your healing. This kind of affirmation has the long-lasting effect of giving you cherished memories and feelings of pride that you can carry with you forever.

The hospital chaplain was so sweet as she looked at Mariah, and we were instantly glad to have her there. She asked what we named her and said she thought it was a beautiful name as her hand touched her heart. To my surprise she then asked if I would mind if she held Mariah. I would have never expected her to ask but it made me feel good. She held her so tenderly and told us that she would cherish that she was able to hold our Mariah. I remember tucking the blanket around Mariah, worrying that the chaplain would get a bloodstain on her church clothes. I could tell she wasn't worried about it and didn't give it a thought. —*Greta*

The nurse who took care of us the night that Thomas died was so tender and caring. I didn't really sleep much that night. I mostly stayed up holding my son's body. She and I talked often throughout the night. As her shift was ending the following morning, she asked if she could hold Thomas. I gave him to her and she sat down and held him in front of her and just looked at him—I mean really looked at him. It was as if she was trying to absorb his very being, even though he was no longer alive. Her whole being was so present with him. Oh my gosh, I was so proud. You know that your baby is already dead, but that's your child. It doesn't matter if they're alive or dead. So to have somebody want to hold him—he'd been dead for 12 hours, he was not looking like a newborn baby—meant a lot. She looked at him like she was admiring a healthy little newborn baby. I can't tell you how wonderful that made me feel. Her actions validated every feeling I had. My son was worthy, he was beautiful, and he mattered! —*Kathleen*

DECISIONS ABOUT YOUR BABY'S BODY

Autopsy

Depending on your baby's condition, you may be asked whether you want an autopsy. If the condition was confirmed before or after birth, an autopsy is generally not necessary. If doctors still are uncertain about the condition that caused your baby's death or if an autopsy might reveal information that could help you make future childbearing decisions, you may wish to consider it. Some religious traditions discourage or prohibit autopsies, so that may be a factor in your decision as well.

Organ Donation

Organ donation from a newborn is possible less often than is popularly believed. For the organs to be of a usable size, babies must be a minimum weight. To donate organs, a donor must be brain dead—most often from accidents or catastrophic neurological injuries—but on a ventilator to supply oxygen to the body. If the body is shutting itself down gradually and the heart eventually stops, as in most natural deaths, vital organs are unusable for transplant. But other tissues such as corneas sometimes can be donated within twenty-four hours of death.[4] A baby with anencephaly does not meet the criteria for brain death until the heart stops beating. Tissue donation might be possible after that.[5]

If it turns out that donation is a possibility and you wish to do so, be aware that you will need to relinquish your baby's body earlier than you may have planned.

Before she was born, we had thought that organ donation was not going to be possible due to her probable low weight. In the evening after her death, we found out that we could apply to have Lily be an eye donor. We had decided to do this if possible when she was first diagnosed. So, even though we had to give her up earlier, we decided to carry out this donation. —*Katharine*

Providing After-death Care Yourself

As discussed in Chapter 6, you can choose to care for your baby yourself in the intimacy of your home during the time between death and cremation or burial. Preparing your baby's body and having a vigil at home can be a reverent, powerful experience. Research has even found that keeping the baby's body for viewing at home helped parents with their grief.[6] Meeting your baby's needs after death is another way of making the most of your brief time together and maintaining your fundamental role as your baby's caretaker.

Caring for the body is mostly as simple as bathing, dressing, and keeping the body cool with dry ice hidden underneath blankets.[7] The baby could be tucked cozily in a bassinet in a room made peaceful with quiet music, fragrant flowers, and candles. Visitors could spend time privately with the baby, with casual conversation and food and drink in other areas of the house. You could even choose to make this a joyful time.

⁓ Before Simon was born, we thought we would have a memorial service for him shortly after he died. But we were so elated about his birth—even though he went on to die—that we weren't ready to move into mourning mode straightaway. We decided to have a party to celebrate his arrival instead. We invited friends and family to come meet him at a celebration in our home, and it was so much more enjoyable for all of us than it ever could have been in a funeral parlor. We genuinely enjoyed that time of sharing our baby with everyone. In fact, all of the days he was with us were amazing. Obviously there were times when we felt extremely sad because we couldn't keep him forever. But when we remembered to just stay in the moment with him, it was beautiful. We had time to hold him and love him and memorize every detail of how he looked. We had time for countless photographs. Very significantly, keeping Simon with us after his death gave our 3-year-old daughter time to really get to know her brother. The bond she feels with him is profound, and we cannot imagine having chosen to try to "shelter" her from experiencing him. To the contrary, we have learned a lot from her relationship with Simon. As we watched her be with her baby brother all those days and saw how in love with him she was—regardless of the fact that he had died—we came to understand that she loved him just exactly as he was. She didn't love him any differently after his death than she had before, and this was so valuable for us to experience. All told, Simon was with us in his physical body for six days after his death. That time together as a family was priceless and irreplaceable, and we cannot imagine having missed spending even one of those moments with him. —*Susan C. and Camilo*

If you choose to let professionals handle after-death care, you'll be asked to relinquish your baby's body to the morgue or a funeral home. If you do after-death care in your home, you'll relinquish your baby's body to its final resting place. As the time nears to surrender your baby's body, you may feel a desire to make the most of your last moments together.

    ⌐ I had one last time alone with my baby. How can you possibly squeeze in all the hugs to last a lifetime? I tried to hold him all the possible ways a mother can, and prayed that I wouldn't ever forget what that felt like. —*Kristin*

    ⌐ The making of one last cherished memory took place a few hours before we had to hand him over to the mortuary representative. I undressed Frankie and put eucalyptus oil on the bottom of his feet, his chest, his hands, and his forehead. I did it so he would smell good when he left to go on his "journey," but now I also think I was performing a ritual, sort of baptizing him. My husband cried as he videotaped me doing this. I don't know if I'll ever be able to watch the footage, but at least I know it's there. —*Susan E.*

    ⌐ The hospice nurse arranged for the funeral home to come to get Anya's body. My wife and I bathed Anya and laid with her in our bed for some time while we waited. —*Steve*

Inevitably, inexorably, the time comes.

    ⌐ I don't think the sadness kicked in until we told them they could take him away. That was the next hardest part after getting the initial fatal diagnosis: wrapping him up and getting ready to tell the nurse to come in and take him. —*Greg*

    ⌐ Handing him over to go to the funeral home was without a doubt the most difficult moment of my life. I could not even extend my arms. My husband asked them to wait outside, and he came to me and took Jordan from my arms. With a kiss, I released Jordan to his father. —*Jenny D.*

A Gift of Time

⁓ Kissing our sweet Lily goodbye was one of the saddest and hardest moments of my life. I was the last one to hold her and leave her in the tearful nurse's arms. I will never forget how special Lily felt and smelled right at that moment. —*Katharine*

Your baby's changing appearance may make it clear that it's time to relinquish the body, even if it doesn't make it any easier.

⁓ Mariah's skin was getting worse by the hour and we didn't want to remember her that way. I unwrapped her just one more time because I knew this would be our last time to see her. As she lay on my bed swaddled again she looked like a doll that we wished could've been squirming and crying. I picked her up and cried and said, "Oh, Mariah." My husband and I cried together as we held her and prayed. We each kissed her forehead and said, "I love you." It felt strange telling a dead baby this but we knew it was the only way we could let her know in heaven. I placed her in her crib and told the nurse she could come and take Mariah. I watched her crib as long as I could as the nurse wheeled her out of our room. —*Greta*

⁓ The time came for us to give up our baby. I think we were ready; she was so cold and started to change color. Everyone lined up for one last look at our baby. They all held her one more time; there were so many people there who loved her. It was our turn to say goodbye. The nurse just stood there waiting for us to hurry up and give up our baby. I felt rushed and uncomfortable. I wanted some privacy, but I felt ashamed to ask, for some reason. So we said our goodbyes with the nurse standing over us waiting to take her away. She put her in her little bed and wheeled her out. As the door closed, I could see our family standing there crying, watching her leave. —*Chelsea*

⁓ We made sure we kept her with us until 3:38 in the afternoon— exactly twelve hours after she was born. Too short. But I somehow started making peace with her death, knowing that her little body was tired and it was the best thing for her, to let her go. —*Kristi R.*

⁓ I lay awake that night just crying at the thought of him lying all alone in the morgue. I struggled with separating his earthly body

Saying Goodbye

from his heavenly one. He wasn't cold or alone, but nonetheless I couldn't shake an intense feeling that he needed me and I had abandoned him. —*Christie*

Many parents struggle with surrendering the body. If your baby dies in the hospital and you want to use a funeral home, you may decide to skip sending your baby's body to the hospital morgue and wait for the funeral director to arrive instead. If you have previously been able to make contact with a funeral director and already feel comfortable with this person, handing your baby over can be a bit easier. You also may be able to go to the funeral home to see the body in the days before the burial or cremation. Doing so offers you an even more gradual goodbye, which lets the reality of your baby's death sink in and facilitates your letting go of the body.

⌒ We met with our funeral director about four times. So when it came time to call him from the hospital, I sort of felt like he was family. It was nice to send Thomas off to somebody we sort of knew. He wasn't a stranger anymore. That was comforting. —*Kathleen*

⌒ It was so hard to take Nora out of our house. We just took a deep breath and did it. Her body needed to be refrigerated from what we knew. And we needed help with making all the arrangements. Our funeral home director was perfect to work with. He had so much respect for the dead. He encouraged one of us to hold her while we talked. I hadn't held her since that morning and she was now cold. I had brought her dress and asked him to help me dress her. He said yes and then just stood there watching. That was all I needed. I just didn't know what to expect. I am so glad I got to do that. —*Kristi F.*

⌒ We were told it would be very difficult for us when the funeral director came to take her body. I was actually relieved when he came. We visited Gemma several days later at the funeral home, and I'm glad I did because it made it clear that she was too sick to live and that she was no longer with us. —*Courtney*

⌒ When the funeral home came to get her, I got very upset. This baby had lived inside of me for eight months and I took care of her.

A Gift of Time

Now, she was in a strange place. I know her soul had gone to heaven. But it was so hard to think about her not being with me. She was all alone. My brother-in-law and sister-in-law went to the funeral home to check on her and to give the funeral home her clothes to wear. I felt a little better after that. —*Allison*

Before her funeral I remember having an evening when I was crazy with sorrow. I called the funeral home and arranged to go to sit with her the next day. That was a very special time for us.

—*Katharine*

Leaving the Hospital

Leaving the hospital can be an emotional event. If your baby's body is in the hospital morgue awaiting pickup from a funeral home, you are leaving your baby behind. Even if you are taking your baby's body with you, you are leaving behind your baby's birthplace and the caregivers who shared this life-changing experience with you.

I was anxious to get out of the hospital and get started planning Noah's service, but I was also torn by leaving the only place Noah's alive moments were spent. I strangely grew attached to my nurses because they too took part in these short, yet very special moments in our life. —*Kristin*

I didn't want to leave the hospital because I knew I had to leave Vayden but also because of the staff—they were amazing. They cared for me, my family, and Vayden so well and they were so sympathetic to our situation. —*Stephanie*

Many hospitals have a practice of transporting new mothers to the exit in a wheelchair. For some mothers, this is the first time they've emerged from their birthing room, where an entire life and death took place. It is a literal as well as symbolic reentry into the outside world. Particularly if you are leaving your baby behind, the ride from your room to the door can seem lonely and long. The contrast between *what might have been* and *what is* can feel especially sharp.

Saying Goodbye

The ride in that wheelchair down those big empty halls—I had a pillow and a plant in my lap. There was a balloon tied to it that said "Congratulations" with tiny baby footprints on it. I felt so empty! No baby. I was so sad. The tears were burning in my eyes, yet I felt nothing. All I had was an incision, some footprints, a baby blanket, rolls of film, and a broken heart. —*Laurie*

I felt so empty-handed, you know, like the feeling that you have forgotten something. I had no baby, no car seat, no fun going-home outfit for the baby. It was so hard to be wheeled through the hall of the hospital like I just had my gallbladder removed or something. I wrapped my hands tightly around the straps of my purse, rested my arms on top to cover my protruding belly, and I prayed the nurse would walk as fast as she could to our van before I had time to break down sobbing in the hallways. —*Kristin*

A nurse came to my room with the wheelchair to take me to the car. She instructed my husband to go get our car and bring it to the exit door. He ran out ahead of us to meet us at the door. That left me to that long wheelchair ride alone. Once again that deep agony returned. I was leaving the hospital with empty arms. My son had died. The nurse continued to walk quietly to the exit as I sobbed as only a mother longing for her dead baby could sob. As we neared the exit the elevator doors opened. Exiting was a happy little family: a new father walking with his wife as she cradled their newborn. She held half a dozen balloons that all said "Congratulations" or "Welcome Baby." I wonder if the nurse's heart understood what that did to mine, as she began to push the chair faster. —*Jenny D.*

You may wish to have your partner or a family member or friend accompany you on this ride. Perhaps the hospital has a valet parking service or your driver might be allowed to park near the entrance and walk to your room to accompany you back to the door.

You may also be eager to leave or feel relieved to go home.

I had Caitlyn at 12:29 in the morning; I walked out the door of the hospital at 2:30. I had been in there for three days by that point, listening to the sounds of baby heart monitors and women in labor. I just needed to get out of there. —*Shayla*

⌐ I cried silently when we left the hospital. I was leaving my baby there. It felt weird. The ride home was mostly in silence and that was good. When we got home, we unpacked and went straight to our room. We checked our e-mails and website postings that we had neglected for three days, cried at the love and outpouring we had, and went to bed. —*Amber*

Transporting Your Baby's Body Yourself

It may be possible to transport your baby's body to the funeral home yourself or to your home first if you wish. You may need to ask your funeral home or your caregivers at the hospital for a temporary license to transport a dead body and have that piece of paper in the car with you. The idea of transporting your dead child in your car may initially seem strange, but it can be gratifying to watch over your baby's body in another practical way.

⌐ The intrinsic value for me was that I didn't have to leave the hospital without my baby. I held him all the way home, and we showed him the house, we showed him the room that would have been his. After about twenty minutes at home, we drove him to the funeral home and we laid him in the casket. No one ever took him away from us, and that has tremendous value to me now. —*Jessica*

⌐ When we got to the car, my wife wanted to hold Alaina, and it was a bit awkward, because I said no one knows she's dead. We're going to be driving down the street with a baby in your lap. We don't want to get pulled over. We decided, screw it. I don't care what people think. This is our time. So we drove home with my wife holding Alaina. —*James*

Taking your baby's body home might be a surprising or even shocking idea at first. It might seem illegal or somehow unclean—neither of which are true. You could simply rock your baby in the room that would have been the nursery or sit quietly together on the sofa as

Saying Goodbye

a family one last time. You also may wish to have family or friends share this time with you.

> *James:* We just had Alaina at home and talked with her and held her.
>
> *Jill K.:* Hospice talked to us about whether we wanted to have anyone else come over and say goodbye, which we would never have thought of doing. So we invited a couple of key friends over.
>
> *James:* Which is really weird in retrospect: Hey, would you like to come over and see our dead child?
>
> *Jill K.:* We were cremating, and hospice said when families don't get to have a casket and see the person again, sometimes it's nice to have that. And it was. It was surreal. We were joking around, and I was holding her in her blanket. It was like everything was normal and so totally not normal.
>
> *James:* I remember everything I did was just heavy—my breathing, walking around. Somber. It's like you're walking with spirits. It's this amazing experience of walking in both worlds for a moment.

FUNERALS AND MEMORIAL SERVICES

⟶ Since only family and the friend who drove me to the hospital were fortunate enough to meet him in person, my husband and I felt like the memorial service was a way other people in our lives could get to know this wonderful baby. —*Heidi*

A funeral, memorial service, or graveside service offers a way to commemorate your baby's life with your larger circle. They are time-honored rituals that help you see how much others really care, give others permission to talk about your baby and offer their support, and provide structure in a chaotic time.

You will need to make or affirm your decisions about your baby's final resting place and to finish making funeral arrangements. Practical matters include choosing a casket, a shroud, or an urn, if you haven't arranged for one already. (See also Chapter 6.)

A Gift of Time

It was my husband who made arrangements with the funeral company, and it was my husband who did all the talking when the phone calls started coming in. When we talked about it later, he said that in doing all that stuff, he felt in control, that he needed to be doing something, to lessen the pain and sorrow. —*Christine*

It was so strange to come home from the hospital and be looking in the Yellow Pages for a funeral director. It was still unbelievable to me. It was definitely unknown territory for both of us. —*Greta*

The funeral home did not have much choice in caskets. They didn't even show it to us; we were just told it was white. I saw it the day before the funeral, small and white. I was very scared going the first time to the funeral home. It was a very strange feeling. I almost wanted to go; this was one of the only things we could do for our baby. —*Chelsea*

You can take this opportunity to add personal touches. You can tuck special items into the casket such as letters from Mom and Dad, stuffed animals, little toys to match toys given to older siblings as a keepsake, jewelry, or other meaningful items. If your baby will be cremated, ask about including meaningful articles to be cremated as well, such as locks of your own hair or a letter from you.

My children used colored Sharpie markers to decorate his casket top with messages of love, which was a wonderful form of therapy for them and so touching for all who saw it. —*Pam M.*

My husband built a simple coffin the day after Sarina died, with his dad and my dad. They brought the coffin home, and we lined it with Sarina's blankets. One thing that we did plan in advance, and I am so glad that my husband took charge of this, is he asked all family members including grandparents, aunts and uncles, and cousins to contribute something very small to be placed in Sarina's coffin. We wanted her surrounded by all of our love when she made the final journey to be cremated. When it was time for Sarina to be taken away, we all got the chance to say our goodbyes

Saying Goodbye

and to place our little message, or photo, or tiny trinket in with her. Our son placed one of his favorite stuffed toys next to her, my sister wrote her a letter, cousins drew cute pictures and had written some touching poems, my mom placed a rose, I placed a photo of our family. When I looked at her one final time, she looked peaceful and cozy. Then my husband closed the lid and screwed it shut. If he wouldn't have taken the time and put in the effort to make that tiny coffin, we would have had to place her in a cloth bag that the funeral service brought along, and that made me sick. He carried out her coffin and helped put her in the van, and then it drove away. —*Christine*

You can also add your own touches to your baby's funeral or memorial service. Through your choices of readings, music, and other details, you can set the tone and help express your baby's life and your feelings about it.

There would be no funeral Mass for Maggie. Instead, we had a Mass of thanksgiving for the miracle that was her life. It seemed much more appropriate. —*Alessandra*

We picked music that was really meaningful for us and not at all traditional. We closed it with The Beatles' "Yellow Submarine" because we liked to dance to it with her. We told everybody that they didn't have to wear black, and if they were comfortable we'd like them to wear colors. We said kids were welcome. We felt like we had to give people permission. All along, we tried really hard to tell people what we needed, because we know that people are nervous about doing or saying the wrong thing, and they're going to either guess and maybe get it wrong or do nothing at all because they're so scared of doing it wrong. —*Jill K.*

The preparations themselves can be therapeutic.

My husband and I had a memorial service for Frankie a couple of weeks after his birth and death. (I was impressed that all five of his siblings flew in for the service!) We had recently bought our house, and my husband busted his rear end to fix it up in time for the service. I remember a few people saying, "You know, no one cares what kind of condition your house is in during the service." And I remember thinking how they didn't understand, that we weren't doing if for "people." We were doing it for Frankie—we were making the house beautiful to honor him. —*Susan E.*

⌐ When Lucy died, we needed to focus our energy and attention on her twin brother. For this reason, we had chosen to have Lucy cremated. We had the memorial service and burial of her ashes two months later. This was the right decision for us. It allowed us to focus on our son for a while, and it was a chance for me to see once again that people really did care about Lucy. —*Jane G.*

Size of Service

Some families prefer a more intimate service, while others may be unsure about how many people to include. Many parents discover that allowing others to attend can be a heartwarming validation of their baby's existence and a powerful show of support.

⌐ After Sarina died, we decided to only hold a small memorial service for close family and a few close friends. I didn't want to hold a whole funeral service and have people who I didn't even care about come and be with us during such a private and overwhelming emotional and sorrowful time. —*Christine*

⌐ We decided to have a graveside memorial service for our daughter, and it was by invitation only. My husband and I both come from large families, and we have lots of friends, but through this whole time, we found ourselves staying away from people. We couldn't bear the pity in their eyes, nor could we stand it if they didn't acknowledge us at all. And so we shared Hope and her service with just a few. Looking back, I would change this—I know now that the more people who had experienced Hope and that she had been made real for, the more people would have remembered and supported us as we grieved. —*Alaina*

When we first started talking about a funeral, my husband wanted to have a small service with immediate family only. I felt that our extended family and friends would really want to be there to support us. He eventually agreed with me and has since said he's glad we did things the way we did. So many people came from our church and from our workplaces. —*Shellie*

We had a funeral two days after Grace died. It was on my forty-first birthday. There were hundreds of people at the service. Grace touched many lives in her short time here. —*Chris*

Your Baby's Siblings

If you have other children, they have shared in the baby's life thus far, and for many families it seems right and necessary to include them in this final commemoration. Being a part of the family, seeing how others grieve, and hearing others talk lovingly about the baby can help your children sort through their own feelings. For parents, having a living child to hold during the funeral—while in no way a replacement—can be a source of comfort and hope.

If you have a wriggly toddler who you are concerned will create a disruption for you or others, you could line up helpers who could be ready to distract your child with crackers or juice or escort him or her out of the room if needed.

Just like you prepared an older child for the birth of the baby, some developmentally appropriate coaching before the funeral is a good idea. You can explain what will happen, and you can offer reassurances that it's normal for grownups to be sad and cry at a funeral and that everyone will be OK.

I tried to prepare my older daughter that today is the day we would say goodbye to Mariah's sick body. She is in heaven now and her sick body would be in a pretty white box that Daddy will carry. It also occurred to me to let her know that all of our family would be there and she may see some of them crying along with Mommy and Daddy. I reminded her that we'll be all right and that it's OK if she doesn't feel like being sad. —*Greta*

Some families opt against the possible distraction of including their toddler, perhaps even asking other guests at the funeral to do the same, as a way to focus solely on the baby.

⁓ We didn't bring our toddler son to the funeral. I didn't know how to explain the casket going down and that we were covering it up. I'm not sure if that was the right decision. But we didn't want the distraction of him there. This was Thomas's day. —*Kathleen*

Visitation

You may be given the opportunity to see your baby privately before the service, perhaps being able to tend to your baby one last time by dressing or wrapping him or her or by tucking something into the casket. You may also wish to include grandparents and siblings and others close to you, or invite them in after you have had time alone first.

⁓ Louise looked so beautiful in her coffin, dressed in her little pink-and-white polka-dotted dress. Originally, I wasn't going to go and see her. It's not something we do in Australia; open-casket funerals and public viewings are not common, and I had never seen anyone in a coffin before. So when the funeral director suggested I come and see her I was actually horrified, but now I wish I had taken a camera. I am so glad I saw her because it is a good memory. —*Tracey*

⁓ I regretted not seeing David's back, so when I was dressing David at the funeral home before his funeral I made sure to look. You could tell there was something wrong, but it didn't look anything like what I expected. I was so relieved. —*Rachel*

Especially if the body was embalmed, it will look and feel different from the last time you saw your baby. Seeing this with your own eyes can be another step in letting go. And now that you have seen the condition of the body, you can decide whether to leave the casket open or closed for the service or for a visitation if you are having one.

⌐ We were able to see Noah's body at the funeral home, and he looked so weird. I wanted to hold him again so badly, but he felt so different after being embalmed. He felt like a cold doll. I knew then that he was safe in heaven. —*Amber*

⌐ Because of the visibility of Elliot's anomalies, we chose to keep the tiny casket closed. The "mother bear" in me needed to continue to protect my child from curious onlookers, well-intentioned as they might have been. I did not want Elliot's appearance to be subject to speculation from others. I needed others to think of him as a baby, as a little boy, and not as a baby with birth defects. —*Karla*

⌐ The plan was to not have an open casket. Prior to the service, the funeral home people asked us if we wanted to see him, so we said yes. Then my husband's grandma said maybe we should keep it open; he was so beautiful. We then decided to leave it open. I think that having an open casket for an infant was difficult for some people, but it was our reality. —*Deanna*

Whether the casket is open or closed, other ways of sharing your baby include displays of photographs and baby items, slideshows looping on a laptop, or slides or video projected on a screen.

Closing the casket is an emotional moment for many.

⌐ Before the funeral started, I picked him up and held him in my arms one last time. My husband and I both kissed him goodbye and I placed him back in his bed. I remember watching the man from the funeral home as he gently closed the lid. It was the last time I would ever see my son on Earth. —*Donna*

Eulogy

Many services include words of remembrance about the person who has died. Especially because most people in the congregation may not have personal memories of your baby, these words take on added significance. The eulogy can serve as an introduction to your baby, a summary of the path you traveled together, an expression of gratitude to those who walked with you, and a testament to the meaning of even a brief life.

Writing out your thoughts ahead of time helps ensure that you will cover the points you want to cover and helps keep your comments to a reasonable length. You may wish to read the statement yourself, have someone else read it, or give everyone at the service a copy to take home as a keepsake.

⟿ My husband and I gave Anya's eulogy. We didn't think we'd be able to do it, but we owed it to her. —*Delsa*

⟿ We typed up what we were going to say, so if in that moment we couldn't say it, our priest had read it ahead of time. My husband was able to say his, but I got up and realized, no, I can't do it, and handed it off. That way I could convey what I wanted to say without worrying about getting choked up. —*Jill K.*

Carrying the Casket

Unlike a funeral for an adult, the casket will not be heavy and pall-bearers will not be necessary (unless you would like to name honorary pallbearers). The funeral director could carry the casket for you, but having the father carry it is profoundly meaningful, a bittersweet counterpoint to the mother having carried the baby until birth.

⟿ My wife and I walked side by side while I carried her casket down the aisle for her funeral. I had hoped I could walk her down the aisle but dreamed of walking down the aisle for her wedding, not her farewell. —*John*

⟿ Just before it was time to take the casket out, my husband whispered to me that he wanted to do it. It was one thing he could do. You know, they're left out. I had our baby, I birthed him. There's not much that dads get to do. My husband gave him his bath; he found the casket. He wanted to do something. —*Kathleen*

Feelings

The swirl of emotions you may feel at the funeral can be overwhelming. You may feel grief, gratitude, relief, numbness, a sense of surreal distance, an extraordinary awareness of the moment—all seemingly at the same time.

Saying Goodbye

I started crying the moment I saw the little casket by the stained-glass window. I was struck again by the unfairness of this all. Why did I have to bury my baby? During the pregnancy, I dreaded this day the most since it would be the final goodbye. How was it possible to simply turn and walk away? Such a thing I could not fathom or visualize. As it turned out, I did turn and leave. I had to. I had no other choice. I opened his casket, held his tiny hand, and kissed him one last time. Tears spilling over, I told him I loved him and that I would see him soon. Never goodbye. This separation is not forever. I walked away, knowing that I had loved my baby with all that was in me and I had no regrets about any time spent or decisions made. —*Karla*

The funeral was beautiful. There were more people there than I could have ever imagined. I remember sitting in the front pew and thinking, *Why am I not crying? I should be a mess. I love my son more than life itself, but I have not shed a tear*. It was an incredible feeling. I felt more at peace during that service than I had ever felt in my entire life. —*Donna*

When I looked out at all of the people who attended his funeral, for a baby that many other people believe should have had his life terminated because of his condition, I was overwhelmed with emotion. All of these people affirmed Colm's life in a way that I couldn't. —*Pam M.*

I was told that Gianna's funeral was beautiful. The priest's homily touched the five hundred plus souls who had come to support us. My eyes stayed upon the priest and I did not want to look anyone in the eye. I was frozen, trying desperately not to cry. The drive to the cemetery was cold and gray. The processional line was long. —*Doreen*

The day of her funeral was sunny and gorgeous, and although I was thankful for it because of the outdoor service, I couldn't understand how the weather could be so beautiful when I had lost so much. —*Alaina*

It was very strange for me. I wanted everyone to leave, so that I could grieve like I really wanted and needed to. —*Chelsea*

After the last words are spoken and the final song is sung, you may feel a sense of relief.

— It felt like a huge weight had been lifted off of me after the service. I knew we did what we could to honor little Mariah's life. —*Greta*

YOUR BABY'S FINAL RESTING PLACE

Burial or scattering the ashes (unless you decide to keep them) is the last step in caring for your baby's body, the final physical goodbye. It may provide a sense of completion and a sense of having carried your baby full circle, from life through death, watching tenderly every step of the way. A gravesite provides lasting physical proof of your baby's existence. Scattering your baby's ashes can be symbolic.

— Once we were at Sarina's plot, we all circled around it and had our chances to express our thoughts through poems, short messages, and songs. It is a nice memory for me, even though I was so terribly sad. Because it was January, the weather was quite cold. The clouds were out that day, but I distinctly remember a moment during our service when the sun peeked out from the clouds and warmed up my cheek. To me it felt like a sign that Sarina was saying goodbye and that she was going to be OK. —*Christine*

— Anouk was our child, even if she only lived nine months in my womb and thirteen short hours in our arms. Her life had the same value for us as the life of any other child. Giving her a full funeral and burial was not only what she deserved as a human being, it was a ritual that gave us as her parents the closure we needed. Her grave is one square meter of official recognition of her existence. We did have a child, she really existed, she is buried here like any other human being who had a life and a death. —*Monika*

— We decided to bury her at sea. My husband and I and the chaplain went out on a sailboat one mile out at sea. The sun was beginning its descent on the horizon; the sea became very calm. It was that transitional time of dusk. The chaplain said a prayer and read

Saying Goodbye

a poem about how children just pass through us. Then he asked us if we would like to spread the ashes. I said yes, then I said goodbye and how much I loved her, and I spread her ashes. For me it was a healing and beautiful transition from life to death to life. It was the beginning of many healings in the years to come. Because I buried Kelley at sea in the Pacific, every time it rains I feel as if she is coming to greet me because the storms come from the Pacific. —*Leslie*

If you are burying your baby's body in a distant place, you may find it difficult to send your baby's body away, but funeral homes and airlines are accustomed to handling these arrangements with sensitivity. You can also transport your baby's body yourself.

⌐ I was very nervous the day his casket was being shipped to where we were going to bury him. He was going on his own. He was going out of LAX. I was thinking, *They lose luggage! What are they going to do with this?* Both mortuaries reassured me that the airlines know what it is and they're very respectful. But I was nervous he was going to be lost or forgotten. A woman from the mortuary in my hometown, who had also lost a baby, went personally to the airport and called me right away to reassure me that she had him and everything was fine. —*Kathleen*

⌐ We had decided that we wanted to be the ones to drive our son across the country to his final resting place. Then we began our first and only car ride with our son. When we arrived in our hometown, we stopped at the funeral home, where there were people waiting for us. We spent a few minutes holding our son and telling him how much we loved him and would miss him and then we said goodbye. —*Donna*

At the gravesite, like your time together after birth, you can also take an active, hands-on role in this final act of caring for your baby. These final acts also can have great symbolic meaning when performed by the father.

⌐ I carried my son to his final resting spot, and there was not a dry eye anywhere. It was an all-too-surreal moment. All I wanted to do was lay my head down on his casket and cry for him to come home to us. —*David W.*

⌐ My husband and I said our last goodbye to her, and my husband closed the casket he had made of cedar. He was the one who screwed down the lid, a gesture that I could tell was something he wanted to do. It is interesting that I housed Nora for her life, the eight months she lived in my belly, and now my husband will house her body in death. Very fitting that we as parents could do that. —*Kristi F.*

You might plan other symbolic gestures such as laying flowers on the casket, perhaps inviting all the baby's cousins or other special people to join you. You may even wish to help return the earth once the casket is in place. Sometimes gestures happen spontaneously. By letting your instincts be your guide, you may inspire others to do the same.

⌐ We released doves at the gravesite. It really represented releasing him to heaven. —*Corie*

⌐ At his burial, my children and some nieces each took a shovel of dirt to cover his casket once it was placed in the ground.

—*Pam M.*

⌐ We held our daughter's body throughout the funeral. We held her beautiful little body all wrapped up in a special quilt my sister had made for her. Everyone got to kiss her sweet little head goodbye, and we held her between us in the funeral car, right up until we got to the gravesite. It was only when we had to, and that it was our final moments together, that we put her in her little white coffin. This was a very gentle experience. We had never heard of anyone holding their baby throughout the funeral, but my husband suggested this to me the night before we had to say our final farewell. And I have to say it was the most beautiful thing we could have done. I felt we were really with her, right up until the very end. —*Elle*

Saying Goodbye

⌐ When the dirt started to fill in the hole, I got on my knees next to the hole to watch each shovelful go in. I watched as she was swathed by the warm dirt. I watched each one, so full of love, embrace her. I watched every single shovelful of love pour into her grave. I helped move the earth when the pile got smaller. I put in a couple of shovelfuls, but I moved more earth with my hands and fingers. Other women got down on their knees and helped. After we were finished, our friend put roses for each member of our family on top. It was hard to know what to do next. We dispersed reluctantly. But we were filled by what we had done and knew that it was right. —*Kristi F.*

TWENTY MINUTES
by Vincent de Tarlé, father of Pierre

Twenty minutes with him, maybe seventeen,
it's not much
but at least I'll keep them and,
at the same time,
it's so long when one only has just that.

Twenty minutes of happiness and tears,
mixed with admiration, love
which for the first time in thirty years is totally uninhibited,
completely free, with no hope of return,
with no hope of satisfactions (or disappointment)
as will be the case for other parents.

Just twenty minutes, just of love like that,
for no reason, as was so well explained to me,
simply because I am in front of this little boy who held on
      to be with us,
this little boy, mine, my son, the first
and he's the most beautiful, it's true.

Twenty minutes, the most intense, the deepest, and for now,
the most beautiful of my life.

Twenty minutes that were so feared,
but when I would have given away all I have

A Gift of Time

that I would have even stolen, a lot and from anybody,
so that I could have twenty-one minutes.

Twenty minutes for him to educate me,
my own son, because he teaches me the important things in life.

Twenty minutes to go from concept to reality, to put a name on
   this face
so often repeated, whispered, murmured with longing.

Twenty minutes to be able to continue to talk to him,
to be able to tell him how much I love him
and be sure that he believes me,
to be able to explain to his brothers and sisters who will come after
and tell them that they too will be loved until the end.

Twenty minutes not to teach him rugby, history, drawing, wine
and all those things that I don't yet know.

At the twenty-first minute there is in the end that peaceful feeling
that we have made the right decision.

And then, a week of difficulties: the administrative formalities,
   the arrangements,
the lack of understanding (that we had to face without being
   aggressive)
of those who explained to me again after the birth of my child
that he didn't have the right to live, that he was not normal, had
   many problems,
that it was no use, that that story had at last finished,
that we could move on to something else.

One week for those people present at those moments to take a
   special place in my life.

One week to say goodbye to him.

Excerpted and translated from the French.
Used with permission of the author.

Saying Goodbye

nine

Continuing Your Journey

After Your Baby Dies

⟶ I woke up the day after the funeral feeling so very sad. I sat in bed for a long time and then got up to read cards and cry a lot. I really felt the loss and was so sad the day of honoring her and planning for her was over. I missed her so much. I just needed to be sad and felt completely filled with Nora. —*Kristi F.*

After your baby dies, you turn a corner in your emotional journey of parenting this child. You will likely feel some relief that the uncertainty of waiting for death is over and perhaps gratitude that your baby's quality of life was what you had hoped for. Your anticipatory grief served as a gradual goodbye, and with careful plans in place, you were in many ways prepared for your baby's death. But you may also feel some regret about certain aspects of your experience. And grief still hits hard.

⟶ Sadness came. For a long time. A deep sadness. A confused sadness. A distracted sadness. There was so much I wanted to do and just couldn't. I had to just ride the wave. —*Kristi F.*

⟶ It's just plain sad. There are no words. Some days it's almost physically painful. —*Jessie*

Anticipatory grieving does not erase your need to grieve after your baby dies. You will likely experience an intense, renewed surge of grief, perhaps not right away, but as the finality of your baby's death sinks in, so does the full scope of your loss. Your focus shifts from looking forward to meeting and embracing your little one to looking back with intense longing. This chapter offers you information and support after your baby dies.[1] You have already learned much about grieving and coping during your pregnancy, and this emotional awareness can serve you well as you continue to grieve. You have already demonstrated your ability to persevere under extraordinary circumstances and your devotion as a parent to your baby. You can tap into this strength and this love to carry you forward.

THE MOTHER'S POSTPARTUM RECOVERY

When your baby dies shortly before or after birth, not only do you feel emotionally devastated, you may also feel physically drained. Your grief may cause you to feel fatigued yet still have difficulty sleeping, and your arms may literally ache for your baby. In addition, you also must recover from pregnancy and childbirth, perhaps including incisions from an episiotomy or a caesarean birth. While most of your sadness and despair can be attributed to your baby's death, you also may experience some degree of postpartum mood swings as your hormones readjust to prepregnancy levels, an adjustment that can exacerbate your grief for several months. (If you are concerned about postpartum depression, don't delay talking to your doctor.) You must also cope with breasts that are beginning or continuing to produce milk. You have all the signs of recovering from pregnancy and giving birth, without the reward of having a newborn in your arms.

Many mothers feel they should be able to recover quickly because there is no baby requiring round-the-clock care. But adjusting to your baby's death is taxing. Particularly if there were complications with the pregnancy or birth, or if delivery required any invasive or surgical procedures, your body needs extra care, as its reserves can be quickly drained by grief. You deserve to take plenty of time and care to recover physically and emotionally.

It was hard for me to "take it easy," as my mom kept reminding me to do. I had no baby to feed, or watch rest on my lap, and no diapers to change. I felt like I didn't have an excuse to be tired; after all, I didn't have anything to show for the very physical labor I had just gone through. —*Kristin*

⌒ My postpartum recovery was painful, as I'd had a C-section. But I think it was good to be forced to stay down by the pain, as that gave me time to fully receive care from other people. If I had not been in so much physical pain I might have felt like I needed to do things and would have not taken the time to experience the immediate weight of grief. —*Susan E.*

Breast Care

⌒ When the milk started to come in, it added insult to injury.
—*Pam F.*

In addition to a postpartum mother's other physical discomforts, having breasts engorged with milk can seem especially cruel. If you'd looked forward to breastfeeding, you will grieve the loss of this special way of mothering your baby. If you had the chance to breastfeed or express milk for your baby, you may deeply miss this nurturing act.

For most mothers, breast milk comes in a few days after birth, or production continues unabated if they've been nursing or pumping. You may find it reassuring to see that your body was capable of nourishing your baby—or you may find it a bitter reminder that there is no little one to feed.

This aspect of a bereaved mother's recovery is sometimes overlooked. If you are experiencing discomfort, you can take ibuprofen or acetaminophen or place ice packs wrapped in cloth inside your bra.[2] Hot and cold therapy gel packs made especially for breast care are available in drugstores. (You may hear about women using chilled, raw cabbage leaves to ease engorgement. This is a folk remedy that studies have found to be no more effective than placebos, but the coolness may be soothing.[3])

If you need more relief, you can remove just enough milk to reduce the uncomfortable feeling of pressure, swelling, or lumpiness but not enough to empty your breasts.[4] You may be able to express by hand, or you could use a simple, manual breast pump. If you haven't already been pumping, electric pumps are too stimulating and efficient when you're trying to reduce milk supply. If you have been pumping, do so at increasingly longer intervals. A warm shower may also help the milk "let down" and relieve the pressure. Leave in as much milk as is comfortable, because a chemical present in the retained milk signals the milk glands to stop production. The need to release some of the milk will vary depending on how much milk you are producing, how long it has been since your baby was born, and if you were on a regular nursing or pumping schedule. You might not need to release any, but you may still need to put nursing pads in your bra for a week or so for any leakage.

Wearing a tight bra or binding your breasts, an old remedy, is not recommended because it can increase your pain and has no effect on reducing milk supply. Restricting fluids doesn't work either.[5] Drugs used to be prescribed for lactation suppression but were found to pose serious safety concerns.[6] Letting your milk dry up naturally is safest.

If you wish, especially if you already have some breast milk in the freezer or if you have a copious supply and want to continue pumping for a time, you might consider donating your milk to a human milk bank. (If you are taking medication, check first to see if it affects whether your milk can be used.) Some bereaved mothers have found donating milk to be therapeutic and meaningful.[7]

The Postpartum Checkup

About six weeks after the birth, mothers should have a pelvic exam and a general physical checkup. These exams can reassure you that your body is healing properly, an important consideration whether you are planning another pregnancy or not. It's also a chance for you to ask questions and get information about continued recovery, sexual intimacy, and attempting or avoiding another pregnancy.

To be sure that medical staff are aware of your situation, you (or someone else) could call ahead to make sure that your chart is flagged, and you can ask to be taken directly to an exam room. Being examined by someone who assumes all is well can sting. When you are treated with compassion, it can feel like a gift.

They never flagged my chart, even after my son had been born and died. When I went in for my six-week postpartum appointment, I assumed everyone in the office would be aware of what had happened. I was wrong. One of the assistants sat me down in a very public place and began to ask me questions about my delivery in a very routine, casual way—how many weeks, my son's height and weight, C-section or vaginal delivery, etc. I remember sitting there realizing that she didn't know what had happened. I started to have a panic attack and kept thinking, *Please don't make me have to say it out loud*. Sure enough, she got to "Are you breastfeeding?" and I had to tell her that my son had died. I could tell she was very embarrassed and felt bad. She finished up without looking at me again and quickly stuck me in an exam room. Once I was alone I completely fell apart and started sobbing. When the physician's assistant came in, I was still upset and crying. She knew what had happened but tried to tell me my emotional reaction was due to postpartum hormones! I wanted to jump up and strangle her. That was the last time I stepped foot in that office, and I have found a new ob-gyn.

—*Kathleen*

The nurse checked me in and was so considerate. She carefully read my chart and offered her sympathy. She sat in front of me and said, "I am so sorry for the loss of your baby. How are you doing?" It brought tears to my eyes, and she handed me tissues. It was so nice of her to ask; she could have easily slipped out of the room without saying a thing. —*Greta*

YOUR GRIEVING PROCESS CONTINUES

After your baby dies, you will probably revisit many of the emotions you experienced during your pregnancy. The difference between then and now is that your baby is gone, no longer nestled in your body or your arms. You may review all those layers of loss that you pinpointed earlier and add the irrevocability of death to this roster. You will mourn deeply.

As explained in Chapter 3, grieving is a painful but necessary process that enables you to come to terms with loss and move forward in spite of it. Grieving is ultimately a constructive process whereby you gradually let go of what might have been, and you adjust to what *is*. As you move through your grief, you can figure out how to restart, recreate, renew, and recover.

This process began during your pregnancy. Now your task is to adjust to your baby's absence. You can recover emotionally by revisiting your memories and keepsakes, by telling your story to sympathetic listeners, or by turning to activities that offer a sense of meaning or renewal. As you move through your grief, you are progressing along a continuum of healing.

Letting Go of What Might Have Been and Accepting What Is

The process of letting go takes time. It began the moment you received your baby's diagnosis, and it continues to unfold as you move forward with your life and gradually adjust to what is. At first, you may focus on any immediate disappointments, such as if your baby's life was even shorter than you had hoped or if your baby was born still.

One of the hardest things for me to think about is the timing of Maggie's life. She was born at 3 a.m. and died a bit after 7 a.m. When the world went to sleep, I was still pregnant. When they awoke, her entire life had come and gone. For some reason, that notion is hard for me. —*Alessandra*

I had hoped that Frankie would live longer, and that I could feel his warmth, could bathe him while he was alive, and maybe even breastfeed him. So I was disappointed that his time was so short. But then again, I was grateful that he lived past birth at all.
—*Susan E.*

I wish I would have gotten to see Isaac breathe or open his eyes or cry. But those are things I can't change, nor are they things I had control over. I feel as though we were as prepared as possible, made the best memories that we could have, and loved Isaac deeply. You can't have any regrets about that. —*Stacy*

Even parents whose time with their baby was relatively long also need to make peace with the amount of time they received.

> *James:* The length of her life was completely our hang-up. Alaina's life was six months. That's all she was ever supposed to live.
> *Jill K.:* I didn't think she was going to die and say, "Shoot, I really wanted to live X amount of time." I don't think that's how her spirit would feel. She would just say, "Wow, I felt a lot of love there."

As time passes, you're not just letting go of your baby, but also all the hopes and dreams you had for your future.

⁓ I think the worst part is letting go of the dreams we had for Ashley. She would have been only two years younger than her older sister. I picture them playing together at the park, two sisters. We planned for Ashley and wanted her so badly. We only had a glimpse of her personality. What would she have done if she had a full lifetime with us? What would she be like? Losing our hopes and dreams for her is really tough. —*Shellie*

⁓ We don't get to see her grow. That's the hardest thing for me right now. The only memories I have are of that snapshot in time. . . . She was such a peanut. I see her clothes now, and I think, was she really that small? —*James*

While you let go of what might have been, you can still focus on the sweetness of the time you did have or on the sheer fact that your baby lived at all. It is possible to simultaneously let go of the previously imagined future and hold on to the memories of your baby's life.

In addition to the tips in Chapter 3, the following sections hold more insights about moving through your grief following your baby's death. Some words of guidance:

- Expect your grief to be complex and intense.
- Have realistic expectations.

- Accept your preoccupation with your baby as a natural expression of your grief.
- Accept your unique experience of grief.

Complexity and Intensity of Grief

After your baby dies, your grief may encompass many of the same emotions you experienced during your pregnancy but sometimes with greater intensity.

⟿ You name the emotion, I experienced it. I was completely unprepared for losing her and for making the grief journey. I experienced anger, bitterness, guilt, questioning, hiding—I rarely recognized myself each day in the mirror. I no longer knew who I was, what I wanted, or where I was going and neither did any of the people closest to me. —*Alaina*

⟿ I felt such helplessness afterward, both physically and emotionally. You're so emotionally drained. I remember saying to my mom, I feel so helpless. Just so helpless afterward. —*Jill N.*

If you have a surviving twin, triplet, or more, you have a complex combination of grief and gratitude.

⟿ My emotions continuously go up and down. I just look at Sarah and cry sometimes because she is our miracle baby. Then I wonder if she knows something major is missing from her life. —*Allison*

⟿ It was so good to hold my surviving baby in my grief—and so hard to hold my surviving baby in my grief. I felt guilt. I felt like it was hard to really grieve well. —*Kristi F.*

⟿ It's difficult when it is implied that Lucy's death somehow "doesn't count" because I knew that she was ill; when people are willing to acknowledge that I had a difficult pregnancy, but not that my daughter died; when it is assumed that Lucy's death does not matter because I have her twin brother, Samuel. —*Jane G.*

Physical symptoms of grief such as fatigue, sleeplessness, a hollow feeling in the chest, or lack of appetite may become more pronounced.

You may find yourself frequently sighing, and your tears may well up at any time—in the shower, in the car, while doing the dishes. You may have experiences that seem real but aren't, such as hearing your baby's cry or feeling your baby move inside you. At times, you may feel like every cell in your body aches.

⟋ The month following Caelyn's death, I felt her move inside me. Each time was exactly like it was when I was pregnant. I even put my hand down to my belly, only to find my belly was no longer there. It happened three different times. —*Chelsea*

⟋ I would dream there was a baby crying, and when I woke up—there was no baby. People told me that was normal. I didn't know what normal was anymore. —*Laurie*

⟋ My heart and arms ache because I long to hold her. —*John*

You may even have passing thoughts of wishing you were dead so you could be with your baby. These are all parts of grief and you can simply let these feelings flow through you. If these thoughts persist, talk with your doctor.

⟋ Sometimes I wish I had died right along with her. How could I go on living? I wanted to be with Caelyn more than anything. I love my husband and my family dearly, but the love I felt for my baby was so much more and so different that I would have given up everything to be with her. I held onto something my doctor told me during a visit after the first signs of trouble. She said that I needed to be strong and healthy for my husband and for my future children. That is what essentially kept me going. —*Chelsea*

Having Realistic Expectations for Your Grief

Grieving is a process that takes time. Throw deadlines out the window. Recognize that your sorrow will ebb and flow, and as your shock wears off, you may feel worse for a while. Over the course of the first few months, feeling worse instead of better can be discouraging, but be aware that this downturn is normal and expect this to happen.

⌐ The first month was the hardest. It was hard to fall asleep, and just thinking about her brought a lump to my throat. There were a variety of emotions, everything from joy to anger. I remembering feeling like this could not have possibly happened and just wanting to wake up and have my baby. —*Gina*

⌐ My emotions have been like a roller coaster. Some days I cry, some days I am fine. It's different each day. It's funny because there are days that I *want* to cry, I want to hear a sad song, and that helps me cope somehow. It might sound weird, but that helps the pain. —*Lizabeth*

⌐ I think I was at my worst about six months after Sarina's birth and death. It was summer by then, and I had focused on making it to summer and somehow thought that by then I would be feeling more like my old self. However, it was the opposite. I felt so down and unhappy and anytime I did have a laugh I would instantly think of Sarina and her not being with us, which ruined the happy moment. By that time, friends had stopped asking about my feelings and I was sick of saying I was still so sad. I just ended up saying I was fine. I felt so fake. —*Christine*

⌐ Some days I would feel OK and think, OK, now I can move on, and then I'd be crying the next minute. I couldn't seem to get a handle on my emotions. Talking with other families who have been through this helped. —*Debbie*

You may wonder if you will ever emerge from the abyss.

⌐ I physically recovered very quickly after the birth; emotionally and mentally it took a lot longer than I thought it would. I was quite depressed for almost a year. I grieved for a long time, and it was a roller coaster of emotions. Sometimes I thought I was fine, and then the littlest thing triggered a breakdown. I got through that year a day at a time. —*Christine*

⌐ The year following Gianna's birth and death were a blur. My days were filled with the routines of my children and my home, yet I was never alone to search within me. I was never alone to let the floodgates open. Oftentimes, I would think of asking a friend if I could escape into their homes when no one was about. I longed to find the solitude. I never was alone that first year—perhaps just in my shower. My children and husband did not want to see me sad, but it is a necessary path to healing. For this reason, it took me well over a year to be interiorly strong again. —*Doreen*

You can also expect your feelings to intensify or resurface during certain times of the year associated with your baby's life and death. These "anniversary reactions" can be especially pronounced during holidays, your baby's birthday, and anniversaries such as your baby's due date. Even if you didn't share holidays with your baby after birth, you may have memories of being happily pregnant the last time a holiday came around, or you had anticipated having a newborn for the next celebration. You are acutely aware of your empty arms. Other dates that may be seared in your memory are the date of your baby's diagnosis or date of death. Even a similarity in the day's weather may cause you to be flooded with memories or feel especially blue. And sometimes you cannot pinpoint why you're feeling down.

Holidays are hard, and seeing my nieces and nephews thrive has been bittersweet. —*Chelsea*

The most painful thing is that after three years, people no longer talk about Nathaniel or how important dates might continue to be hard for me, i.e., Mother's Day, the anniversary of his birth and death. It makes it seem like he did not exist and that the profound impact his life and death have on me is not important. —*Annette G.*

The situations that I expected to be hard (her first birthday, seeing other newborns, etc.) haven't been as tough as I thought. It's the unexpected time that sorrow bubbles through that catches me off guard. —*Alessandra*

Healthy grief eventually subsides, although traces can linger. Don't be alarmed if it occasionally sends a sharp pang when you least expect it—even years later—perhaps when you see a toddler the same age as your baby would have been, or if you realize that today is the day your child would have started school.

    ⌐ The death of a child is a dynamic and changing loss. I grieved the loss of her kindergarten graduation; this year, I will grieve the absence of her entrance into second grade; and in the future, I will grieve the absence of every milestone she misses. *—Dana*

These ebbs and flows of your grief are normal. Over time, your reactions will become less intense. For instance, someday you may even look at the calendar and realize that a significant date came and went. This is not forgetting your baby; this is honoring your baby by living your life.

Preoccupation with Your Baby as a Natural Expression of Grief

During your pregnancy, you became accustomed to thinking constantly about your baby. After your baby dies, this preoccupation may intensify as you are filled with yearning for this baby who is no longer with you.

    ⌐ In the first couple of months following Elliot's death, I thought that I would drown in the missing of him. *—Karla*

You may feel scattered and distracted, and daily tasks can seem trivial. You may wonder how everyone else can keep going after your world has come to a screeching halt.

    ⌐ I have found it difficult to concentrate on work. *—Steve*

    ⌐ I took five weeks off of work. I didn't want to go back to work, I just couldn't. It was hard enough going back to work for two days a week. I cried the entire hour to work and most of the day. It felt so crazy to go to work and do things when my baby died. *—Chelsea*

Even though your bond has been altered by death, you still have powerful biological urges to nurture and protect your baby. Particularly if you're the mother, biochemical postpartum changes in your body put you in parental overdrive. Both mothers and fathers may feel protective of their baby but have nowhere to focus their parental energies.

⟳ Right now the hardest thing for me is having so much love and no outlet for it. It feels as if there is nothing I can do with the love I have for her. My breast milk is gone; my bruises from my blood draws and IV are gone. I barely have anything tangible to show I had a baby, and that is very hard. —*Kristi R.*

⟳ I had a very strong urge to try to protect Anya somehow although she had already passed. The thought of her being alone is difficult, and I often wonder what she is experiencing now. —*Steve*

⟳ It has been painful to feel all kinds of mothering instincts inside of me that have nowhere to manifest as they were intended.
—*Susan E.*

Your preoccupation is a way to hold onto your baby and to continue your gradual goodbye. Viewing photographs, holding your baby's blanket, writing your baby's story in a journal, wearing a special piece of jewelry, or reviewing your memories are ways to affirm your baby's existence and feel connected to your little one.

⟳ When I am especially sad and longing for him, I look at the pictures, his hospital clothes, the locks of hair, or his handprints and footprints. They are tangible reminders of my little boy that I so love and miss. The nurses let us have his little undershirts and newborn hat. They still smell like him, and I feel a tingle in the back of my head every time I smell them. —*Heidi*

⟳ Those plaster molds are without a doubt my most precious keepsakes I have from Jordan. I can still stroke his tiny fingers and kiss his tiny feet. I place more value on them than any silver or gold I could ever own. —*Jenny D.*

⟳ I have two drawers of preemie baby clothes, blankets, and booties that my daughter actually wore. I have tons of pictures, six hours of videotape, footprints, handprints, a lock of hair, baby bracelets. I have presents people brought for Grace. I have a special necklace with her picture as a hologram on it and it is inscribed. I wear it every day, close to my heart. All of these things validate the fact that Grace was real and she was here. She had an impact on the people that held her. She was my daughter—not a diagnosis. —*Chris*

⌐ I have all the beautiful letters we received, and the ones I cherish the most are the ones that say "Congratulations"—I think that those people really "get it." They realize that we were all lucky to have each other and that her physical absence from our lives doesn't negate her rightful place in our family. —*Alessandra*

Photographs are particularly treasured keepsakes.

⌐ The photos mean a great deal to me. I looked at them often in the beginning—like every other hour. —*Susan E.*

⌐ Sometimes, everything just seemed so incredible—did I really have a baby? The pictures were a tremendous help, to be able to see my daughter. —*Monika*

⌐ A few months after our son's life and death, we received a package in the mail. It was a CD of 232 photos from Jordan's time with us. I cannot possibly express the joy I felt in receiving these photos. We had thought all of the joy of his time was in the past, and then out of the blue we get this gift of a moment looking at these photos for the very first time, new photos of our son. —*Jenny D.*

⌐ My most prized possessions are the photographs I have of all my three children together. There are two that are very special: one of my two boys holding her, where you can see Maggie looking right up at her brother; all three of them look as though they were just meant to be together. The other was taken the moment they met her. Our 5-year-old's eyes are full of delight and our 7-year-old has his arm raised in victory. That picture describes the tenor of her life better than any words—we celebrated every second she was with us. —*Alessandra*

⌐ The photographs are priceless. Before this loss happened to our family, I used to think that having pictures around the house was kind of weird. Well, it all changes when it happens to you. I now have framed pictures of our family of five and one on my refrigerator. I want to talk about all three of my daughters every day. —*Allison*

⌐ The pictures mean the world to us. I don't think I would remember exactly what he looked like if it wasn't for the pictures. Somehow they also make him seem more real. He really did exist. He was not a figment of our imagination. No one can ever deny him. —*Kathleen*

If the photos are disappointing or you wish you had more or better keepsakes, this is another loss to be grieved. But having even one good image can help you remember what your baby looked like. Photographs and all of your other keepsakes validate your grief and your love for this child.

If your baby's body was buried, visiting the gravesite can be a way to satisfy your preoccupation—or it can feel like a desolate reminder. You may even have fleeting thoughts about wanting to dig up your baby. These thoughts may make you question your sanity. But you are not insane; you are simply missing the one who would give meaning to your protective feelings: your sweet baby.

⌐ The gravesite is like an official acknowledgement of her existence, even if I don't go there often. —*Monika*

⌐ Going to the cemetery is hard. I know my baby is in heaven, but the same bones that kicked in me are lying there in the ground.
—*Allison*

As the months go by, your preoccupation will fade and you'll achieve a new balance. For now, accept yourself where you are.

⌐ As time went on, I knew I had to put everything away. I didn't get tired of seeing my photos and keepsakes; I just knew it needed to

be done. I had two feelings about it. In a way I felt like it was a dis-
honor to her, and in another it was moving on and healing. —*Greta*

Your Unique Experience of Grief

Your path through grief will be as unique as you are and perhaps
very different from your partner's path. (There will be more on your
relationship with your partner later in this chapter.) As introduced
in Chapter 3, there are intuitive grievers and instrumental grievers.
You may tend to be an intuitive griever, who feels your way through
grief. You may yearn and rant and cry over what you have lost. You
may benefit from talking with others or writing about your emotions.
As you release feelings, you are coming to terms with your baby's
death.

Or you may tend to be an instrumental griever who expresses grief
largely through immersion in activity. You may focus on your work,
devote yourself to a cause related to your baby's condition or experience, delve into sports or hobbies, create a lasting memorial or legacy
for your baby, or immerse yourself in religious or spiritual undertak-
ings. You may benefit from engaging in activities that are meaningful
to you, that aim toward self-improvement, or that honor your baby's
life. As you work toward your goals, you are adjusting to life without
your baby.

You may be a mixture of both, perhaps spending the first year
overwhelmed by emotion followed by a burst of energy devoted toward your work, self-improvement, or charitable activities. Or you
may shift back and forth between immersing yourself in emotions
and immersing yourself in activity. Whether you tend to be intuitive
or instrumental, you still benefit from facing and moving forward
through your grief.[8]

IDENTIFYING YOUR FEELINGS

By naming your emotions, you can get a handle on them. Knowing
what you're feeling can help you make sense of your grief. Separate,
identifiable feelings can seem more manageable than a tangled mass
of undefined pain. In addition to your obvious feelings of sadness, the
following is a brief summary of some of the other common feelings

Continuing Your Journey

that parents experience after their baby dies. Some coping strategies are summarized as well.

Shock, Numbness, and Denial

Immediately following your baby's death, you may not feel much of anything. Particularly if your baby's death happened suddenly or sooner than expected, you may need some time to absorb it. Early on, any semblance of normal activity can seem unreal.

⌐ I was in shock before the birth, during, and some time afterward. . . . I believe I finally realized what I lost about a week or two after the birth. I couldn't get enough cards, although each card that came in and every piece of mail made me get anxious. It was almost as if that card might bring Caelyn back. On some level, I thought I might be going crazy. I felt like ordering her pictures, making a scrapbook, receiving sympathy cards and other gifts might in some way bring her back. But they were actually confirming that she was gone. I would hurriedly open the cards and then realize they too said how sorry they were for our loss, instead of "Oh, didn't you know, you are in a very bad dream. All of this was a mistake. There is no way your baby died." —*Chelsea*

Responsibility and Guilt

⌐ I had a really hard time and kept questioning and second-guessing everything we did. "What if we did this or that?" would constantly be in my mind. Even though I knew she wouldn't live long and I have knowledge of the medical field, I still could not understand why she died. —*Debbie*

⌐ I have felt somewhat responsible for Frankie not having kidneys. In my darkest, deepest moments, I find myself crying out to him, apologizing to him that I couldn't give him kidneys. (The condition comes from my side of the family, doctors are pretty sure.) —*Susan E.*

If you faced difficult medical decisions regarding aggressive intervention, it may help to remember that you didn't choose death; you chose what you believed would give your baby the best possible life. Your decisions were right for your baby's particular circumstances and the information at hand. Most important, they arose out of your love for your baby.

If you feel guilty for feeling relief that this ordeal is over—not only for your child but also for yourself—remember that your wish wasn't for your baby to die. You accepted that a short life was your child's destiny. Your wish was to protect your baby and allow a peaceful death. So when your baby does die peacefully, it's natural to feel some sense of gratitude and relief.

Anger

You may feel frustrated, impatient, and irritable, because your baby's death is so very unfair and your life has changed in unexpected and crushing ways. Helplessness is another common source of anger: You may feel angry because your baby had a fatal condition, and there was nothing you could do about it. You may have anger about how your baby's life and death turned out.

⌐ During the pregnancy I often said, "I have peace about the outcome. I know it is God's will and we will be OK." I want to take that back. I don't like it at all, and there is no peace. I feel like I've been robbed of the most precious gift. —*Chelsea*

⌐ Many times after we got our son's diagnosis and after he died, people would comment about how strong I was, how brave they thought I was for not terminating, and what an inspiration Thomas was to them. I would just want to scream when I would hear those things. I didn't want to be a role model for strength and morality. I didn't want my son to be an inspiration to others. I just wanted him to have a boringly normal life. —*Kathleen*

⌐ There were times when I was very bitter and angry, times when I fought the pain of grief. I knew how horrible it was to be tossed in the sea of grief from our previous loss, and I fought the pain more this time. But it still came. I felt my family had been robbed of the joy of childbirth. —*Kelly G.*

Continuing Your Journey

⟿ The anger has been most difficult. Sometimes I'm just so enraged that this happened to me and my husband. Why us? It's so unfair. We are good parents who work so hard to have a good family life. Why did we have to lose our baby? —*Jennifer*

⟿ My anger has been the hardest to deal with. I was so angry for so long. I think it is because all I ever wanted was to meet her alive, and that was denied. —*Jamie*

⟿ I had so many people ask me what they could do to help. They would do anything I wanted. I wanted to scream at them: "I don't want anything but my baby back, all I want is Caelyn. NO! I don't want to eat or go do things, I want my baby. Can you do that?!" I held my tongue and merely said, "Thank you, but I don't need anything right now." —*Chelsea*

You may also feel let down by a lack of support from friends and family, particularly if they don't acknowledge your baby's death or down the road when they think you should be feeling better.

⟿ I received hundreds of cards congratulating me on Samuel's birth. Less than 10 percent of them have mentioned his twin sister, Lucy. This has been incredibly difficult. —*Jane G.*

⟿ We have an enlarged picture of Dominic in our living room. We hosted Thanksgiving here a year and a half later, and not one of the twenty-seven people said anything about his picture. They don't ask us how we are or bring up his name at all. I am so sad. —*Tami*

⟿ It can be hard when people stop mentioning your baby's name and acknowledging this loss in your life. They've moved beyond it, and you're moving forward, too—yet it is always with you. —*Missy*

As you adjust to your baby's absence and regain feelings of confidence and control over your life, your feelings of anger will naturally fade. For now, remember that people who really do want to help will welcome your feedback and suggestions. As you work through this feeling, any lingering anger can become a source of power rather than a drain.

⌐ I will say this for my anger: It contributes to a sense of power, if not control. When I let the anger come, life seems clearer and I'm more willing to tackle it head-on, whatever shape it takes. I guess I would say that my courage comes from a balance of gratitude and healthy anger. —*Susan E.*

Emptiness

You may feel that your heart, your body, your home—everything— is empty. Wandering in a world that seems oblivious to your grief can drain it of color and light.

⌐ It feels very empty. Family pictures feel empty, the dinner table feels odd—vacations we take and everywhere we are together feels empty. —*Tami*

⌐ It was hard to go to church the first time after the funeral service. Before, Anouk was with me, first in my womb and then in the casket. Now she wasn't there anymore. —*Monika*

⌐ The most difficult emotion for me has been how lonely and isolated I feel. I feel so alone without Jonah. Whenever we'd go somewhere in the car, I'd feel empty-handed as we'd leave the house without a car seat and diaper bag. For months, it just felt like something *huge* was missing. —*Heidi*

⌐ I wanted to cry, but mostly I walked around with a hole in my heart. I always hurt and felt a void. A piece of me was gone forever.
—*Kristi F.*

Vulnerability to Tragedy

Your baby's death may make you hyperaware that tragedy can strike at any time and that none of us are truly in control. You may worry about your other children, your partner, or your own health— and your worries may swell far out of proportion to any actual risks you may face.

⌐ I feared for my older son and his health—I feared that he had something that I didn't know about. I feared for my husband; would he get knocked off his bike? How could I cope alone? —*Elle*

Continuing Your Journey

⟶ I am constantly worried that something will happen to one of my other children. I think about death a lot. I am afraid to die and to lose my children. I am afraid of the pain they would feel if they lost my husband or me. —*Brooke*

These kinds of fears are normal, but you don't have to be ruled by them. While taking reasonable health and safety precautions, try also to keep in mind that most fears never materialize. Distinguish between real and imaginary fears and only pay attention to those based on the reality in front of you. Ignore the ones that lurk in your mind or are triggered by overwrought media stories. As you grieve and adjust, your feelings of vulnerability can fade. You can strike a new balance between maintaining control and trusting that whatever the outcome, your life can be lived well.

When you identify your feelings, you needn't analyze them or justify them or struggle against them—simply name them and experience them. This mindful acceptance can help you to process what you've been through and what it means to you, and this is what leads to healing, personal growth, and increased self-awareness. Remaining unaware of your emotions or striving to avoid them can doom yourself to repeating this emotional process and staying stuck, which can be far more painful in the long run. Your feelings are a normal part of this journey that has been painstakingly and successfully navigated by many bereaved parents before you.

MORE TECHNIQUES FOR COPING

In addition to the suggestions in Chapter 3, here are some others that can come into play now that your baby has died:

- *Set aside time for yourself and your grief.* Touch your keepsakes, visit the cemetery, organize your baby's photos. Take time to cry.
- *Take care of yourself physically and emotionally.* Attend to your health, and be gentle with yourself as you grieve. Find respite in activities you enjoy.

- *Talk about your baby.* Telling your story to anyone who will supportively listen can be very therapeutic.
- *Let others support you,* even if they don't do it well. Understand that many people are doing the best they can with a situation that is foreign to them. Tell them what you need. If they are true friends, they'll be glad to know.
- *Write letters to whomever you wish*—the rude neighbor, the kindly stranger, your doctor, the hospital, God, Mother Nature. Don't necessarily send them; the writing is for you. Particularly if you have regrets, write a letter to your baby, and then if you wish, imagine or write your baby's reply.
- *Read about grief, personal accounts of loss, or medical or spiritual issues.* Be open to advice that seems helpful and pass by whatever isn't.
- *Lean on the parts of your spiritual beliefs or religious faith that comfort you.*
- *Try to recognize anything positive*—discovered strengths, new growth, enlightened perspectives, meaningful pursuits, better relationships. Although it can be a struggle to find treasure in adversity, doing so can help you to heal and to honor your child's memory.
- *Make a conscious decision to survive.* After a while, you can decide whether to remember your baby and move forward with what you've gained or remain stuck with what you've lost. Many parents mention that eventually they reach a point where they just decide to start learning to live with it. When you are ready, you can do that too.
- *Remember that your grief is normal and you are not alone.*
- *Have faith that eventually you will feel better.*

In spite of the unpredictable ups and downs, you can expect your grief to slowly soften over a period of several years. This may seem interminable, but as the months pass, the ups do become more frequent and longer lasting. Eventually you will discover that you can remember your baby without keenly feeling the grief. You may always feel twinges of sadness, but eventually you can also accept this journey with a sense of peace that comes from knowing that you gave your baby a life full of nurturing and love.

⌐ I don't feel in denial or angry. I'm very sad but not depressed. Sometimes I even feel a sort of peace that we were able to do what we did for Ashley and to spend that beautiful time with her. There is some level of acceptance that it wasn't meant to be. Ashley was just too sick. —*Shellie*

Your life will never be the same, you'll always bear scars, but your broken heart can heal and you can settle into a "new normal." Eventually, when you are ready, you can see the meaning of this experience and the strength and wisdom you have gained. You can integrate your baby's life and death into your own life's journey, and you can remember the riches and joy your baby gave you. You move forward, holding your baby forever in your heart.

⌐ I do not mean to say that I am better because she suffered and died. I am better because she lived. I have a choice each day, as do each of us in grief. Do I want to be mournful, sad, and depressed? Because of my pain, do I want to stay inside of the darkness of grief? Or, do I want to celebrate the life my child lived and rejoice in the knowledge that she chose me as her mother? —*Dana*

For more reflections on healing and finding peace and acceptance, turn to Chapter 10. Wherever you are in your journey, you can benefit from seeing that other parents have not only survived this experience but thrived. You can too.

REGRETS AND MAKING PEACE WITH THEM

The grieving process typically includes reviewing and making peace with regrets. As you think about anything you wish had happened differently, you are identifying and grieving additional losses associated with the death of your baby. The most common regret is not being able to carry out certain plans before your baby died. Especially if you acquire more ideas after it's too late, you may find yourself obsessing over the bath you didn't give, keepsakes you didn't collect, one last kiss you didn't bestow. In can help to remind yourself that even the best-laid plans can be derailed by the fatigue and drugs associated with labor and birth. Also, there was only so much you could reasonably compress into your limited amount of time.

⌐ Sometimes I find myself forgetting how challenging the time was and thinking of unreasonable regrets—like why didn't I take the family to a professional photography studio?! For the most part, I have a lot of peace that while I may wish I had done more to make memories, Lucy really did have the best life a little girl could have. —*Jane G.*

Ironically, in light of the hesitation many parents initially feel about taking photographs, a common regret is not taking *enough* photographs or not including more people, especially siblings.

⌐ I didn't even bring a camera because I thought for sure I wouldn't want pictures. I regret that now, as I would have loved a picture of her hands. I deeply regret not allowing our other children to come to see their sister in person. —*Shayla*

⌐ I wish I had taken a picture of her and me together where you could see both of our faces. I wish we had better pictures of all four of us. —*Jane G.*

⌐ By the time our older son came to the hospital, he was two hours beyond bedtime with no nap, and Thomas had already died. I just didn't think that it was best to bring this exhausted, overwhelmed child and thrust his dead baby brother onto him, just so we could snap a picture. Now I wish we had. —*Kathleen*

Another common regret is not spending more time alone with the baby, before or after death. Many parents wish they'd done more to explore and appreciate the wondrous creation that was their baby.

⌐ I wish that I had been comfortable exploring that little body which I had carried within me for months. —*Doreen*

Continuing Your Journey

I wish I had changed Lucy's diaper so that I could have looked at her girl parts! —*Jane G.*

The only regret I have is not spending more time with Nathaniel alone before others came into the room. By the time everyone left and I had him to myself again, I was very tired. —*Annette G.*

My biggest regret is that I didn't hold Dominic longer after he passed away. I was in shock. If someone would have gently told me to stay with him, because it would be the last time forever on this earth, I would have embraced that. The nurse took so long to clean him up that by the time she called us back to his room it was 2 a.m. and I was a wreck. I wish I could go back to that moment so much. I try to make peace with it by remembering how much I held him while he was alive. —*Tami*

I wish I would have undressed her and looked at her body more carefully. There was always someone around (too many visitors) and I wanted to be alone to do this. I do know that I did all that I thought was right at the time. You can't turn back time. —*Sherry*

Some parents regret their attitude or emotional condition during the pregnancy. It may help to remind yourself that you did the best you could with the support you received and the information you had.

Despite our very deliberate attempts to make no mistakes so there would be no regrets, I still have them. I regret that after the diagnosis I took little joy in my pregnancy because I was so afraid of this experience and all of the "what ifs" that were going through my mind. Today I look back and think, boy, if I had just known that this was going to turn out to be one of the greatest blessings in my life, I could have just relaxed and enjoyed what I could of it and made the most of the experience. I am still coming to terms with this. I tell myself that we did the very best we could for Michael and that he had a family that loved him very much. —*Missy*

I regret that I didn't want this child at first, but I am human, and I did want him after the shock of finding out I was pregnant went away. I did everything for my child that I humanly could, and that I cannot regret. How can I regret a beautiful life given to us? How can I regret the joy and spiritual blessings he brought us? —*Sue*

As with grief, the way to come to terms with regrets is to mindfully accept and move through your thoughts and feelings about them. As your grief softens, your perspective can change. You can recognize that you persevered through an incredibly challenging and extraordinary time and forgive yourself for any perceived shortcomings. Eventually, you can shift your focus from what you weren't able to do or the experiences you weren't able to have, to what you *were* able to do.

My only regrets were not having flowers, not taking early pictures with her and her older brother, and not having time alone with her. None of these things matter to me anymore. I have so many special memories with her. —*Katharine*

I have no regrets—or the little ones I do, I don't beat myself up over them. I wished we had bathed her, but we didn't. There is no sense beating yourself up for the "what ifs" or "could haves" or "should haves." We did everything we could as parents for her and we made decisions other parents never have to make regarding the care of their children. We also had to let go, something all parents must learn to do. But our letting go was just of her physical self— not her spirit—not what she gave to us and what she still gives us and teaches us. —*Elizabeth D. P.*

You nurtured and protected your baby. The rest—the particular experiences, the photographs, material mementos—are meaningful but ultimately peripheral. Your love for your baby is what matters and what endures.

YOU AND YOUR PARTNER

Our marriage has been made stronger. We had moments that were rough, and we had to learn that we both don't handle grief in

Continuing Your Journey

the same way. We had to communicate why we felt certain ways and express our individual feelings. —*Annette H.*

My husband and I talked a lot. We took a week-long driving trip through the Blue Ridge Mountains to get away. —*Delsa*

I remember one day, about a month after Sarina passed away, I was crying in the living room while our son was playing, and my husband said to me, "I just want the old Christine back," and he cried too. It seemed to me that he was better at coping, he didn't show his emotions like me, and that often made me feel angry. I wanted him to be more expressive. I wanted him to tell me when he thought of Sarina. I wanted him to be more sad. He told me that just because he wasn't as expressive on the outside as I was, that he too lost Sarina and that he too was hurting, he just didn't show it like I did. This was a difficult time in our marriage, but I do believe it has brought us closer together. —*Christine*

All couples struggle to support each other through their shared grief. Because each person's grief is unique, you and your partner will have different ways of expressing, coping with, and moving through grief. As discussed earlier in this chapter, one of you may tend toward intuitive grieving, while the other may be more instrumental. What you may find supportive, your partner might find intolerable or inconsequential. After the six-week postpartum exam, you may get the green light for sexual intimacy, but partners may differ in how eager they are. Sex can be a painful reminder of the conception of your baby, or it can be a loving and tender reunion—or both. If you and your partner have different styles or are otherwise out of sync, it can help immensely to simply accept your differences, communicate without judgment, listen without trying to fix, and encourage each other to do what each of you need to do.

When you have differing needs, it can be a challenge to find the middle ground. While some couples seem able to take turns offering comfort to each other, most couples need to find additional sources of support. Consider other people in your life who can offer support—and not just those who will cry with you. Perhaps there are people who make you laugh, who will exercise with you, or who will simply listen. You can think of all those people as spokes in your wheel of support.[9] Seeking support elsewhere doesn't mean that your partner isn't enough or that your marriage is in trouble; it's acknowledging that when you are both sinking, it can be hard to hold each other up.

⌒ It was especially hurtful when my husband got sick of my grief. That was difficult, but we continued to try to work on that and time has taken care of a lot. —*Sue*

⌒ My husband doesn't have near the support network I do, yet it's hard for me to be a big help to him since we are both still grieving so. He has one friend that is a great support to him; otherwise, even his parents don't know how to handle all this. Avoidance seems to be their way, which just hurts my husband even more. —*Heidi*

Some couples grow more distant, if this experience widens a wedge that already existed between them. Other couples retreat into themselves at first but come back together again, stronger than before. And some couples manage to stay close, drawing together in the face of adversity and gaining new respect for each other. Whatever your pattern, it is a chance to grow for each of you.

⌒ Life changed for my husband and me. There was a new understanding between us. One that was pulled from the depths of the past and the present. We got to know each other on a new level, again. —*Kristi F.*

⌒ One thing that I can say is that my husband and I have grown so much stronger in our marriage. I could not imagine going through all of this without him, as well as sharing my "Kevin moments" with someone other than him. My husband and I feel the same pain but deal with it differently. With a lot of communication and heartfelt conversations, we are now able to help one another through our toughest of toughest times. He is my heart and soul. —*Amy*

Continuing Your Journey

⁓ Staying close to my husband has been a big support for me. He is my best friend. He is the one I talk to when I am sad and when I miss Aubrielle. He is very understanding, and he just lets me talk. —*Holly*

⁓ It has been very difficult but I feel that our marriage has become stronger. —*Steve*

You may have heard that bereaved couples have a high divorce rate. Statistics vary widely, with some studies suggesting a higher risk of breaking up and others finding that the divorce rate is actually *lower* than among the general public.[10] As a couple, you can make a commitment to survive this shared experience together.

⁓ My husband and I have a great marriage, and I didn't want to lose that on top of losing our baby. I later found out that those divorce statistics are usually overstated, and my husband and I are closer than ever. I don't see how you can look into the depths of absolute heartache and despair with someone and not come out with a more intimate understanding and appreciation for each other. I love my husband now more than ever. —*Kathleen*

⁓ I see my husband differently now. He's my best friend. We have been to hell and back together, and we survived. In fact, our marriage is stronger than ever because of it. —*April*

How you and your partner weather this storm can largely depend on the relationship skills you already hold or are willing to learn. Be patient with your grief and each other and get extra help and support if you feel the need. And if you do decide to part, this can be yet another painful but priceless opportunity for personal growth.

YOUR OTHER CHILDREN

How your other children respond will mostly depend on what they understand about death, their relationship with their baby sibling, their reaction to your grief, and the support and reassurance they receive. As discussed in Chapter 3, giving children simple, reassuring, straightforward answers helps them cope, and communication will continue to be important now that your baby has died.

⟞ I believe that for my older children it was of biggest importance that they were able to see Anouk. It made her real in their eyes, and they were able to see with their own eyes that she was not to live. They never asked later why Anouk did not survive. They saw and understood. And none of them ever had nightmares or was disturbed. —*Monika*

Just as your expression of grief is unique, so is your child's. Their sense of loss will naturally be different and not as intense as yours. Children often express feelings through creative play, so pretending or drawing about death is normal. Very young children are often affected most by disruptions in the family's emotional climate and routines. Older children may express a desire for a living sibling, which can add to your heartbreak. Key to supporting them is keeping your baby's life and death an open topic. You've already experienced the benefit of openly accepting your baby's life and preparing for death during the pregnancy, and your children can benefit from continuing open communication about remembering this baby and processing their experiences and feelings, now and as they grow.

⟞ It's been painful for me to watch my daughter envy her friends who have sisters and know that she will also forever have the void in her life. I have dealt with those moments simply by hugging her or letting her know that I am thinking about her and her own pain. —*Shayla*

⟞ Our older daughter is only 2, so she doesn't understand much about what happened and why her parents are sad. But she did meet Ashley in the hospital. We talk about Ashley and show pictures of her. It was tough when about a month after Ashley died, my older daughter asked me, "Where's As-lee?" It was the first time she asked me this. I didn't think she would ask me that at such a young age. Then she lifted up my shirt, pointed at my tummy, and said, "As-lee." I told her Ashley was not in my tummy anymore. I said she has gone to heaven and that she died. Of course a toddler can't understand that concept. She asked a few more times where Ashley was. I wish I could have helped her better understand, but she is so young. I believe it is best to be open and honest about death, and we will continue to tell her about her sister as she gets older. —*Shellie*

Parents often are amazed at how naturally their other children integrate the baby's life and death into their own lives. Their actions and words can warm your heart and affirm your baby's life and place in your family.

After watching a particularly pretty sunset, our daughter turned to my husband and me and said, "I hope Jonah got to see that one from heaven!" About two weeks after Jonah's memorial service, she made a picture that she said was for Baby Jonah. She ran outside and stood on her tiptoes with the picture as high over her head as she could reach. She then asked me if I thought Jonah could see it from heaven. At night as we tuck her in bed, she likes to yell, "Goodnight, Baby Jonah. We love you!" so he can hear us all the way up in heaven. I cherish these kinds of things that she does because she's such a good big sister even though her little brother isn't here to reap the rewards. —*Heidi*

Our 4-year-old son has been amazing. I am so proud of him. He talks about his brother Brayden so proudly and often loves to just go outside and yell up to him. He has so much love for a baby he never knew and has been so strong in dealing with this. We have done everything we can to help him cope by talking about Brayden often, getting books, and taking him to a class with other children his age dealing with loss. He has been a great support for us as well. Just hearing him talk about or to Brayden melts our hearts and reaffirms that Brayden's life, no matter how short, had so much impact and purpose. —*Camille*

One day my older daughter and I went for story time at the library. We ran into someone I knew who recently had her second daughter. As we stood and talked, I bent down to ask her oldest daughter how she likes to be a big sister. Instead, my daughter was quick to respond proudly, "I just love being Mariah's big sister." Oh, if she would only know what a great sister she would've been. —*Greta*

⟶ I had been a little worried about my older daughter. I really should not have worried. I think children understand and accept things better than adults. She was prepared for five months for the birth and death of her baby sister. She sang to her every day that I was pregnant. She would tell her that she would go to heaven and everything would be OK. It was so sweet. She still talks about Aubrielle, how she is in heaven, and how she has no more "owies." —*Holly*

⟶ Our other children still talk about Rose. It is very comforting. My biggest fear was that we would all forget about her, and that has not been the case. —*Debbie*

As time passes and your family recovers its balance, memories of this experience will continue to surface from time to time. As your children grow, their questions and sense of loss will change, and your ongoing openness will continue to benefit all of you.

DEALING WITH THE OUTSIDE WORLD

Some of the challenging social situations you'll face include informing others of your baby's life and death; deciding what to tell people, if anything, about your experiences; and being around others' babies.

Letting Others Know

Whether you shared your situation widely while you were pregnant or not, you will likely want people to know that your baby has been born and what happened. Birth announcements are a traditional way of sharing the news of a new baby with family and friends; it is certainly appropriate to send announcements letting people know about your baby's birth and death.

⌐ We sent birth announcements to our friends and family. It said, "We are heartbroken to announce both the birth and death of our son, Thomas." It had his date of birth, weight, and length. It also had one of the pictures of him that was taken in the recovery room. I wasn't sure how people would take it when they received it. But, honestly, I didn't really care. He was born, and I wanted everyone to know it. He was going to be deprived of so many things: no welcome-to-the-world presents, no first birthday . . . the list goes on and on. I was determined to at least give him a proper birth announcement. All of the responses that I got were positive. Several people said that it really tore them up to read it, but they thought it was a beautiful thing to do. My best friend has kept it on her refrigerator. That has meant a lot to me. He's right up there where he should be, with all the other babies and kids that she knows. —*Kathleen*

If you've been keeping family and friends informed through a website or blog, naturally you'll want to update your site. If you live in a small town with a local newspaper that is widely read, you might consider placing an announcement in the paper.

⌐ After the announcement was published, I couldn't believe the response. We received so many flowers and cards and so much food. It was so touching. All of those thoughtful gestures and words were what I held onto during those first few weeks. It validated that Sarina was thought about and that people cared enough to let us know. —*Christine*

For work colleagues, an e-mail message can be an appropriate way of explaining your situation and framing it the way you want.

Unfortunately, official notice of your baby's birth may also be sent automatically to school districts and companies that sell baby formula or diapers. Finding a free sample of formula in your mailbox amidst the sympathy cards is a juxtaposition that can feel like a punch to the gut. You can remove your name from mailing lists by contacting the Direct Marketing Association.[11]

As you begin to reenter your world, you may find it difficult to begin socializing again. Some people may be uncomfortable talking about your baby and your experience of continuing your pregnancy. Fatal conditions and death are sensitive topics, and well-intentioned people may attempt to keep your mind off your baby or say nothing for fear of saying the wrong thing.

⌐ People didn't know what to say, so I felt like they kind of tried to avoid us. In social situations, I felt like the elephant in the room. Meanwhile, I yearned to talk about Jonah—his life, even his death. I felt like most moms get to proudly show off their new babies. I didn't have a baby to show them, but I had a beautiful story to share. I just wanted them to ask. —*Heidi*

⌐ We found it very difficult that everyone was so focused on the fact that he was gone. They were not with us through each step of Timothy's life and did not understand how happy we were to have been blessed with Timothy. We tried to help them see that while our son was with us he made us the happiest parents in the whole world. —*Donna*

⌐ It was less than a week after I lost my baby girl and the rest of the world was moving on. It really surprised me when it hurt so badly. I saw a friend and was with her in a group setting for a few hours. I waited for her to say something about Mariah—anything— and she didn't. I know she probably just didn't know what to say or didn't want to bring it up and make me sad. But I was thinking about it anyway and I didn't mind talking about it. —*Greta*

⌐ One of the hardest things while carrying Anouk and after her death was that many people did not recognize her life. They thought that because she didn't have a brain (that's the meaning of the word anencephaly, but that's not what anencephaly really is) she wasn't a real human being. Isn't the brain what makes a human being? So a body without a brain is just a body, not a real person. And because I just lost a body (in their eyes), and not a real child, why would I be so affected by her death? Plus, anencephaly is hard to look at; in many medical sources, affected babies are still referred to as "monsters." In many people's eyes, it is impossible to love such a baby. So I ended up not telling people about the anencephaly anymore but just mentioned that she had "a fatal birth defect." Not because I would have been ashamed of her, but because I was so tired of getting hurt again and again by the thoughtless comments about my daughter. —*Monika*

⌐ I met an old neighbor in the supermarket about two months after Rose died. She said she had heard about my "mishap." I wanted to scream at her: My baby was not a mishap, she was my child, my daughter. —*Elle*

⌐ While most people handled interacting with me very well, a few people never said anything at all to me. Not even, "I'm sorry about your loss." That was really painful to me. I would just keep my mouth shut and then go home and cry my heart out. —*Susan E.*

Like most grieving parents, you may have longtime friends or close family members who disappoint you when they don't acknowledge your grief. A shifting of friendships is normal when you veer away to a different path. With the passage of time, you may find that some relationships can be repaired.

⌐ What has caused me a great deal of sadness is the loss of so many friendships. I am not the same person I was before I heard the word "anencephaly." For the most part, the people that I count as good friends now were people that I hardly knew one and a half years ago. —*Jane G.*

⌐ My mother-in-law told me that she was very glad she wasn't there when it happened because she didn't want to see him. She said it would have been too hard. This is your grandson! He's going to be born. He deserves for you to see him. His own grandmother didn't want to see him. I understand where that feeling is coming from, but I don't want to hear that. I think had she been there, it would have been different. I was scared too. But when you're there, it just seems natural and OK and it's not scary. —*Anna*

After the funeral, my brother was so angry and didn't understand why we didn't try to save Bethany. I e-mailed him and explained to him exactly what Trisomy 13 was and that had we tried to save her, we would just have been prolonging the inevitable. He still was very angry and wouldn't talk about it or acknowledge it. However, on her birthday this past year, he did send me an e-mail and apologized for his behavior and how proud and amazed he was at how we handled the whole thing. —*Angel*

Meeting new people can present special challenges. Even if you don't plan on telling your story, casual questions about children come up. You may want to think ahead of time about how you would like to respond. Some parents always mention the baby who died, while others quickly assess the situation to decide whether the questioner needs to know.

The hardest thing for me is answering the question, "How many children do you have?" I always want to acknowledge her but sometimes don't want to get into the whole explanation with people. —*Katharine*

Most of the time I say I have two children, but I find that I'm more willing to share the story now than I was right after it happened. It's a hard thing because our language doesn't have a way to refer to a child you had who died. There isn't a term. It's an awkward thing to explain. You don't want to make the person you're talking to feel uncomfortable so you don't talk about it, but then you end up feeling like you've marginalized your own child, so you end up being the one who feels bad. —*Missy*

You may have renewed appreciation for those who reach out to you or aren't afraid to listen. You can learn to rely on this oasis of support and forgive those who cannot be there for you.

Our families were a godsend. They were there for us whenever we needed anything. But more importantly they were there to offer love, a shoulder to cry on, someone to talk to, and help dealing with the emotions that come with such a loss. —*Donna*

Continuing Your Journey

⌒ My aunt sent us some flowers with the most wonderful card. It said "Thomas was here just briefly, but he is loved." He *was* here, but he *is* loved. That says it perfectly. It means the world to you when someone else acknowledges that. —*Kathleen*

⌒ The night that we buried Gianna, we found a single pink rose on our front door with a note that said, "Every time you see the lights burning in our windows, please know that we are thinking of you during this time and have your family and Baby Gianna in our prayers." All the neighbors on our street had a single candle burning in a window. It was a beautiful gesture. —*Jennifer*

Others' Pregnancies and New Babies

If you are in your childbearing years, chances are you have friends and family who are too. Whether it's in your circle or in public places such as stores and restaurants, you are going to be faced with other pregnant women and newborns. You may feel as if you are surrounded or find yourself attuned to babies in ways you never felt before. Seeing babies born around the same time as yours can be especially difficult. You may resent people who take their children for granted. You may want to avoid baby showers or holding babies for a time. These are all normal reactions that will fade as you heal.

⌒ You can't go into the grocery store or post office, get gas or a movie, it seems, without finding another woman who has what you so desperately want. —*Alaina*

⌒ My company has a day care, and there are many infants and small children. At lunch I see them playing with their parents, and it is very difficult. —*Steve*

⌒ I haven't mustered the courage to hold other babies yet. I know that when the time is right, I will. I want to, but not yet. Mostly, I want to hold them and cry for Jonah while I do. —*Heidi*

⌒ Seeing other baby girls with dark hair born around the same time Gianna was born is really difficult—especially seeing them being nursed or a circle of admiring people around them. They are darling babies, but I wish I had my baby too! —*Jennifer*

A Gift of Time

It was hard to see other newborns with a perfect round head and the parents who just take it as normal to have a healthy baby. But I remember that before Anouk's diagnosis, I was just the same: Why would a baby die? They're made to live, not to die. —*Monika*

Honestly, other people's babies really don't bother me too much or pull my heartstrings. They are not my child; they are not my baby. I don't want their child and I don't want their lives. I just want my child back, and I can't have her. And I wouldn't swap my life for theirs, because I had my baby for just the shortest of times but to me I feel blessed that she came to us. That she chose us, and she knew we would do what was best for her. I am honored she chose us to be her parents. We were so lucky to have had her. —*Elle*

The other day as I was getting out of my car, I heard a baby crying down the street and my whole body warmed up, or reacted, did something I can't explain. It's been seven and a half months since I lost Frankie—are the hormones still coursing through my body? Or is it that given the intense but brief time of motherhood, my system fundamentally changed? —*Susan E.*

SUBSEQUENT PREGNANCIES

The question of whether to try for another baby looms large for many couples. Many are ambivalent. You may feel a sense of urgency because you want to have living child in your arms, but you also know that another baby doesn't fill the void left by the baby who died. You may also dread what might lie in store for you if you embark on another pregnancy.

One day I was certain we had to get pregnant immediately; the next day I was certain I was never going to willingly put myself in this position again. —*Alaina*

We get a lot of "Oh, you two, don't worry, you can have another baby," as if having another baby would replace our Noah. Like it would take away our loss and grief. Having another baby would bring joy to us and we would love that baby with all of our hearts—

Continuing Your Journey

335

just as we loved Noah. But another baby would not be Noah or replace him. —*Jenny A.*

Trying again brings its own challenges. If you have trouble conceiving, this adds to your grief. And if you do get pregnant, your innocence is gone.

As my period came each month, sometimes early, sometimes late, I felt hope ebb away and was left feeling empty-handed, broken, unloved, and forgotten. Each period represented one more month without a new baby and accentuated my sense of loss over Elliot. —*Karla*

I tried to have a subsequent pregnancy after Grace but unfortunately suffered three more miscarriages over the years. Each time, I wrestled with the loss of Grace and felt that I needed to have a healthy baby to move on in my life. After all of this struggle, I have come to accept that Grace was my last baby. That has been difficult: The promise of having another baby to hold and fill my empty arms was not to be. To end my reproductive years with a loss has been difficult. —*Chris*

As I write this, I am 17 weeks pregnant with another baby. So far, after fairly sophisticated and extensive testing, this baby seems to be totally healthy and showing no signs of the chromosomal abnormalities that took Maggie from us. This subsequent pregnancy has been hard for me; the worrying is so burdensome. I hate that my naiveté is gone, that pregnancy is no longer an optimistic, hopeful, exciting experience. That seems like another one of the things we lost when we lost our Maggie. I hope this baby is born healthy—I am not sure I can survive this experience twice. —*Alessandra*

Your baby's condition may have revealed genetic information about you and your partner that has implications for possible future babies.

The doctors and genetic counselors now believe my husband and I carry a recessive gene causing Lillie's and William's conditions. It brings a 25 percent chance with every child. We have one healthy child. We want more children. Do we even risk trying again and possibly facing another loss? Our families have started to suggest adoption. They've been hurt too much too. —*Pam F.*

⮑ We know now that my husband and I are both carriers of a recessive gene and that, if we have another baby with the same condition, it is always fatal. It's a good thing to know, but heartbreaking. Now what do we do? We want to have a baby so badly. Would it be wrong to try again, knowing our chance of it happening again is one in four? My husband and I have decided to try again someday. I have often said that it just has to be OK; there is no way this could happen again—it just can't. —*Chelsea*

⮑ My husband came up with these two questions to answer: What is the worst that could happen? We could have another sick baby that dies. Can we deal with this? That answer was no for a long time, and then it was yes. —*Behka*

You may explore adoption—or you may decide to be content with what you have. Whether you eventually have another child or not, the process of coming to terms with your reproductive destiny is part of your movement toward peace and healing.

⮑ I thought I would want to have another baby after Thomas died. But I don't. I have this sense that my husband and I are just supposed to "circle the wagons" and count our blessings. Whenever I think about not trying for another baby, I get this deep feeling of inner peace. I wish I didn't. I really *want* to want another one. But I just can't deny that inner peace feeling. I think most of our friends and family really want us to have another baby. I think there is this real sentiment that we would be "OK" if we just had another baby. I found lots of books about the stresses and difficulties involved with trying again. I haven't found much out there about the stresses and difficulties that come with deciding to *not* try again. It has been a lonely journey. —*Kathleen*

As you come to terms with your reproductive fate, your baby also may have granted you a sense of acceptance and greater appreciation for whatever future pregnancies may bring—another gift from your little one to you.

⁓ Sidney prepared me to raise a special-needs child. I do not fear that, and in fact look forward to it if I ever have the opportunity to do so. I would have given anything to raise her, problems and all. —*Laura W.*

⁓ My next pregnancy was so hard (my sister called it my "pregnancy of denial" because I wouldn't even allow myself to believe it could ever work out), but I feel proud and brave that we went for it. I am delighted to have this lovely little person to love and nurture. I am a better person and parent because of Maggie, and that is Maggie's gift to the lovely sister who came after her and to the brothers who miss her daily. —*Alessandra*

⁓ This whole process of gratitude, acceptance, and listening to my intuition heavily informs how I handle the possibility of our conceiving another baby with Potter syndrome. On good days—when I feel such gratitude—I envision the period when I carry another baby as a time of joy, whether or not she or he will be able to live outside of my womb, similar to how it felt to carry and love Frankie. It's possible that we'll have to go through this all over again if I do get pregnant—and I most definitely will carry to term. —*Susan E.*

ten

Reflections

⟶ I am so glad that we welcomed her to our family with love. Of course, I wish that she were still alive today. But I do not regret the experience or wish that it had never happened. —*Katharine*

⟶ Though this experience has definitely been the hardest time in my entire life, I have no regrets about carrying Elliot, loving him, grieving him, or missing him. —*Karla*

⟶ As heartbreaking as it was at the time, it was so significant in my life and my husband's life and the lives of my family members. I wouldn't change it. I wouldn't change it at all. —*Missy*

⟶ She was always wrapped in loving arms with a warm heartbeat near her. It comes down to that. She came, she lived, she felt love, and then she died. She smelled our farm and our house. She felt the sun and wind on her face. She opened her eyes and took us all in, but she was never far from the place from which she came. The spirit world. Heaven. From God in its many forms. And there she returned. And it hurts so much. A hurt that I know will never go away. But she was worth all the hurt, and I am so thankful that she came into my life. —*Kristi F.*

⟶ She didn't bring sadness. She brought joy, utter joy. —*James*

After the worst of the storm has passed, you will have time to reflect on what it was like to be battered by the winds and darkness of your grief over your baby's diagnosis and death. You will notice that your own sky is brightening, and the torrents of tears become occasional puddles glistening in the sunlight. This final chapter holds words of encouragement about adjusting and moving forward. Parents reflect on their experiences, including spiritual beliefs and struggles, finding meaning in their journey, as well as their personal transformations.

REFLECTIONS ON YOUR JOURNEY

⌒ It was worth it. He was worth it. —*Tracy*

Once you're on the other side of your baby's birth and death, you may be surprised by how gratifying your time together was.

⌒ The first weeks after Luke's diagnosis, never in my wildest dreams did I imagine how wonderful and rewarding this journey would be. Yes, it was painful and sorrowful, but I could not imagine the joy that would also be a part of this. Luke has left us with so much more. I am so blessed to have lived and experienced this little life. —*Sue*

⌒ I can honestly say that if God gave my husband and me the option to have never done this; to never have even been pregnant with Austin and to never have even heard the word anencephaly; if God said it's either Austin with anencephaly or no Austin at all, we'd choose Austin. It was not easy and at times the most difficult thing we'll ever face, but knowing what we know now, I'd do it all over again, just for that one chance to hold his hand and cry while he went to heaven. I'd take nothing back and I have no regrets. —*Jo*

⌒ Initially, I resisted this experience and wanted it to end. While I was living it, it alternately broke my heart and made me angry. From the perspective I have today, I see this experience as one of the greatest blessings in my life. It shaped me, clarified my values, and revealed a level of strength I did not know I possessed. —*Missy*

⌒ I always refer to the journey we shared with Maggie as being bittersweet. Everyone understands the bitter: You plan for and expect a child and then you find out that she is too sick to live and that there is absolutely nothing you can do about it. That is about as bitter as it gets. But the bitter is only part of the story. There are so many moments of sweet—the sweetness you feel when you finally meet the child you adore so deeply, the sweetness you feel when you take advantage of the opportunity to mother her in the ways that she needs you to, the sweetness that exists when your other children are able to understand that love is worth it, the sweetness that surfaces when people share their kindnesses and compassion so lovingly, and the sweetness that exists when you feel no regret at the choices you made. —*Alessandra*

This journey was beautiful because we were able to celebrate her life and not look at it as a tragedy. All our baby daughter will ever know is love. —*John*

Reflections on Knowing the Diagnosis before Birth

Knowing your baby's condition before birth can be both blessing and burden. Most parents say that in retrospect they are glad they knew. While it makes for a more sorrowful and complicated pregnancy, the knowledge lets you absorb the shock of your baby's condition before birth, provide comfort and palliative care instead of unnecessary intensive care, and make the most of your baby's short life.

If I hadn't gotten an ultrasound, I would have innocently carried on with the pregnancy. And then our first moments with him outside the womb—not to mention Frankie's own moments—would have been an agony, because when the doctors would have seen that he couldn't breathe, they would have yanked him from us and frantically put him on respirators, etc. When I imagine this alternative scenario, I am so, so relieved that I had that ultrasound done that revealed what was to come. Having known his fate actually makes me feel like I had extra time, even though I would have had three remaining months whether I knew or didn't know that he would die. Since it wasn't the quantity of time that had changed, I guess it must have been the quality of time that had changed: I was able to really be present with him and more aware of him during those last months. —*Susan E.*

A father whose baby had died told me, "The finding out is worse than when it actually happens." What he meant was that the devastation of learning the diagnosis is worse than the actual experience of the child's death. This helped to decrease my fear of her death. And I found it to be true. I began grieving the day I learned her diagnosis and later, as difficult as her death was, I was ready for it and it didn't break me. —Jill K.

The five months of "knowing" were not easy, yet I am forever thankful that I knew. The time I had allowed me to prepare so that we could enjoy each and every second we had with Daniel. Our time with him wasn't filled with that initial shock and devastation of finding out. We were filled with such joy and love. In a very bittersweet way, those days with Daniel were certainly the best in our lives; we were a complete family. —Kim

Reflections on Continuing Your Pregnancy

You may find peace in knowing that your decision to continue this pregnancy allowed your baby to live as long as his or her body could sustain life, yielding to the natural course of life and death rather than forcing it.

I have a tremendous amount of peace that I did the right thing and that Lucy was able to live the days ordained for her. I have come to peace about her death. —Jane G.

For me it felt more manageable to know that I had let nature take its course. And I gained a lot of strength and joy from the days I had with Alaina. Having it end sooner would not have decreased my suffering. And having it end later did not increase my suffering. It was maybe just a different kind of suffering. —Jill K.

I am very certain that we did the right thing by letting Lily live her life in the way that she did. I know that I wouldn't be where I am emotionally if I had terminated her life early. —Katharine

A diagnosis of marginal placenta previa was what put a halt to our original decision to induce at 24 weeks, and for that diagnosis I will forever be grateful. We felt great peace once we stepped out in faith to let things happen naturally, to let Frankie develop as he must. —*Susan E.*

⟶ If we had decided to terminate this pregnancy I would have dealt with pain, suffering, loss, and regret. By carrying Brayden until natural death I was able to love him longer, give him everything I could, and there is zero regret. You cannot avoid the pain, suffering, and loss either way. —*Camille*

⟶ I really have peace that we carried her to term. I know in my heart that I have given my daughter all that I could and loved her every day of her life. —*Annette H.*

⟶ At Grace's funeral, the priest said that people thought we had taken the "hard road," but my husband said it was just the opposite. We had no "what ifs"—we knew what she looked like, smelled like, and felt like. We knew the ending of our story, and we did it with love. My husband said we had taken the easy road because we had no regrets or guilt. He was right. —*Chris*

⟶ By giving my son the protection of my body to face the announced death, I was giving him life, all of his life, so that it would be recorded in our family, in all of our history, and in the hearts of each of us. It wasn't a morbid walk but a formidable surge of love. —*Isabelle*

Back when you were making your decision, you and others around you may have been doing the math, calculating the time you'd spend pregnant and the amount of time you may or may not get with your baby after birth, and questioning whether the investment of time could possibly be worth the fleeting moments of life outside the womb. You may feel that you now have your answer.

⟶ The thirty-three hours we had with him made all the anxiety, confusion, and depression during my pregnancy worth it. As soon as we saw him, we knew without a doubt that we had made the right decision five months prior. —*Heidi*

I would not trade those four hours for anything. It was worth all the physical pain. And even if I had to go through it all over again with my next pregnancy, it would be worth it. —*Holly*

It has meaning and it wasn't a waste of time. All the effort that we went through—going to doctors' appointments, the delivery, the funeral—it may seem like more work to do all that stuff, but we're glad we did it. —*Greg*

A perinatologist said things to us like "the outcome will be the same" even if we didn't induce prematurely. Now that I'm stronger emotionally, I know that the outcome would *not* be the same. We would not have had all of the special time to share with Gianna during her life in my womb. We would not have been able to share some amazing, precious moments with our baby and our sons. —*Jennifer*

You may also have a profound and renewed appreciation for the value of the time you spent pregnant, realizing that it's not just the time after birth that matters. Looking back on the months of pregnancy that once seemed agonizing and interminable, you may see it now as precious and like no time at all. Ultimately you discovered that rather than adding to your grief, carrying and giving birth to your baby added to your joy.

What changed was the way I saw my baby during pregnancy. Before, I was just impatient for the moment my baby would be born. The pregnancy didn't count. The diagnosis made me realize that my baby was already important, that I had to enjoy every moment of her life because maybe there would be no "after." —*Monika*

When Lucy was first diagnosed, I hoped that I would miscarry her quickly. It was difficult for me to feel a great bond in the womb. Through my pregnancy, I began to desire to meet her alive, and as difficult as they were, I really treasure the three days that I was able to spend with her. —*Jane G.*

I can't even count the times I cried in bed, completely begging God to take this burden from me. But time healed so much pain. Toward the end of the pregnancy, I was still sad for the outcome, but my pain and heartache were turning to excitement to see our baby. His birth day was not about his diagnosis—it was about who Austin was. I don't even think of that day as the day he died; I think of it as the day he lived! —*Jo*

It was a blink of an eye. It wasn't long enough. If I could—and I said this then—if I could have carried him for the rest of my life just to keep him safe and keep him going and could have known that he would have been happy, I would have done it. Even though I was terribly uncomfortable and huge and I could hardly breathe and I definitely couldn't sleep, I would have done it for him. Yet it was his time to go. —*Jessica*

You may have a sense of fulfillment as parents, in that continuing the pregnancy gave you more time to be a mother or father to your little one, even if it was in ways you didn't expect when you first learned that you were pregnant.

As a mother, I have always felt that it was my job to identify what my children need and give it to them. Sometimes those needs are simple and straightforward—clean laundry, a healthy meal, a hand to cross the street safely. Maggie's needs were not like those of my sons. She needed us to give her a safe and peaceful transition from one world to the next. Carrying Maggie to term did that for me—it gave me the opportunity to "mother" her until she didn't need me anymore. That knowledge made it infinitely easier to make peace with her death. —*Alessandra*

Parents often say they'd do anything to keep their kids safe. For us, we feel like we were powerless in keeping Jonah alive, but to our best ability and our best understanding of the situation, we kept him as safe and as comfortable as we could. We were the best parents we could be for him. —*Heidi*

Perhaps you were harboring hopes—maybe secretly, maybe up until the end—that your baby would be a miracle that would prove the doctors wrong. Even if your hopes were crushed, you may still find comfort in knowing that you didn't close off that chance.

⌐ The reason I am glad we didn't terminate is that David Michael deserved a chance, even the fraction of a chance it was. Godspeed, son. I love you. —*David W.*

Reflections on Medical Decisions Made for Your Baby

Now that you have seen how events played out, you may feel that your decisions about medical intervention were validated and any doubts have lifted.

⌐ Having Noah placed directly in my husband's arms after birth was the best decision. He did not go to the NICU. He did not leave our sight or our presence. He was with us from the start of his life. He was with us at the end of his life. —*Jenny A.*

⌐ I am so grateful we opted simply to hold and love him. Perhaps sending him to the NICU might have allowed his lungs to be more adequately suctioned or a ventilator to be hooked up, but we would not have been able to love and caress him like we did. And I don't think doing either of those things would have lengthened his life significantly. —*Heidi*

⌐ I am so glad that we took her home, that she was always with us, and that we didn't give her to doctors to operate on. I couldn't imagine her all alone, hooked up, and invaded. We kept her cozy and comfortable, and we got to hold her and love her for every moment of her life. —*Christine*

⌐ The neonatologist later told me that she was convinced that had she attempted to intubate Isaac, he would have been in great pain and would have likely passed away even sooner. —*Stacy*

⌐ Despite the pain, there is true beauty in allowing a child to live the days that were naturally ordained for her. I have read many stories of babies with fatal anomalies being sent to the NICU. I am just so glad that my daughter was able to live almost all of her sixty-four hours of life in someone's arms, knowing that she was greatly loved. —*Jane G.*

Even if you are confident about your decisions, you may find yourself needing to reflect about them, talk them through again, or retrace them in your mind. You may have questions about what transpired or concerns that would be eased by checking back in with your caregivers.

⌐ I do sometimes wonder what it would've been like if we'd chosen a different path, what would've happened to Sarina if we'd opted for surgery. I sometimes let myself fantasize about what Sarina would be doing and what she would look like if she had been born healthy and with a whole heart. I always dream of her that way, a healthy little girl, not what life would have been like for her in reality. —*Christine*

⌐ I wish hospice would have talked to us about why she wasn't eating before she died—I feared later that we had starved her—and they could've helped us understand that she would go peacefully and that we were equipped to handle it. I have had to make peace with this and think that I have. —*Kristi F.*

Your subconscious may do some of this processing for you.

⌐ Almost a year after Nora died, I had a dream that she was still alive. She was still a tiny baby but growing and seemed normal. We started to feel like maybe she wouldn't die. I thought we should take her in to check her heart again, and I started to feel like I wanted to do anything to keep her alive. Strange dream. One of those you want never to end. It gave me a perspective on that feeling of wanting to keep a baby alive no matter what. —*Kristi F.*

Reflections on Perinatal Hospice Support

Parents who had perinatal hospice and palliative care support express deep gratitude and appreciation for it, even if they resisted the idea at first.

⌐ I had to be broken from my stubbornness to discover how truly amazing perinatal hospice really is. They are a gift of comfort and mercy when no one else understands and a friend and educator when nothing in the world makes any sense. If only I could have known earlier, I could have been saved from so much stress and worry and I could have spent more time cherishing my moment as David's mother. —*Rachel*

⌐ When you first get this diagnosis that you're going to have this baby who's going to die, you see yourself somberly walking into a hospital and dumping off your baby and going home. But having all these things in place, having that support, made the experience a whole lot better than it might have been. —*Greg*

Parents who did not receive perinatal hospice or birth planning support but learn about it later may feel cheated, even angry, and feel that they were provided substandard care.

⌐ I didn't find out that perinatal hospice existed until eight months after our son was born and died. I was quite angry when I discovered this. Why didn't my doctor bother to find out about this? Our lives could have been so much easier with the help and support of a hospice. —*Kathleen*

⌐ During my pregnancy no one had mentioned having a birth plan. This was a term I learned months after her birth. Looking back on it, I do regret the confusion I experienced at her birth. The situation had been taken out of my hands. For months I was her sole provider and all of a sudden she was being examined and monitored, for no reason. —*Doreen*

Some parents respond to the lack of services by becoming involved in implementing a program in their area. Others go back to their physicians and let them know that perinatal hospice coordination would have helped immensely. As perinatal hospice becomes the standard of care, know that you were one of many brave pioneers who gave this movement its momentum.

Whether you had formal perinatal hospice care or not, you may feel a special connection to your caregivers because they are among the few people who shared this experience intimately with you and witnessed the arrival of your child.

⟋ We are so thankful for our doctor. Our doctor chose to take on this challenge, despite being at a small hospital. Without him, we'd have probably delivered at a large hospital hours away, away from my desperately needed kids and family. This was the first baby he's ever delivered with anencephaly. He commented to us a few weeks later about how we had impressed him and thanked us for letting him be apart of Austin's life. —*Jo*

If you experienced resistance or lack of understanding from some caregivers during your pregnancy, you may need to come to terms with that. Perhaps you had other practitioners who stepped up for you, and as you heal, your focus can turn to that instead.

⟋ I guess I've always had it in my head that once people in the medical field see death, they essentially have to distance themselves from it so it doesn't tear them up inside. That is why I can't really be angry with my other doctors who made me so mad in the beginning. But the nurses on duty during the birth put their hearts on the line when they helped me. They were so loving and so caring, and even though that is what I hoped for, I never imagined I would get it. —*Rachel*

Reflections on Facing Fears

For many parents, fear was an overwhelming emotion during the pregnancy. You may have harbored fears about what your baby would look like, that your baby would suffer, that your baby might survive severely disabled, that death would be difficult to witness. Given the situation, these were normal fears, but in hindsight, your fears may have loomed much larger than the reality. You may even feel a sense of accomplishment for conquering your fears or facing them as they dissolved. You found your baby beautiful in spite of visible anomalies; you gave your baby a life of comfort; you unconditionally loved and accepted your baby for the very being he or she was; you accepted death with grace.

⌒ One thing that's hard for me to admit, but it's important for me to admit: I was afraid of what he would look like. When he was born, of course, there was nothing to be afraid of. He was just a very small baby, probably the size of a baby at 20 weeks' gestation, a little peanut. He was still perfectly proportioned, just very small. He did have some facial characteristics that were unusual, like his left ear came far down his face, the spacing of his eyes, his mouth. But there was nothing to be afraid of. I think it's important for women in this situation to know that it's OK to be a little bit afraid. That's a hard emotion to feel, to be pregnant and to be afraid to meet your baby. —*Missy*

⌒ Our biggest fear was that Noah would suffer. My husband and I did not want him to suffer during the birth process, during his life, or during the dying process. We went to great lengths to keep him comfortable at all times. We succeeded in every measure. He had a happy ten weeks here with us. —*Jenny A.*

⌒ I am a pediatric nurse, and I would see families come in with children having disabilities and I would think, *I couldn't do that.* Now I know after having Rose that even though she was severely handicapped, I loved her as much as my other children. Even if the only thing she ever did was open her eyes and look at me, that would have been enough for me to keep her forever. —*Debbie*

⌒ I was so scared to think of Ashley dying in our arms. I didn't know what that would be like. The brief time with Ashley breathing slowly in our arms was so beautiful as well as sad. The experience of letting Ashley die in peace with her family there was so profound and powerful. I didn't expect to feel some acceptance—some peace—about what happened but I do feel that way. —*Shellie*

Even if you felt a generalized anxiety about all the unknowns, you may see now that the worst part was the anticipation, and that actually living through each moment turned out to be much more manageable.

A Gift of Time

⁓ Throughout this whole experience, everything we thought we couldn't do, when we got to that point, somehow we found the strength. Everything I worried about, the worry was so much greater than what it really was like. I worried about making it through the funeral, for example. But when you're sitting there doing it, it's so different than thinking about it and anticipating it. —*Kathleen*

⁓ It wasn't as scary as I thought it was going to be. In the beginning, it was the fear of the unknown: Am I going to make it to term? If you make it to term, are you going to have a stillborn baby? If your baby's born alive, are you going to have all these medical issues you're going to need to deal with? Are you going to have to make decisions? It's just that fear of the unknown. In today's society, you like to know that you're going to be here from 2:00 to 4:00 and after that you're going to go to the next thing. It was out of our control how it was going to play out. But it wasn't scary. She was calming. —*Bianca*

Reflections on Witnessing Death

⁓ All I knew about death came from TV. Well, it wasn't like on TV at all. It wasn't a scary moment, but a moment filled with peace. —*Monika*

This may have been the first time you have ever witnessed someone dying. Obviously it is a profound, life-changing experience that gives you much to ponder. Many parents say their baby has taught them to not fear death. You may be more philosophical about death and the meaning of life, and you may have more confidence and a better understanding of how to face and cope with the death of a loved one.

⁓ Death is a part of life and I am no longer afraid of it. Every life, no matter how short or how limited, has a purpose. Sometimes it is hard to understand that purpose, but it is there. Our children touch so many lives in their short time with us. —*Sue*

⌐ I didn't want her to die at home. I didn't want our house to feel it had a dark cloud over it. Now I don't think it would have. Death wasn't sad; it was life. It was the end of a life, the end of having her to hold. But she's still with us, and we still communicate with her, and we still look at her photo every day and kiss her. We just don't have that physical touch. —*James*

⌐ I learned that death is a part of life, not something to be avoided and hidden but rather to be embraced if it is affecting someone that you love. The love will take you through the difficult times and bring you into a place of light and life even when you think that will never happen. —*Chris*

⌐ Now I know that death can be peaceful and right—and that hiding from it is often harder than facing it head-on. I also think that the sorrow of love is much less powerful than the force of love. —*Alessandra*

SPIRITUAL BELIEFS AND STRUGGLES

⌐ I felt inadequate. I wondered why this had to happen more than once to our family. Did I not have enough faith? Was there some lesson that I had to learn? —*Kelly G.*

Whether you began this journey as someone with strong faith in God or a higher power, someone with doubts, or someone who looked primarily for earthly meaning and purpose, wherever you began is likely not the same place you are right now or will be as time goes on. Wrestling with existential questions about the meaning of life and death is something that most people do as they mature, but your quest may have been accelerated and made more urgent by your experience with your baby.

Perhaps you look to goodness in this world rather than faith or religion to sustain you.

⌐ I grew up in a nonreligious household. Therefore, I have never felt any strong connection spiritually and do not hold any strong beliefs. I like to think there is a higher being, and that somehow there is an afterlife, and that I will one day meet Sarina again, but I am not sure about that. Sometimes, I feel that death is the end. What has helped me get through this experience is the love of my family, my husband, my son, and my friends. I feel I have become more compassionate. During the whole experience, when I felt angry, when I thought, *why me?* I would then think, *why not me?* Terrible things happen to people all the time; I am lucky to have what I do. I try to remind myself of the good things in my life, and that I need to be grateful for what I do have: health and love and family. I feel so sad that Sarina's life was so short, that she was never able to experience all the joyful things in life, but she did live and she was loved. *—Christine*

For some parents who are religious, their faith is strengthened. It is a rock to which they are able to cling while a flood-swollen river rages against them, anchored until the river subsides.

I remember being so scared and alone on the diagnosis day and not thinking I had the strength to continue. My faith was there, but it hadn't been tested like this before. Now that I am on the other side and have survived this, I realize that my faith is stronger because of this trial. My faith continues to be my life raft during difficult times. It doesn't change the loss, but it does help you move through the most difficult times in life. *—Chris*

The only thing that has changed is how close I feel to heaven now. I do not feel as if it is so far away. *—Holly*

I get emotional at Mass when all of the angels and saints are called upon, because this is as near to her I can be for now. I hope I never get over these emotions. *—John*

My husband and I are still working on finding peace in this whole thing, but the one thing that has helped has been our faith. If we didn't believe that Jonah is in heaven, in the presence of his Creator, and that some day we will be reunited, then losing Jonah would be unbearable. *—Heidi*

Reflections

Some parents find their faith shaken deeply. You may wonder why you and your baby were not spared. Anger is a normal element of grief, and some direct their anger toward God.

⌒ My faith has never been tested so much as it has in this past year. I often said during my pregnancy that this must be God's will, and I really tried to do the right thing by going to church and praying. It has helped some, but I feel so alone sometimes. I haven't been able to pray much or go to church since her death. —*Chelsea*

⌒ Because of this experience I am, as of right now, quite uncertain in my faith. I am hoping to come full circle and be once again strong in my beliefs, but I have to wonder why things like this are allowed. People keep telling me that "God needed another angel." I find this hollow. I have to stop myself from snapping back at them. God didn't "need" another one. I am not a big fan of the "angel makers." —*Jamie*

⌒ I am still bitter and angry at God. I do not want to be, but I do not know how to resolve it. I hope that someday I will find peace and will again trust the Lord. I went from a strong belief in God's love to almost none. I believed that God was going to give us a miracle because my husband was becoming a believer. Now he is not and I am faltering. I pray that God will forgive me for being so angry and blaming him for my pain. —*Brooke*

⌒ There is this underlying river of anger flowing through my soul. I still feel angry with God. —*Kathy*

⌒ I still cry out to God on occasion and say, "I don't understand!!!" —*Tami*

As you move through your grief, you may develop a deeper, more nuanced approach to faith. It may mature from an innocent belief that a strong faith results in prayers being answered the way you would like. You may become more conscious, devoted, or philosophical about your spiritual life.

My beliefs did not remove my grief or sense of loss. I still miss her deeply. But my understanding of where she is now and what she is doing has deepened. I have a different concept of faith now. Faith is not getting what you want because you believed hard enough. It is believing that God has your best interests at heart and continuing to do right, even when you do not get what you want. It was a hard lesson, and still is. —*Laura W.*

I think my faith is different after this experience, perhaps stronger in some sense. I was maybe on "autopilot" when it came to faith and religion, but this experience made me look at things in a new way. I think of it like a nudge to stop hitting the snooze button and to be more engaged with my spiritual side. I truly feel like I had a glimpse of the divine as I held our daughter. —*Shellie*

I've had a fairly easy life up until now and I've often wondered how I would react in the face of a serious trial. Would my faith sustain me? Would I run to God or run from him in the face of adversity? So far, thankfully, it has been the peace and comfort I feel when I seek God that keeps me going back to him. He didn't "zap" us with this just to punish us or teach us some lesson we were blindly missing all these years. He is far too loving to have those motives. Instead, I like to picture it that he is cradling Jonah in one arm and our wounded souls in the other. He will see us through this, and I don't want to stray from him in the meantime. —*Heidi*

I have never struggled with "Why would God let this happen?" because I feel that his death is a necessary part of life. Also, others have questioned why God would allow our baby to die, as opposed to a young crack addict hooker's baby. I think while this is natural, I don't deserve a baby any more or less than that hurting crack addict mother. (The innocence of the baby and what the baby deserves is another matter.) On my good days, when others are asking, "How could God do this to you?" I think, *I am the luckiest person in the world.* And what about Frankie, anyway? I hope that maybe right now he is experiencing all of the love that I have had, or will one day if he makes it back to earth. —*Susan E.*

Reflections

Reflections about Miracles

During your pregnancy, you or others around you may have prayed for a miracle. Many parents find that their definition of what constitutes a miracle has changed.

⌐ Some of our friends had been praying for a miracle: that her diagnosis was wrong, that she would live. When I met Maggie, I knew the miracle they had been praying for had been granted— it wasn't the one they had intended, but it was miraculous, nonetheless. —*Alessandra*

⌐ A friend who had experienced a lot of loss in her life wrote me a card. She wrote, "Be on the watch for miracles because they can be disguised in many ways." I remember at the time almost feeling a little bit resentful toward her for that comment, because I felt that there were no miracles at work in my life at that point. I didn't see any beauty in my dad dying, and to know that my son was basically dying a slow death inside me I didn't feel like there were any miracles at play. It wasn't until I had the benefit of hindsight that for me there was no denying that it was meant to happen just the way it happened. —*Missy*

⌐ People kept saying, "Maybe she'll be a miracle." I took offense to that but didn't know why. I finally figured out why I didn't like it, and here's how I described it in her eulogy: "Alaina has taught me to believe in miracles, but I've had to change my definition of what a miracle is. James and I have made a point of never wishing that she would live a certain amount of time. We didn't want to define the success of her life by how long it was. I guess it's because I didn't want to think that she would be a miracle only if she lived a long time. I believed that she was already a miracle. And then I start to think, *Well, what about all of the other babies in the world, aren't they miracles too? And then, what about adults?* And I am left with the realization that we are all miracles, but we just don't recognize it. And miracles happen all around us, but we just don't see them. I guess it takes a very special little girl like Alaina to show us that we are all very special, and miracles are occurring all around us all of the time." —*Jill K.*

A Gift of Time

Similarly, beliefs about life after death may be tested. What once may have seemed like an abstract question becomes more urgent and concrete. You're no longer just vaguely curious about whether souls exist beyond death—you need to know about *this* soul. Does your baby's spirit still exist in some form? Where is your baby now? Like so much of your journey, the question of the nature of your child's spiritual existence is another mystery that cannot be answered in this world. For many parents, a belief in some form of existence after death provides consolation.

Before Nathaniel was born, my focus lay primarily with the physical nature of this world, but afterward my heart followed him, and I now see beyond this physical sphere to the spiritual realm where he is. This new, broader outlook permeates my life and gives it shape and meaning. It reminds me that I, too, am an eternal being and the choices I make here reverberate in eternity. —*Annette G.*

I believe that we will see Ashley again someday, when we die. To me, even if our time on Earth ends up being all there is to our existence, the belief that there really is more to it than that makes my life better. My spiritual beliefs enhance my life and give me some peace about losing Ashley. —*Shellie*

Even when she was alive, I focused on being connected to Alaina's spirit as it existed separately from her body. Now I continue to feel her presence around me. Here's what I said about this in the eulogy: "When she did stop breathing, we didn't panic or cry, we just held her and I felt her there with us, saying, 'It's OK, I'm right here. I'm not in that body anymore, but I am right here with you.'" Her spirit was so real in that moment, I will never doubt whether souls continue to exist after this life. —*Jill K.*

Right after Thomas died, I had a hard time believing in heaven and life after death. I really, really wanted to, but I just couldn't. I had never questioned those concepts before my son's death. But, now I was. My baby was dead, and I couldn't imagine him being anything but dead. I couldn't picture him anywhere but in the ground. It was a very difficult time for me. Now I think of heaven in more spiritual and less religious terms. My beliefs about God have changed and have become a little less specific and more universal. —*Kathleen*

⌐ Prior to all of this, I believed there was a God, a heaven, and that we leave our life here when we die and live in an eternity of peace and love. Since losing Kevin, I have often questioned this belief. Is there really a place called heaven? Or is this something that was created to help people with their grieving process? —*Amy*

⌐ I don't know exactly what form Frankie takes right now. I know that energy itself doesn't die—one just has to refer to the law of conservation of energy in the field of physics to start: Energy just changes form. So Frankie's energy is out there in some manner. Strange as it may seem, I do take a bit of comfort in that. Because what is energy? It's not just our physical being; it's also our consciousness, our intelligence, our emotions, and our awareness. Yes, my spiritual philosophies are wrapped up in science, but I'm not such a hard-core rationalist that I won't consider that we humans don't know all that there is. Our minds have a limited capacity and therefore can't know all that there is. So perhaps there is a greater intelligence than all of us? Or one that connects all of us? Are we part of that great intelligence? And therefore Frankie and I are tied to one another on a most intimate level, that we are still part of one another. I can't deny that my body misses his body, though, and I really would like to believe that our bodies will meet again. —*Susan E.*

Feeling Your Baby's Presence

Some parents are comforted by an unmistakable sense of their baby's presence and a transcendent feeling of peace. It may be dramatic or just a quiet feeling. Perhaps you have a vivid dream or notice a butterfly that seems to linger longer than usual. If something like this happens to you, know that you are not losing your grip on reality.

⌐ During the night before Josiah's funeral, I woke up feeling like my heart was *huge* and outside my body, like a three-foot square.

There was so much love I couldn't keep it in my body. I kept asking myself, "What is this? Can I keep it?" —*Behka*

⌐ I woke out of a sound sleep. One of the kids was standing by my bed and needed something. This happened often; whoever it was would stand there looking at me until I woke up. For some reason they never touched me and I usually woke up before they spoke, so this night was no different than usual. I rolled over and no one was there, yet someone was. I felt him. I think Luke came to tell me he was OK. Then he was gone. —*Sue*

⌐ I was sitting here one day at the computer, mourning the death of a friend's baby, and I thought, *Caitlyn, I miss you so much.* Suddenly it felt as if someone touched my neck. I literally turned around to look and no one was there. I was filled with such peace as I really feel I was touched by her presence and that she is now somewhere in which she is healthy, happy, and waiting for a hug from me. —*Shayla*

⌐ My peace with him was established in a dream I had the night after he died. He told me he loved me. —*Scott*

⌐ The week Remi died I was lying on the couch watching television, trying to relax, and all of a sudden I felt a sort of pressure on my belly—the kind of feeling like you have a baby lying on your belly and chest when they are so little and warm. It was so significant that it took my attention immediately away from everything else and I just knew it was Remi—immediately. I knew she was letting me know she was still with me and around me though I can't physically hold and kiss her anymore. I tried not to move a muscle, as I was fearful that the feeling would leave. A month or so later I had the same experience while trying to fall asleep in my bed. This has happened a handful of times since her death. I will be just doing other things and it really almost stops me in my tracks. An overwhelming feeling of warmth and love, like Remi is hugging me, all over—a complete feeling. It could even be compared to grief as well. Things will be going fine and then it hits out of nowhere. Same thing. —*Jessie*

Reflections

Every day since Alaina died, more special moments have occurred. We've been running into people that we haven't seen for years; we've made wrong turns and stumbled upon special messages from Alaina. Through these experiences my adult brain is telling me that these things just happened randomly and there are rational explanations for all of them, which is true, there are rational explanations. And my brain starts telling me that I am looking for meaning in random experiences as a coping mechanism. But if I tell my brain to be quiet for a minute, and I let my guard down, let go of the fear of sounding crazy, and I listen to my gut and my heart, I can see Alaina's spirit right here with us, interacting with us all of the time. —*Jill K.*

Some parents desperately wish for some kind of message from their baby, some proof of continued existence—a dream, anything—yet nothing seems to come. This can feel like yet another desolation. It is a mystery why some parents have these experiences and others do not. If you have not and are longing for some kind of contact, consider that every thought of your baby, every ache of your love and grief, is a form of contact more mystical and profound than anyone in this world can know. Consider also that if another parent has had a dream or an experience that to them is convincing proof of their baby's continued existence, it means much more than that their baby's spirit still lives. It means that *your* baby's spirit lives too.

LONG-TERM REFLECTIONS ON GRIEF AND HEALING

It has been three years since Nathaniel's death. Losing Nathaniel was by far the most painful thing that I have ever experienced. At times it is like a deep black pit and at other times it is like wandering in a wasteland. The pain has been unbearable at times, but the crucible has refined me, profoundly changing me in important ways. —*Annette G.*

It is hard to believe that fifteen years have passed since we had Daniel here with us. While I will always wonder what he would be like now and how our family dynamics would be different, I no longer feel the raw grief that I used to. What helped me heal? Allowing myself to grieve fully. I found other parents who were going through the same thing and together we got through those dark and difficult days. If I had tried to pretend it didn't happen, I think it would have been much harder. I really, really actively grieved and then finally and gradually I felt peace. And the peace felt right, just like the grieving felt right before. I believe that Daniel is OK now and we are OK now. What happened is tragic, but I do have a happy life. It just takes time to heal. —*Kim*

Working through grief and incorporating your baby's death into the narrative of your life is a long road. Unlike common misconceptions about "closure" or "getting over it," healthy grief is a process of enfolding your loss experiences into who you are while also reentering the fullness of life. Instead of closing a box and walking away, you move forward, embracing the memory of your baby's life, the insights acquired, and the lessons learned.

With the passage of time, intense sorrow fades and healing emerges from the love that remains. The fiery test of saying goodbye to a beloved child burns away the chaff and leaves behind a love that is indelible and clear.

Finding Peace and Meaning

It has been almost three years since that day, but I no longer feel sad. Gianna was a special gift. It was an honor to bring her into this world and send her to the next. —*Doreen*

I have gone from asking the question, "why?" to which there is no satisfactory answer, to asking, "how?" By this I mean I am no longer dwelling on why his death occurred but am asking how his life and death can be used for good in the world. I am pondering what things I can do to honor him, and also help others, as a way to keep his memory alive, and so keep a connection with him. —*Annette G.*

You may find comfort in believing there is a purpose to your journey, even if it still isn't clear to you—and may never be. Even if you can't understand why, you can still arrive at a sense of peace about what happened.

⌐ God didn't create Jonah with too many chromosomes to punish us for something. For some reason, our little boy was meant to just be with us for a little while. But we know there is a purpose for it. While it hurts and it doesn't make sense to us, I need to trust God now and keep believing that someday we will see Jonah again. —*Heidi*

⌐ I tend to question why, and I don't have an answer yet, but I know I will sometime. Sometimes I feel that Maryann was here to teach others love and compassion. —*Annette H.*

⌐ I don't think I have found a meaning to her passing, but I do think I am making steps toward having some peace with it. There are moments where I still can't believe this happened and how much it has shattered the dreams we had. I know we did our best, and that Anya knew she was loved. —*Steve*

Reminiscing about positive memories also can help you find peace.

⌐ I see him in my mind everywhere I go. I feel him in my heart. When I wake up in the middle of the night, I still see him, asleep, on a mound of pillows in between my husband and me. I still see his smile; it is etched in my mind. I still know the touch of his soft skin. I still can feel my lips kiss his and feel my cheek slide across his. I can still smell the lotion that I slathered on him. I can still see my husband feed Noah his bottle so carefully and so lovingly. I can hear my husband sing to him and I can see Noah cradled in his arms. Noah is everywhere. We will never be without him. He is a part of us. —*Jenny A.*

⌐ I felt such peace to have been able to meet her, talk to her, see her eyes, have her see us and hear us. We loved her so much and she loved us right back. It was also excellent to see how in charge of her own life she was—she had such a strong will and spirit.

It was palpable. Someone said that God was in charge; I'm not sure that was true. I think Maggie was in charge—God helped, of course, but really, it was her show. It was extraordinary. She was amazing. —*Alessandra*

You may find meaning in honoring your baby's memory. You have experienced a depth of commitment and love that knew no bounds, and you may feel a strong desire to channel that excess energy into something productive. Perhaps you wish to memorialize your baby in ways that help others. Or you may decide to embrace other aspects of your life with more fullness and gusto, whether it's family, friends, work, or something else you have a passion for.

Some parents wish to extend a hand to other parents traveling the same path, offering their hard-won insights and a listening ear.

If this appeals to you, you could start by plugging into existing organizations and support groups. A word of advice: For your own healing, as well as to offer the best possible assistance to other parents, it's a good idea to wait a while after your own baby's death before jumping into the fray. While grief doesn't operate on a predictable timetable, it does take time. You'll need time and energy to process your own grief so it isn't compounded by the grief of others—and so their grief isn't made worse by yours.

You don't need to do anything to give meaning to your baby's life; your baby's life has intrinsic meaning. But it may give you a rewarding and renewed sense of purpose.

Ultimately, many parents find peace and meaning in what endures: love.

The main thing I learned is that we are made for giving and receiving love. This is old news; does it really take thirty-six years to learn this?! I have had an experience that I would not ask to repeat. One that is common, in that nearly all of us have experienced loss. But one that is unusual in that a lifetime's worth of pain, loss, love, and joy were compressed into a few brief moments. In the short time that has passed since Lily's death, the experience has come to feel like a great gift, one that has given me a profound sense of one aspect of our being. Thank you, Lily, for giving me such a clear and deep awareness of our innate fitness for loving. —*Mark*

⁓ I loved Keiran from the moment I knew she existed. Nothing changed that when I found out that she would die. If anything, I loved her more. I tried to fit a lifetime of love into nine months. She was always loved, always warm and safe inside me. We should all be so lucky that all we know is love. —*Jamie*

⁓ I continue to work on my faith that the universe is ultimately based on a principle of love. And the love I have had for Frankie, it is profound. I wouldn't change having him for anything in the world. —*Susan E.*

Your Baby's Place in Your Family

One facet of the intrinsic meaning of your baby's life is that he or she is a permanent member of your family. If you were able to include other family members during the short time your baby was alive, this can help them recognize and affirm your baby's importance. Siblings sometimes are more open to talking about the reality of their baby brother or sister than adults are.

> *Greg:* I was very glad that everyone was able to be there and able to hold him and see him in person, not just in pictures. We all had that shared experience of what his life was, that as short as it was, we all were there for it. Today I don't feel uncomfortable mentioning his name to people. His grandma and grandpa have pictures of him in their house.
>
> *Jill N.:* Our older son recently had to color a school bus at kindergarten, and then the teacher told them to draw some people in the windows to give the picture more details. So Joel drew a face in each of the five windows, and when he brought it home and was showing it to me, he said it's our family: "Greg, Jill, Joel, Josh, and Jada." I just thought that was so awesome that he would include Josh on his school bus of our family. We aren't the only ones who remember—Joel does too. And our new baby girl will get to remember her big brother too.

This acknowledgement of your baby's place in your family offers reassurance that moving on is not disloyal. Your family can move forward while holding your baby in your memories and your hearts. This "remembering and moving on" is a hallmark of healing.

⸻ Silly thoughts, like the idea that I will never be able to take a family picture that is totally complete, make me feel a bit disloyal to Maggie. How can the family change without her? Part of me thinks that I will just never take another full-family photograph again— that way her absence won't feel so acute. We'll see. Perhaps time will change my perspective. *—Alessandra*

⸻ My husband, our son, and I went on vacation, and I didn't have feelings of guilt or even sadness over going without her. I actually felt OK because I just knew she was with us. I can't explain it, can't rationalize it. I just know she is "around." It's really a beautiful thought. *—Jessie*

Your Baby's Impact on Others

As you gradually emerge from your intense concentration on your baby and begin reawakening to the larger world, you may be awed to realize the effect your baby has had—and will have—on others. The ripples will extend farther than you may ever know.

⸻ I think it's really incredible that a life that only lasts for twenty or thirty minutes can have such an impact on so many other lives around us. People still talk about his story. I wouldn't trade it for the world. *—Missy*

⸻ We know that our baby has called many people—including us—to greater holiness in a very unique, special way. If she had been a perfectly healthy baby girl, she wouldn't have been capable of touching the hearts of so many in the special way she did. We have heard from so many people that her little life strengthened their faith and helped them become better parents, spouses, and people in general. She taught others to not take their loved ones for granted. *—Jennifer*

Perhaps your example broke through your caregivers' biases against continuing a pregnancy and caused them to reconsider.

⌐ One of the nurses told me that Carina and our whole experience touched so many people. She said, "I know of a lot of people who've changed their viewpoints about a lot of things because of it." —*Bridget*

⌐ Our perinatologist said we should be prepared for resistance by members of the medical team to our decision to continue. He warned us of that, and he was right. I love my gynecologist, and I respect her immensely, but she is a scientist. She initially was puzzled as to why we wouldn't just terminate the pregnancy. And as the weeks wore on, she never pressured me but she continued to dangle it out there: You could just be done with this, I see how hard this is on you, that window is closing so we would have to make a decision about it soon. Incredibly, when he was born and he let out a cry, she looked at me and she said, "I never expected that," and she just bawled. Afterwards she told me, "I'll never forget that experience. I'll never forget that cry." So I think she learned something in it too. I would like to think that she did. She's a great lady, but she was coming at it from more of a science perspective, and I was coming at it from a spiritual perspective. —*Missy*

⌐ I remember in the recovery room, we were praying aloud, and all of a sudden I became aware of quite a few voices praying with us. I saw a least half a dozen people, mostly nurses, praying with us. I was quite shocked and touched when I spotted my doctor. The man who pushed for us to terminate our son—and could never really understand why we didn't—had hung around after hours and was praying with us. That was quite a moment. I often wonder how he will respond to the next couple who face a similar painful experience. Will he understand and be more supportive? I will never know. I would like to think that that might be part of Thomas' legacy to this world. —*Kathleen*

Your journey and your baby may also have gently challenged those close to you who privately—or explicitly—disagreed with your decision to continue.

A Gift of Time

My entire family wanted me to terminate (I still can't bring myself to write "abort"). They thought it would be easier on me. In the end everyone was so glad that I decided to continue. We all fell in love with her. —*Jamie*

Some family members had implied that they felt it would be best that we "take care of this," and they continued to feel that way throughout my pregnancy. Their tune changed as soon as they were holding him. They were very apologetic and admitted they were wrong for thinking that continuing the pregnancy was nothing less than a gift. —*Jo*

PERSONAL TRANSFORMATION

You may have a sense of pride about how you handled your journey, and you may have surprised yourself by strength you didn't know you had.

Being almost a year away from it I can say that I am proud of myself. I feel real pride in my decision and how I handled everything. It was the hardest time of my life, and I have learned so much. I had my moments of weakness and self-pity, but I don't necessarily see that as a bad thing, just a human thing. The whole situation has completely changed my priorities. The dynamics of my relationship with my family and friends has changed. All in all, I am a better person because of my little girl. —*Jamie*

It's certainly bittersweet, but it's much more sweet than bitter. The proudest moment of my life to that date was giving birth to Eli. —*Jessica*

I have been called a saint for carrying Luke. I have been told by many that they couldn't do what I did. I am not a saint, and you don't know what you can do until you are faced with it. —*Sue*

When I (we) decided to carry to term, so many people were incredulous that we had the strength to do that. If it was an incredulousness that any woman could carry a baby to term who she knew was going to die, or if it was that I showed them that I was stronger than they thought, I don't know. I suppose it's both. —*Susan E.*

Reflections

Mothers may feel a sense of pride in the power of their bodies and their capacity to nurture and give birth to another human being. Even women who give birth to healthy babies need to revisit and reprocess memories of this intense, life-changing experience. Especially if it's your first delivery, you may feel a sense of achievement and fulfillment in accomplishing something that only a woman can do.

⌒ Perhaps my carrying to term became sort of an unintentional metaphor for the full development of me as a female. —*Susan E.*

You may find that your perspective about what is important—and what is no longer important—has matured.

⌒ Why get upset because there is a long line at the store? Why behave horridly because someone cuts you off in traffic? There are better battles to fight. I know I can survive anything and that if I survived her life and death, anything else life throws at me is a walk in the park. —*Elizabeth D. P.*

⌒ I've learned a lot about letting go, and faith, and trust. It was a lesson learned for life in general. —*Bridget*

⌒ I have grown so much since the day that Ramona was diagnosed. I feel like I am 28 going on 40. —*Rebecca J.*

⌒ Life is short. It's a cliché, but we often overlook everyday blessings. My husband and I always considered ourselves fortunate. This situation has proven that. We are fortunate to have such wonderful, supportive family and friends. We were fortunate to receive the diagnosis prior Anya's birth. We were fortunate to have forty-four hours to celebrate our daughter's life. We are fortunate to have one another. We are fortunate to have the future ahead of us. —*Delsa*

You may experience significant growth borne of how this experience has changed you. Friendships may be lost and new ones gained. You may seek a new balance, become more assertive and more compassionate, and feel a deeper appreciation for the miracle of life. You are not only living in a new normal, you have *become* a new normal.

A Gift of Time

When I first learned of our bad news, I was so determined to not let this experience define me. Now I realize that perspective is flawed. If I let this experience define me, as long as I'm coping in a good way, I will forever live and love a much richer life. —*Jennifer*

My beliefs, ideas, and feeling about the situation and my life all have taken a new perspective since my pregnancy and Katherine Elizabeth's death. I am not the same person. It seems that in a matter of three months, from when we found out about her diagnosis to when she was born and died, a part of my life has just stopped and a new one has begun. I hold my kids with more love, I treasure our family more, I am building stronger relationships with my friends and establishing new even more. I feel as if my life has a new purpose that was not there before. —*Lizabeth*

I learned that life is precious, especially when it comes in a fragile imperfect package. There is value to a life that others say is disposable. I learned that parental love is unconditional—and not dependent upon a doctor's diagnosis. —*Chris*

As hard as it was, I wouldn't change a thing. I am a different, a better woman than I was before Zachary. I am a better mom to my children. The little things that used to irritate me now bring great delight. I look at them more, listen to them more, hug them and kiss them more, and I love them more. —*April*

One of my friends who lost her son to extreme prematurity commented that her son's death has made her a better person. I am not quite there yet, but I can see how Lucy's death has made me a better mother—much better able to accept the things that I cannot change, and more compassionate to others who are hurting in many different ways. —*Jane G.*

My soul has grown and matured. Even though Nathaniel was taken away from me, he has given me some beautiful gifts. His life has taken me in new directions and given me a larger, more patient, and understanding heart. I am more focused on relationships as the most important thing in life. I feel I live more purposefully and deliberately than I did before. —*Annette G.*

Reflections

⌒ Our family is stronger. We have a stronger sense of unity and love. Our children are bonded to each other because together they have endured something hard, twice. Our faith is stronger. We are better people. —*Behka*

⌒ I wouldn't trade my time with Emily even if it meant I could have a healthy baby instead. I've learned more from her than I ever believed it possible to be taught by one little girl. —*Jane T.*

You may also experience a spiritual sort of awakening that enriches your life. You may have a greater awareness and appreciation for the blessings of the natural world, as well as the magical experiences and the mystical connections that are part of your life.

⌒ I have seen the world through magical, clear eyes. Right after Frankie's passing everything around me seemed colorful, so alive.
—*Susan E.*

⌒ The other day my husband and I visited the cemetery. As we were leaving, the sun was setting. The sky was red. The sun was behind a cloud and the cloud was outlined in fire. The cloud couldn't hide the power of the sun. It was beautiful. As I admired this awesome sight, the impression came that our clouds have a silver lining, too. The opportunity to have Jacob and Josiah in our family is a blessing that I don't understand the magnitude of yet. —*Behka*

⌒ One of my most cherished memories before Jonah's birth was during a family getaway to Aspen. We were hiking on Independence Pass at about 11,500 feet, surrounded by gorgeous 13,000-foot peaks with glistening snow melting into an alpine lake. I was in awe at the view around me, and I was overtaken by a feeling of peace that if God could create this kind of splendor, He could certainly take care of our son for us. It was almost a moment of resignation that regardless of what was to happen, Jonah was going to be in wonderful hands. We'll take whatever time we get with him and after that, he will be OK. My mind often goes back to that moment. When we see a beautiful sunset or a rainbow, my husband and I are often reassured that the same God who made that happen is now enjoying our son for us. —*Heidi*

⌒ I am much more focused on the spiritual side of things. Having a stillborn baby did something deep in my soul that is difficult to put into words. I knew that Nathaniel lived. I felt him move and grow within me, and yet when he emerged from my womb, he had died, but somehow I knew even as I cradled his lifeless body in my arms that his soul still lived. I always knew death was not the end, that our souls are eternal. But having the transition of Nathaniel's soul go from his body to an eternal dwelling place happen inside my body caused a major paradigm shift for me. At his birth, there was a deep and sacred silence that enveloped the room. The stillness and silence he ushered in with him remains with me as a cherished part of my soul. In that stillness and silence I have connected with a merciful God who tenderly cares for me, and in that relationship I have found hope. Nathaniel has linked me to the Mystery that lives in and among us and transcends space and time. He opened my eyes to a greater reality. —*Annette G.*

IF YOU COULD REACH BACK IN TIME . . .

Rather than asking parents if they have any advice to offer to you, we asked them this question instead: "If you could reach back in time and say something to yourself on the day of the diagnosis, what would you say?" Here are some of their hard-earned insights:

⌒ You still have the opportunity to love this child. You *can* do this. She loves you and wants to be with you. She needs you to help her—that is your responsibility as her parent. —*Katharine*

⌒ This will be the hardest thing you may ever do, but it will show you amazing things about yourself, about God, and about the true nature of miracles that you may never learn in another way. —*Annette G.*

⌒ You are about to have one of the choicest experiences of your life. Look for the good and the beautiful and you will find it. Notice the details. You will not walk this road alone. Have faith. Make sure to take care of your other children too. —*Behka*

Celebrate your daughter for who she is; don't hide away because she's not what the doctors think she should be. Just because the miracle you pray for doesn't happen, doesn't mean that a miracle didn't happen after all. —*Alaina*

Esto vir, Latin for "be a man." You are about to receive the most gracious gift. Receive it joyfully. She deserves that. —*John*

Love her. Get to know her. Love the child, not the syndrome.
—*Martina*

It is possible to bond, to care more than you ever imagined, to experience unconditional love in its truest form, and to allow your baby's life to transform you in ways you hadn't imagined. —*Jane T.*

I would say this will be hard but it will be worth it. You will learn more about yourself and life and you won't be the same person—you will better and wiser and able to reach out to more people than you ever could have imagined. And you will love your baby no matter what. —*Debbie*

It is OK to live your life and be happy after this type of experience. Because you are happy does not mean that you have forgotten your child or you do not love him or her. You can honor your child through living a good life—a life that will enable you to say, "I did my best," so you can be with your child again. —*Holly*

If I could go back and tell myself one thing, it would be: "You will be OK." —*Jill K.*

MOVING FORWARD WITH GRATITUDE

I will forever be grateful to Frankie for the lessons he taught me about how to really love, how to appreciate life in all its forms, and how to live a life of joy and faith. One thing that has helped me survive is feeling the gratitude that I have had Frankie in my life at all. A little time is better than no time. —*Susan E.*

As you move forward, you will discover that your baby's life has a deep, positive, and lasting effect on you. You can accept, even embrace, what *is*. You protected and parented your baby in profound ways, allowing your little one to live out the life that was his or her own unique destiny. You are your baby's parent, always. Death is not powerful enough to erase your bond or the fact that your baby *lived*.

      I didn't voluntarily return her to God; I had no choice. I did have a choice in how I could love her, honor her, share our journey and her life with those people that we loved and knew us. We are all better for having followed our daughter's lead in this story. She was a gift and I am grateful, every day, that we allowed ourselves to receive it. —*Alessandra*

APPENDIX
Sample Birth Plan

Your birth and care plan can be as unique as your baby is, but most plans need to address some similar topics. A valuable beginning is to state your overriding wishes for your baby's life. For example, one family's statement was, "Our overriding wish is that our son's brief life be free of pain and filled with love." The details of your birth plan will flow from your broad vision.

A typical perinatal hospice birth plan includes these other main areas.

Essential Information
– Your baby's name (if you have already chosen one)
– The parents' names
– Contact numbers for your obstetrician, pediatrician, clergyperson, or other key caregivers
– A brief summary of your pregnancy and your baby's diagnosis

Wishes for Labor and Delivery
– Caesarean birth or vaginal birth
– Fetal heart monitoring during labor
– Comfort measures and pain relief for the mother
– Cutting the umbilical cord
– Support people you wish to be present

Wishes for Your Time with Your Baby
– Family and friends
– Other siblings
– Spiritual rituals
– Photographs and video recording

- Keepsakes such as footprints, handprints, locks of hair, crib card, ID bands
- Bathing your baby
- Being with your baby during the dying process and after death

Medical Decisions

If medical intervention is possible and you have already reached some decisions, these should be specified in your plan. Possible topics include

- Suctioning and oxygen after birth
- Delaying routine procedures or providing them while your baby is in a parent's arms
- Resuscitation
- Ventilators
- Feeding
- Medications
- Additional testing
- Taking your baby home if possible

Plans for Your Baby's Body

The plan can also include information about your wishes if your baby dies in the hospital, such as

- Keeping your baby with you
- Autopsy
- After-death care for your baby's body, such as funeral home information or details about transporting your baby's body yourself

It is essential to consult with someone at your hospital to confirm that your plan is workable, to revise it if necessary, and to ensure that any special arrangements can be made. For more discussion of birth planning, see Chapter 6.

This document is a way to share your decisions and hopes with your caregivers, who can use it as a guide as your baby's birth, life, and death unfold. Your birth plan is not set in stone; you can modify it and be flexible as circumstances change. You can let your baby lead you.

— *For more resources for parents and caregivers, visit*
www.perinatalhospice.org.

NOTES

1. Quotations translated from the book *Un enfant pour l'éternité* (A Child for Eternity) by Isabelle de Mézerac (Éditions du Rocher, 2004) and used with permission of the author. De Mézerac is the founder of Soins Palliatifs et Accompagnement en Maternité (SPAMA) or Palliative Care and Support in Maternity Wards, a support association based in France. Their website is www.spama.asso.fr.

CHAPTER 2. What Now?

1. The U.S. Supreme Court's *Roe v. Wade* decision allows states to restrict abortion during the third trimester (after 24 weeks) but requires exceptions for the life or health of the mother. *Doe v. Bolton*, the companion case to *Roe*, defines health as "all factors—physical, emotional, psychological, familial, and the woman's age—relevant to the well-being of the patient." *Roe v. Wade* 410 U.S. 113 (1973), *Doe v. Bolton* 410 U.S. 179 (1973), www.findlaw.com/casecode/supreme.html. Third-trimester abortions performed under this broad definition of health are legal. If the mother's health is not at risk, many states ban abortion after viability, but a fetus with a terminal prenatal diagnosis might not be considered viable.
2. For more information, see C. Lammert. "Rights of parents when a baby dies: choices or mandates?" *Caring Notes*, professional newsletter of Share Pregnancy and Infant Loss Support, Inc., November 2009, www.nationalshare.org/rights-choices-or-mandates.html. See also J. M. Lamb. "Parents' needs and rights when a baby dies." *Health Progress*. December 1992; 73(10):52–55, 57.
3. Although some researchers found that seeing and holding stillborn babies can be traumatic for some mothers, it's important to note that these same mothers reported being coerced rather than supported into doing so. There

is far more evidence that when parents are supported in making autonomous and informed decisions, seeing and holding the baby is associated with fewer anxiety and depressive symptoms among mothers of stillborn babies than not doing so. J. Cacciatore, I. Rådestad, J. Frederik Frøen. "Effects of contact with stillborn babies on maternal anxiety and depression." *Birth: Issues in Perinatal Care.* December 2008;35(4):313–320.

4. Doctors Byron Calhoun and Nathan Hoeldtke began providing perinatal hospice support in 1995 in their obstetric practice at Madigan Army Medical Center outside of Tacoma, Washington. See B. C. Calhoun, N. J. Hoeldtke, R. M. Hinson, K. M. Judge. "Perinatal hospice: should all centers have this service?" *Neonatal Network.* September 1997;16(6):101–102.

5. World Health Organization, "Palliative care," www.who.int/cancer/palliative/en

6. C. Saunders. "Care of the dying: the problem of euthanasia." *Nursing Times.* 1976; 72(27):1049–52. See also St. Christopher's Hospice, www.stchristophers.org.uk

7. "American Board of Medical Specialties establishes new specialty certificate in hospice and palliative medicine," news release from the American Board of Medical Specialties, October 6, 2006. www.abms.org/News_and_Events/downloads/NewSubcertPalliativeMed.pdf

8. WebMD.com, "Vacuum aspiration," http://women.webmd.com/manual-and-vacuum-aspiration-for-abortion

9. WebMD.com, "Dilation and sharp curettage (D&C) for abortion," http://women. webmd.com/dilation-and-sharp-curettage-dc-for-abortion

10. "Outpatient second-trimester D&E abortion through 24 menstrual weeks' gestation," by W. M. Hern, Boulder Abortion Clinic, www.drhern.com/outptsecondtriab.htm

11. M. Haskell. "Dilation and extraction for late second-trimester abortion." Presented at National Abortion Federation Risk Management Seminar, Dallas (TX), September 13, 1992. Available at www.nrlc.org/abortion/pba/Haskellinstructional.pdf

12. C. Goldberg, "Shots assist in aborting fetuses; lethal injections offer legal shield," *Boston Globe,* August 10, 2007; W. M. Hern. "Laminaria, induced fetal demise and misoprostol in late abortion." *International Journal of Gynaecology and Obstetrics.* December 2001;75(3):279–286. The Humane Society of the United States considers the use of potassium chloride for euthanizing dogs and cats to be "inhumane." For more information, see their website, www.animalsheltering.org/resource_library/policies_and_guidelines/statement_on_euthanasia.html

13. W. M. Hern. "Selective termination for fetal anomaly/genetic disorder in twin pregnancy at 32+ menstrual weeks. Report of four cases." *Fetal Diagnosis and Therapy.* May–June 2004;19(3):292–5.

14. *Carhart v. Ashcroft*, U.S. District Court transcript, vol. 6, April 6, 2004, p. 168.

15. Personal communication with caregivers, March 25, 2010.

16. Children's Hospital of Wisconsin Fetal Concerns Program, "Anencephaly." www.chw.org/display/PPF/DocID/34371/Nav/1/router.asp

17. B. C. Calhoun et al. "Perinatal hospice: comprehensive care for the family of a fetus with a lethal condition." *Journal of Reproductive Medicine.* May 2003; 48(5):343–348; M. D'Almeida, R. Hume, A. Lathrop, et al. "Perinatal hospice: family-centered care of the fetus with a lethal condition." *Journal of American Physicians and Surgeons.* Summer 2006; 11(2):52–55, www .jpands.org/vol11no2/calhoun.pdf

18. Maternal deaths related to induced abortion are 3.4 per 100,000 at 16–20 weeks gestation and 8.9 per 100,000 at 21 weeks gestation or more. A. Bartlett et al., "Risk factors for legal induced abortion-related mortality in the United States." *Obstetrics and Gynecology.* April 2004; 103(4):729–737. That compares with deaths related to pregnancy, childbirth, or the postpartum period of 7.5 per 100,000: Centers for Disease Control and Prevention. "Maternal mortality—United States, 1982-1996." *MMWR.* September 1998; 47:705–707.

19. C. H. Zeanah et al. "Do women grieve after terminating pregnancies because of fetal abnormalities? A controlled investigation." *Obstetrics and Gynecology.* August 1993;82(2):270–275.

20. A. Kersting et al. "Grief after termination of pregnancy due to fetal malformation." *Journal of Psychosomatic Obstetrics and Gynaecology.* June 2004; 25(2):163–169.

21. M. J. Korenromp, G. C. Page-Christiaens, J. van den Bout, E. J. Mulder, J. A. Hunfeld, C. M. Bilardo, et al. "Long-term psychological consequences of pregnancy termination for fetal abnormality: a cross-sectional study." *Prenatal Diagnosis.* March 2005;25(3):253–260.

22. A. Kersting et al. "Psychological impact on women after second and third trimester termination of pregnancy due to fetal anomalies versus women after preterm birth—a 14-month followup study." *Archives of Women's Mental Health.* August 2009; 12(4):193–201.

23. B. C. Calhoun, N. J. Hoeldtke. "The perinatal hospice: ploughing the field of natal sorrow." *Frontiers in Fetal Health.* May 2000; 2(5):16–22.

24. "Operations, treatments, and medications that have as their direct purpose the cure of a proportionately serious pathological condition of a pregnant woman are permitted when they cannot be safely postponed until the unborn child is viable, even if they will result in the death of the unborn child." U.S. Conference of Catholic Bishops' *Ethical and Religious Directives for Catholic Health Care Services,* June 2001, 4th ed. IV: *Issues in Care for the Beginning of Life.* www.usccb.org/bishops/directives.shtml. "Jewish law permits abortion to save the life of the mother—in fact it insists on abortion if

this is necessary to save the life of the mother. This is because the mother's life takes precedence over the life of the fetus. The danger to the mother must be clear and substantial, and the abortion cannot be done in the very last stage of pregnancy. The Mishnah states that where there is danger to the mother's life, an abortion can be performed at any stage from conception until the head of the infant emerges." Source: www.bbc.co.uk/religion/religions/judaism/jewishethics/abortion_2.shtml, updated July 15, 2009. "Islam allows abortion to save the life of the mother because it sees this as the 'lesser of two evils' and there is a general principle in Sharia (Muslim law) of choosing the lesser of two evils." Source: www.bbc.co.uk/religion/religions/islam/islamethics/abortion_1.shtml, updated Sept. 7, 2009.

CHAPTER 3. The Emotional Journey

1. For further reading, see *Finding Life beyond Trauma,* by V. M. Follette and J. Pistorello (New Harbinger, 2007); *The Mindfulness & Acceptance Workbook for Anxiety* by J. P. Forsyth and G. H. Eifert (New Harbinger, 2008); and *The Mindfulness & Acceptance Workbook for Depression,* by K. D. Strosahl and P. J. Robinson (New Harbinger, 2008). See also www.goodtherapy.org
2. American Art Therapy Association, www.arttherapy.org
3. "What Is a Child Life Specialist?" Child Life Council, www.childlife.org/The%20Child%20Life%20Profession/
4. See *Talking with Children about Loss: Words, Strategies, and Wisdom to Help Children Cope with Death, Divorce, and Other Difficult Times,* by M. Trozzi (Perigree Trade, 1999). Trozzi directs the Good Grief Program at Boston Medical Center, www.bmc.org/pediatrics/special/goodgrief/overview.html
5. Many people find comfort in the book *When Bad Things Happen to Good People,* by Harold S. Kushner (Anchor, 2004).

CHAPTER 4. Waiting with Your Baby

1. See www.caringbridge.org or www.carepages.com
2. To learn about doulas, see the website of DONA International, www.dona.org
3. D. B. Chamberlain, "Life before birth: the fetal senses," www.birthpsychology.com/lifebefore/fetalsense.html

CHAPTER 5. Making Medical Decisions

1. For more discussion of medical interventions and your baby, see T. K. Koogler, B. S. Wilfond, L. F. Ross. "Lethal language, lethal decisions." *Hastings Center Report.* March–April 2003; 33(2):37–41.
2. For a list of questions to ask your baby's caregivers, see *Loving and Letting Go* by D. L. Davis (Centering, 2002).

3. Although Trisomy 18 is often considered universally lethal, a "small but significant percentage" can survive six months to a year, according to C.-C. Hsaio et al., "Changing clinical presentations and survival pattern in Trisomy 18." *Pediatric Neonatology.* 2009;50(4):147–151.

4. World Health Organization, "Palliative care," www.who.int/cancer/palliative/definition/en

5. For more information, see the following articles: A. Catlin, B. Carter. "Creation of a neonatal end-of-life palliative care protocol." *Journal of Perinatology.* April–May 2002; 22(3):184–195; N. J. Hoeldtke, B. C. Calhoun. "Perinatal hospice." *American Journal of Obstetrics and Gynecology.* September 2001; 185(3):343–348; S. Leuthner, E. L. Jones. "Fetal Concerns Program: A model for perinatal palliative care." *MCN: The American Journal of Maternal Child Nursing.* September–October 2007;32(5):272–278; D. Munson, S. R. Leuthner. "Palliative care for the family carrying a fetus with a life-limiting diagnosis." *Pediatric Clinics of North America.* October 2007; 54(5):787–798; L. H. Sumner, K. Kavanaugh, T. Moro. "Extending palliative care into pregnancy and the immediate newborn period: state of the practice of perinatal palliative care." *Journal of Perinatal and Neonatal Nursing.* January–March 2006; 20(1):113–116.

6. Hospice Net, "Preparing for approaching death," www.hospicenet.org/html/preparing_for.html

7. D. S. Diekema and J. R. Botkin. "Clinical report—forgoing medically provided nutrition and hydration in children." *Pediatrics.* August 2009;124(2):813–822.

8. "Catheterization, umbilical artery," http://emedicine.medscape.com/article/1348931-overview

9. R. Carbajal, A. Rousset, et al. "Epidemiology and treatment of painful procedures in neonates in intensive care units." *JAMA.* July 2008;300(1):60–70; L. Szabo. "Study: Needle-poked newborns in need of pain relief." *USA Today.* July 1, 2008, www.usatoday.com/news/health/2008-07-01-babies-pain_N.htm

10. K. J. Anand and P. R. Hickey. "Pain and its effects in the human neonate and fetus." *The New England Journal of Medicine.* November 19, 1987;317(21):1321–1329.

11. Joint position statement from the American Academy of Pediatrics and the Fetus and Newborn Committee of the Canadian Paediatric Society. "Prevention and management of pain in the neonate: an update." *Paediatrics & Child Health.* 2007;12(2):137–138.

12. R. W. Cohen. "A tale of two conversations." *Hastings Center Report.* May–June 2004;49.

CHAPTER 6. Getting Ready

1. For more information, see A. Catlin. "Thinking outside the box: Prenatal care and the call for a prenatal advance directive." *Journal of Perinatal and Neonatal Nursing*. April–June 2005;19(2):169–176.

2. Birth planning information from Annette Klein, RN ICCE, perinatal loss coordinator for the Birth Center of United Hospital, Saint Paul, Minnesota. Material copresented with Amy Kuebelbeck at a plenary session at the National Society of Genetic Counselors 26th Annual Education Conference, Kansas City, Missouri, October 13, 2007.

3. Thanks to Mara Tesler Stein, Psy.D., a Chicago-based clinical psychologist and author who specializes in pregnancy crisis and parenting, for these insights.

4. For example, Now I Lay Me Down to Sleep is a national network of professional photographers who volunteer their services to families experiencing the death of a baby. www.nowilaymedowntosleep.com. See also Touching Souls: Healing with Bereavement Photography, www.toddhochberg.com. Todd Hochberg is a Chicago-area photographer whose work, funded by grants and donations, is free of charge to grieving families.

5. J. H. Fanos, G. A. Little, and W. H. Edwards. "Candles in the snow: ritual and memory for siblings of infants who died in the intensive care nursery." *Journal of Pediatrics*. June 2009;154(6):849–853.

6. For more information, visit Crossings: Caring for Our Own at Death, www.crossings.net; the Funeral Consumers Alliance, www.funerals.org; and *Caring for the Dead: Your Final Act of Love* by Lisa Carlson (Upper Access, 1997), a comprehensive funeral guide for consumers.

7. Funeral Consumers Alliance, "What you should know about embalming," www.funerals.org/frequently-asked-questions/funeral-arrangements/48-what-you-should-know-about-embalming

8. For detailed information, see *Resource Guide: A Manual for Home Funeral Care* from Crossings: Caring for Our Own at Death, www.crossings.net/resourceguide030109.pdf

9. See Green Burials, www.greenburials.org

10. Trappist Caskets, New Melleray Abbey, Peosta, Iowa, www.trappistcaskets.com/childs_caskets.asp

11. Funeral Consumers Alliance, "Scatter-brained: all about cremation and what's left." www.funerals.org/frequently-asked-questions/cremation/376-scatterbrained

CHAPTER 7. Welcoming Baby

1. See the position statement by the Pregnancy Loss and Infant Death Alliance, "Infection risks are insignificant for bereaved parents who have close

contact with their deceased baby's body." www.plida.org/pdf/infection Risks.pdf

2. D. R. Genest, D. B. Singer. "Estimating the time of death in stillborn fetuses: III. External fetal examination; a study of 86 stillborns." *Obstetrics and Gynecology.* 1992;80:593–600.

3. For example, see "Breastfeeding disabled or handicapped babies," La Leche League International, www.llli.org/NB/NBdisabled.html

CHAPTER 8. Saying Goodbye

1. Hospice Net, "Hospice: preparing for approaching death," www.hospice net.org/html/preparing_for.html

2. Thanks to Annette Klein, perinatal loss coordinator for the United Hospital Birth Center in Saint Paul, Minnesota, for this insight.

3. Pregnancy Loss and Infant Death Alliance position statement and practice guidelines, "Infection risks are insignificant for bereaved parents who have close contact with their deceased baby's body," 2005, www.plida.org/pdf/infectionRisks.pdf. For bereaved parents, the risk of contracting infection from their deceased baby's body is insignificant, even if there is suspected infection in the baby's body, or if the body is at room temperature for extended periods. For anyone other than the parents, including health care professionals, the risks are still low, and their gentle touching and holding of the baby is affirming, validating, and comforting to the parents.

4. The Gift of a Lifetime, "Understanding death before donation," www .organtransplants.org/understanding/death/

5. Organ Procurement and Transplantation Network/United Network for Organ Sharing Ethics Committee Report, June 26, 2007. www.unos.org/CommitteeReports/board_main_EthicsCommittee_9_4_2007_13_1.pdf. Also "Use of anencephalic newborns as organ donors" position statement from the Canadian Paediatric Society Bioethics Committee, which said, "Infants with anencephaly require the same respect for life given to other human beings." *Paediatrics & Child Health.* 2005;10(6):335–337; www.cps .ca/ENGLISH/statements/B/b05-01.htm

6. L. Wijngaards-De Meij et al. "The impact of circumstances surrounding the death of a child on parents' grief." *Death Studies.* 2008;32(3):237–252.

7. For many helpful specifics and information about legal requirements, see the *Resource Guide: A Manual for Home Funeral Care* by Crossings: Caring for Our Own at Death, www.crossings.net/resourceguide030109.pdf, or the Funeral Consumers Alliance, www.funerals.org

CHAPTER 9. Continuing Your Journey

1. See also *Empty Cradle, Broken Heart: Surviving the Death of Your Baby* by D. L. Davis (Fulcrum, 1996) for comprehensive information and additional support.

2. See "Weaning after infant loss," Children's Hospitals and Clinics of Minnesota, www.childrensmn.org/Manuals/PFS/Nutr/027491.pdf

3. D. B. Moore, A. Catlin. "Lactation suppression: forgotten aspect of care for the mother of a dying child." *Pediatric Nursing.* September–October 2003; 29(5):383–384.

4. Moore and Catlin.

5. Moore and Catlin.

6. Mayo Clinic.com. "Labor and delivery, postpartum care," www.mayoclinic.com/health/lactation-suppression/AN01456

7. To find a milk bank, contact the Human Milk Banking Association of North America, www.hmbana.org. Their January 2006 newsletter, www.hmbana.org/downloads/2006Jan_newsletter.pdf, includes a bereaved mother's account of pumping and donating breast milk.

8. For more discussion about instrumental and intuitive grieving, see *Men Don't Cry, Women Do: Transcending Gender Stereotypes of Grief* by T. L. Martin and K. J. Doka (New York: Brunner-Routledge, 1999); *Grieving Beyond Gender: Understanding the Ways Men and Women Mourn* by K. J. Doka and T. L. Martin (New York: Routledge, 2010).

9. Thanks to Annette Klein for this concept.

10. "Only 16 percent of bereaved parents divorce, new study reveals," press release from The Compassionate Friends, Oct. 12, 2006, www.compassionatefriends.org/CMSFiles/X101206Press_Release_Survey,_Divorce-National.pdf; "Couples more likely to break up after pregnancy loss, U-M research finds," University of Michigan Health System press release, April 5, 2010, http://www2.med.umich.edu/prmc/media/newsroom/details.cfm?ID=1535

11. Direct Marketing Association, www.dmachoice.org

INDEX

Index

386

Index

journaling, 38, 76, 96, 137–38, 310. *See also* poetry

joy, 53, 57, 193, 206, 208, 209–14, 222–25, 229–31, 240, 263. *See also* love for baby

keepsakes, 24, 376; collecting, 136–38, 177–81; importance of, 177, 224, 230, 265, 310–12. *See also* journaling; photographs

labor, 198–206; emotions during, 201–3; last-minute changes in plans, 204–6; monitoring of baby during, 171; pain relief for mother, 171, 203–4; premature, 194–95; when baby has died in utero, 197–98. *See also* birth; birth planning; caesarean birth

life support: decisions about, 147–48, 157; discontinuing, 257–59. *See also* medical decisions; medical ethics; neonatal intensive care

longing, 207–8, 299, 306. *See also* grief

love for baby, 339–73; after birth, 226–27, 229–31, 238–39; at birth, 73, 193–95, 206, 208, 212–20; captured by photographs, 179–81, 272; since conception, 103–5; after death, 264–66, 267–71, 275, 276–77, 323, 371–72; while dying, 248–63; expressed by children, 182, 229–30, 277, 285; expressed by others, 225, 230–31, 279; expressed in birth plan, 167–68; expressed in medical decisions, 20, 28, 32–33, 149–50, 156–57, 161, 164, 231–33, 259, 346–49; and grief, 209–10; during pregnancy, 93–94, 113, 130, 133–36, 139; unconditional, 349–50, 369, 372. *See also* baby: bonding with; emotions: joy

marriage. *See* couples

medical decisions, 140–64; ambivalence about, 148–50; after birth, 220–21, 231, 244; coming to terms with,

232–33; discontinuing intervention, 257–59; guilt associated with, 155, 314–15; postponing, 152–54; pressure to intervene, 144–46; reflections about, 341, 346–47. *See also* DNR (do not resuscitate) order; life support; medical ethics; neonatal intensive care; perinatal hospice and palliative care; resuscitation

medical ethics, 32, 41, 140, 151–52

mementos. *See* keepsakes

memorial services. *See* funerals

memories, 133–35, 174, 238–40, 264, 267, 329; importance of, 54–55, 274, 303–4, 310–12; reminiscing about, 362–63. *See also* keepsakes; memory-making

memory-making: as coping strategy, 75–76, 130–31, 133–36; after death, 267–70; at home with baby, 233, 238–40, 276–77, 283–84. *See also* keepsakes; photographs

midwives, 27, 115, 117, 125, 205, 208

mindful acceptance, 74–75, 318. *See also* coping

miracles: hopes for, 19–20, 109–10, 153, 259; reflections on, 106–7, 146–47, 152, 219, 224–25, 226, 227, 354, 371–72

miscarriage, 10, 24, 90; wishing for, 19, 40, 60, 149

mothers, 368; and maternity clothes, 61; perspective of, 77, 220–21. *See also* birth; breast care, postpartum; breastfeeding; continuing pregnancy; couples; parenting: instincts; personal growth; postpartum recovery; pregnancy

multiple birth, 63, 132, 236, 305

naming the baby, 132–33, 175–76

neonatal intensive care, 24–25, 172, 174, 178, 183; seeing baby in, 221–22, 226. *See also* life support; medical decisions; medical ethics numbness and shock, 60–61, 197, 199, 207, 214–15, 221–22, 314

nursery, last-minute stocking of, 184, 237

nurses: and birth plans, 166–67, 174, 200; guidance from, 27, 31, 204, 207–8, 249; hospice, 238; learning about perinatal hospice, 122, 159, 366; performing baptism, 176; rushing parents to relinquish baby's body, 24, 269, 279, 322; supportive, 116–17, 124, 158, 160, 200–201, 205, 208–9, 223–24, 230–32, 251, 256, 265, 269–70, 272–75, 282, 302, 349, 366

nutrition and hydration, 159–60, 259. *See also* breastfeeding; feeding; feeding tube

organ donation, 276

pain relief: if needed for baby after birth, 32, 155, 160–62; for mother during labor, 171, 203–4. *See also* palliative care

palliative care, 32, 105, 148, 233, 245; philosophy of, 155. *See also* perinatal hospice and palliative care

parenting: of a dying baby, 247–63; instincts, 232–33, 235–36, 260–61, 264, 309–10, 335. *See also* baby; children; fathers; love for baby; mothers; subsequent child

perinatal hospice and palliative care, xi–xii, 26–29, 32–33, 47, 70, 115–18, 121–25, 127, 142, 378n4, 381n5; decisions regarding, 154–64; feelings about, 166; proceeding without a formal program, 116–18; reflections about, 37, 347–49; resistance to, 21, 116, 120, 144, 158. *See also* medical ethics; palliative care

perinatal loss, outdated practices regarding, 24–25, 188–90

personal growth, xiii, 54, 86, 323, 325, 326, 367–72. *See also* acceptance; adjustment; coping

photographs, 24, 177–81, 290; after birth, 228–29; after death, 271–73; importance of, 178, 182, 310–12; during pregnancy, 136; professional, 179, 180–81; regrets about not having enough, 321, 323; tips for taking, 179–81. *See also* keepsakes; memory-making; ultrasound: images

poetry, 296–97

postpartum depression, 68, 299

postpartum recovery, 299–302; breast care during, 300–301; checkup, 301; emotional aspects of, 299. *See also* caesarean birth; parenting: instincts

pregnancy: complications of, 128–29; coping during, 93–124, 129–31; monitoring of baby during, 129; nutrition during, 127–28; prenatal care during, 125–29. *See also* baby: bonding with; continuing pregnancy; perinatal hospice and palliative care; subsequent pregnancy

premature induction, 34–35; deciding against, 38; ethics of, 40

premature labor. *See under* labor

prenatal care. *See* pregnancy: prenatal care during

prenatal decision-making. *See* continuing pregnancy; medical decisions

prenatal diagnosis: receiving, 6–13; researching baby's condition, 29–33

prenatal testing, 4–6

reframing. *See* coping

regrets, 320–23

relatives. *See* children; friends and relatives; grandparents

relief. *See* coping; death: relief upon

religion: and abortion, 38–42; anger at God, 154, 214, 354; and burial, 188;